APR 28 01			
APR 16 02			
MAY 06			
JAN 02 04			

ABORTION IN THE NEW EUROPE

ABORTION IN THE NEW EUROPE

A Comparative Handbook

EDITED BY

Bill Rolston & Anna Eggert

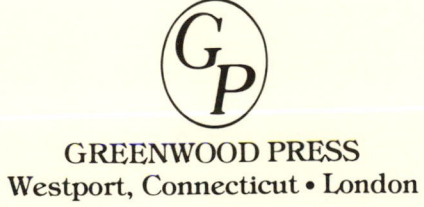

GREENWOOD PRESS
Westport, Connecticut • London

Library of Congress Cataloging-in-Publication Data

Abortion in the new Europe : a comparative handbook / edited by Bill
  Rolston and Anna Eggert.
       p.   cm.
    Includes bibliographical references and index.
    ISBN 0–313–28723–6 (alk. paper)
       1. Abortion—Law and legislation—Europe.   2. Abortion—Europe.
  I. Rolston, Bill.   II. Eggert, Anna.
  KJC8377.A883   1994
  344.4'04192—dc20
  [344.044192]   93–44510

British Library Cataloguing in Publication Data is available.

Library of Congress Catalog Card Number: 93–44510
ISBN: 0–313–28723–6

First published in 1994

Greenwood Press, 88 Post Road West, Westport, CT   06881
An imprint of Greenwood Publishing Group, Inc.

Printed in the United States of America

The paper used in this book complies with the
Permanent Paper Standard issued by the National
Information Standards Organization (Z39.48–1984).

10 9 8 7 6 5 4 3 2 1

CONTENTS

Contents

Contents

TABLES AND FIGURES

TABLES

FIGURES

Finland

Norway

INTRODUCTION: ABORTION IN EUROPE, PRESENT AND FUTURE

Bill Rolston and Anna Eggert

ABORTION RIGHTS: OPTIMISM OR PESSIMISM?

This book is in response to debates about changes in Europe at the end of the 1980s.

In the aftermath of the collapse of the socialist states in Eastern Europe and the ending of the cold war, there were many commentators who were optimistic about the possibilities of progressive change in Europe, especially in relation to the advancement of democratic processes and human rights. At the same time, many were predicting that the arrival of the single European market at the end of 1992 would herald an economically stable and affluent Europe, a Europe of increasingly unrestricted movement of capital and labour.

On the other hand, others were less optimistic. They pointed to the growth of racism and of ethnic conflict, especially but not only in Eastern Europe. They emphasised the strengthening of "Fortress Europe" with its control of immigrants and increasing interstate cooperation in security matters. Their conclusion was that a Europe delighting in being postsocialist, postmodernist, and postfeminist would be one where openings exist for the resurgence of repressive politics and legislation.

Now that a few years have passed, there is much to verify the fears of the pessimists. Old wounds have been reopened in the former Yugoslavia and the former Soviet Union. Racism and the Right have grown in alarming proportions in the unified Germany. And the hopes for the European Community have been revealed as at least premature, with dissension over the Maastricht Treaty, divisions over strategies to handle pressure from the United States to diminish agricultural subsidies, and the precarious existence of the European monetary exchange union, the ERM.

What of the specific issue of abortion in terms of this ongoing debate? At the end of the 1980s there was optimism on the issue. For example, Gottlieb (1989, 157) put great faith in the liberating potential of technology, namely the RU 486 abortifacient pill, and concluded that its widespread availability throughout Europe would mean that abortion could be individualised, the ultimate in democratic control. As a result, " 'pro-life' protesters will have nowhere left to protest and the movement will wither away." On the other hand, it was already apparent by the end of the 1980s that there were powerful countercurrents in various European countries. Poland was already in the process of totally reversing its liberal abortion legislation and practice, and a number of societies that had recently liberalised abortion—such as Spain and Portugal—had only done so in a very cautious manner. Powerful right-wing forces were active in many countries, not least Ireland, where they were confident of further restricting highly restricted legislation and practice. The reunification of Germany was set to ensure a number of negative consequences for the former German Democratic Republic, not least in relation to women's rights in general and the availability of abortion in particular. In this vein, the few "success stories" of the new Europe—in particular Romania—seemed outweighed by the examples of societies in which the right to choose was in question. Would the end of the millennium see the decriminalisation of abortion in Europe or its recriminalisation?

Ultimately the answer to that question rests on a detailed study of each European society. Such a study is necessary as a preliminary step to careful comparative analysis.

PUBLISHED SOURCES

There are, of course, published sources on abortion in Europe, but there were problems, we felt, in relying solely on them as a base for this analysis. Some of the best published sources exist only in German—for example, Eser and Koch (1988) and Ketting and Van Praag (1985). Others concentrate on only one aspect of the question—for example, IPPF Europe Region (1989), which looks only at late abortions. There are some overviews that are remarkably comprehensive but allow for little in-depth coverage of each of the countries considered—for example, Cook (1992) and Jacobson (1990).

Finally, given the rapidity of change in relation to abortion legislation in a number of European countries—Ireland, Germany, Poland—these sources are destined to become outdated quite rapidly; see, for example, Lovenduski and Outshoorn (1986) and Tietze and Henshaw (1986).

For these reasons, we felt that there was room for a reference book in English on abortion in the new Europe. The plan was to consider Europe country by country in relatively brief but concise chapters. We wanted to find authors who could tell us succinctly and clearly about the current legal, medical, and social situation regarding abortion in each of their countries; the history of how that situation came about; and the political forces mobilized for and against a woman's right to choose, historically and currently.

AUTHORS' BLUEPRINT

The authors of the chapters that follow were given a detailed blueprint of questions to be answered and topics to be considered in relation to their country. The instructions are grouped in four main areas.

1. The law in each country: what is legal and what is not, the penalties laid down, and a brief history of the origins of the current legal position.
2. Abortion in practice: facts and figures on legal and illegal abortions, a statistical profile of women choosing abortion, the extent of penalties actually inflicted on women or abortionists, and the attitudes of the medical profession.
3. The politics of abortion: social attitudes about abortion and towards those women who choose abortion, the balance of political forces on the issue, and the ideology and political practices of those groups organised for and against choice.
4. The future: the possibilities of change in public opinion for or against a woman's right to choose, and the possibilities of consequent legal change.

More specifically, authors were given a comprehensive list of questions, as follows.

1. The law in your country. What is the current legal position as regards abortion? Are abortions legal? If so, under what circumstances? What are the punishments for illegal abortion—both for the woman and the abortionist? As briefly and succinctly as you can, can you summarise the history of how this current legal situation came about? If abortion law reform occurred at any time since the 1960s, how did this come about? Was it through the action of political parties, government, pressure groups, or some other mechanism? What have been the challenges to further reform the law, or to restrict it, since the current law was established?

2. Abortion in practice. Can you provide some useful statistics on the extent of abortion in your country? How widely available is legal abortion in practice? Despite formal legal availability, is it in fact restricted to certain classes, regions, age groups, ethnic or religious groups, or to certain gestation ages? Are there illegal abortions? If so, can you provide any information on the number, how they are obtained, how they are carried out, and what if any are the consequences for the women and the abortionists? Has anyone—woman or abortionist—suffered imprisonment or legal prosecution recently as a result of an abortion? What are the attitudes of doctors and other medical practitioners towards abortion? How do women pay for their abortions? Are abortions available on the health service or through insurance? In practice, do women who have abortions keep it secret from friends and relatives?

3. *The politics of abortion.* What is the level of public acceptability in your country of a woman's right to choose? What is the general attitude towards matters of sexual morality? What is the balance of political forces as regards the issue of abortion? Currently what groups are organised for and against abortion? Who are they, what do they argue, and what influence, if any, do they have on decision makers? What are the political activities and practices of these groups?

4. *The future.* Is the climate of public opinion changing as regards abortion? If so, is it changing for or against a woman's right to choose? Is there likely to be any major challenge in the near future to the current legal position as regards abortion? How is that likely to come about?

TRENDS IN ABORTION IN EUROPE

The authors were not expected to answer all of these questions equally fully. Indeed, in some cases they were unable to; for example, authors from countries where the law had changed very recently would sometimes find it difficult to make accurate assessments of future developments. But inasmuch as the authors were able to follow the detailed blueprint provided, this book becomes a valuable tool for comparative analysis. Thus, countries can be considered on the grounds of whether abortion is legal or illegal, and if legal, whether abortion is allowed on the basis of an indications model or a term model. The *term model* allows abortion on request (with or without further requirements, such as the obligation to undergo counseling) up to a specified time limit in respect to gestation; thereafter, abortion is allowed on the basis of an indications model. The *indications model* states that abortion is allowed on the basis of a number of indications—medical, eugenic (foetal abnormality), rape and incest, and socioeconomic. The extent of the indications that allow abortion can be classified as *narrow* (usually medical reasons only) or *broad* (usually up to and including socio-economic indications). The countries considered in this book can thus be categorised as portrayed in Table 1.

Other comparisons are possible on the basis of the data provided. Some countries are superficially similar, but in fact law and practice on abortion differ markedly. For example, the former USSR and the Netherlands both

Table 1
Abortion in Europe—Term Model and Indications Model

Term Model (up to 12 weeks, unless specified)	Indications Model		Illegal
	Broad	Narrow	
Austria	Britain	Poland	Ireland
Belgium	Finland	Portugal	
Bulgaria	France	Spain	
Czech and Slovak	Hungary		
Republics	Switzerland		
Denmark			
Germany			
Netherlands			
Norway			
Sweden[1]			
USSR[2]			

1 = up to 18 weeks
2 = up to viability

have abortion on demand, but there the similarity ends. The former Soviet Union fluctuated between pro-natalist policies and a very broad indications model, ending up with a reliance on abortion that is exceptional:

The ratio of 770 abortions per 100 births in the rural areas of the Central Economic Region of the Russian Federation is statistically valid and has no parallel worldwide. This figure is 30 times as high as in the United Kingdom, and 12 times as high as in Hungary. The area of the Central Economic Region is slightly less than that of France, at 485,000 km². (Popov 1990, 6)

This reliance is explained by the unavailability of reliable contraception, making abortion the favoured method of family planning.

The Netherlands, on the other hand, has prioritised safe and widely available contraception and widespread sex education, with the result that, despite having one of the most liberal abortion regimes in the world, it has a remarkably low abortion rate.

To take another example, some countries in which the majority of the population is Roman Catholic have legislated on abortion in starkly different ways. The Republic of Ireland has traditionally outlawed abortion entirely, in line with Catholic moral teaching, although forthcoming legislative change will allow abortion on strictly medical grounds. A similar commitment to conservative Catholic teaching has been part of the inspiration behind Poland's recent rejection of socio-economic grounds as sufficient for abortion. On the other hand, Belgium is a Catholic country with a liberal abortion law; moreover, a major element in the establishment of this law was the direct action of opponents of the former restrictive law who set up illegal abortion centres.

Some countries—for example, Britain and Sweden—have few illegal abortions, and in fact the abolition of illegal abortion was one of the purposes of abortion law reform; while others—for example, Portugal—rely heavily on illegal abortions. In some countries—for example, Ireland and increasingly in Poland—"abortion tourism" is prevalent; while in others—for example, Britain and the Netherlands—legal abortion is available not merely for the citizens but for women from other countries. The law as regards abortion in some countries has undergone change recently—for example, Germany, Hungary, Poland, Belgium, France; in others, the law on abortion has remained relatively unchanged for many years—for example, Austria, Britain, Switzerland, and Northern Ireland.

It is thus possible to see clear patterns emerging from the information in the chapters that follow. First, the Nordic countries have an almost identical experience of abortion law and practice. Abortion is available on request. There are differences depending on the success of contraception and sex education programmes, but overall there is a relatively high take-up of abortion services in these countries.

Second, there are strong similarities among Eastern European countries, including the European republics of the former Soviet Union. At times, there was a strict policy of pro-natalism that reached its low point in Romania:

Ceausescu proclaimed that "the fetus is the socialist property of the whole society. Giving birth is a patriotic duty, determining the fate of our country. Those who refuse to have children are deserters, escaping the law of natural continuity". . . . A special unit was established within the Romanian State Security Police (Securitate) to investigate allegations of illegal abortions. Securitate representatives were posted in every maternity ward and obstetrical/gynecological clinic or service. . . . Employed women up to age 45 were asked to undergo monthly gynecological examinations in their workplaces. Those who refused to appear, or who could not provide a medical certificate of exemption, were denied their rights to dental and medical care, pensions, and social security, and were also declared ineligible to spend their holidays at the resort maintained by the workplace. Whether or not factory physicians received their full monthly salaries depended on plant employees achieving a state-stipulated monthly birth quota. (David 1990, 9)

Little wonder that one of the first acts of the postcommunist government in Romania was to enact a new law on abortion on 25 December 1989, ensuring abortion on demand up to 12 weeks and for health reasons thereafter.

Romania was an exaggerated form of an approach that had the USSR as its role model in this respect. There, policy fluctuated between being pro-natalist and pro-abortion, the end effect being that abortion became the chief form of birth control.

Despite such patterns, it is important to stress that no two countries are identical as regards abortion, no matter how similar the laws are on their statute books. Practice is never identical, and the manner in which the laws emerged differs. For this reason, the details of each country's story are crucial to an understanding not just of that country but of the picture of abortion in Europe overall, complete with its complexities and nuances. Some of the details of each of the countries considered in this book are summarised in Table 2.

SCOPE OF THIS BOOK

Despite its comprehensiveness, this book does not consider a number of European countries. We made no attempt to consider abortion in Malta, Iceland, and Luxembourg. While we had suggestions for authors in Albania and Yugoslavia, we did not manage to find an author in either of those countries, and contacts with authors in Greece, Italy, and Romania for one reason or another were unable to elicit suitable chapters. The exclusion of Romania in particular, not to mention the underrepresentation of the countries of the Mediterranean, is particularly unfortunate.

We did find authors for chapters on Austria, Belgium, Britain, Bulgaria, the Czech Republic and Slovakia, Denmark, Finland, France, Germany, Hungary, the Netherlands, Norway, Poland, Portugal, Spain, Sweden, Switzerland, and the former Soviet Union. We undertook to write the chapter on Ireland ourselves. Some of the authors are medical professionals, others from a legal background. A number are academics in the fields of law, medicine, or sociology. Many are feminists. None is anti-choice in relation to abortion.

ACKNOWLEDGMENTS

Finding the authors in each European country to write definitively about their countries involved what can only be described as detective work. Our search was greatly aided by a number of strategic contacts.

Rebecca Cook, Assistant Professor in the Faculty of Law at the University of Toronto, led us directly to authors of two chapters (Hungary and Switzerland) and indirectly to the authors of three others (Britain, Czechoslovakia, and the former USSR).

Karen Newman, in the International Planned Parenthood Federation's Europe Region office in London, guided us directly to the authors of four chapters (Belgium, the Netherlands, Portugal, and Sweden), and indirectly to the authors of two other chapters (Finland and France).

Both the editors are members of the European Group for the Study of Deviance and Social Control. Through approaches to other members of the group we managed to solicit six chapters (Austria, Denmark, Germany, Norway, Poland, and Spain).

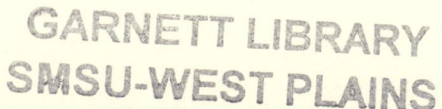

Table 2
Selected Data on Abortion in Various European Countries

Country	Austria	Belgium	Britain	Bulgaria
Year of current law	1975	1990	1967	1990
Grounds for abortion	a. up to 3 months on request. b. from 3 months to full term if woman is minor, her life is in danger, or foetal abnormality.	a. up to 12 weeks on request. b. after 12 weeks if danger to life of woman, foetal abnormality, or likelihood that foetus will not survive.	If risk to life of woman, or physical or mental well-being of woman or existing children, or foetal abnormality (up to 28 weeks in last, later amended to 22 weeks).	a. up to 12 weeks, on request. b. up to 20 weeks, for medical indication (includes e.g. likelihood that pregnancy ends in caesarian section). c. after 20 weeks, if danger to life of woman or foetal abnormality.
Conditions	Medical consultation.	Medical consultation plus six days reflection time.	Agreement of two doctors. Abortion in state hospital or approved private clinic.	
Incidence of abortion	30,000 - 100,000 p.a. No central statistics.	20,000 - 30,000 p.a.	196,000 p.a.	Half of all pregnancies end in abortion. Abortion as important method of family planning.
Cost	Medical insurance pays if medical indication. In some states, public welfare if woman is disabled, a minor or in serious financial difficulty.		Free only if medical indication.	Payment according to income, free if medically indicated, rape, or woman is a minor.
Current politics	Majority of population support current law.	Majority of population support current law despite strong Catholic ethos and opposition of church.	Majority of population support current law. Numerous attempts in parliament to restrict law, all unsuccessful.	Democracy has encouraged emergence of anti-abortion groups on Western model.
Future	No legal change likely.	No legal change likely, but practitioners must follow law exactly to avoid prosecutions and subsequent backlash.	Right will make further attempts to restrict law, probably unsuccessfully.	Need for effective contraception. Unlikely that abortion will continue to be free of charge.

Country	Czech and Slovak Republics	Denmark	Finland	France
Year of current law	1987	1973	1970	1975
Grounds for abortion	a. mini-abortions up to 45 days (if first pregnancy), 55 days (if later pregnancy). b. up to 12 weeks, on request. c. beyond 12 weeks, for health reasons.	a. up to 12 weeks, on request. b. after 12 weeks, on basis of decision of medical committee for medical reasons, rape, or foetal abnormality. For medical reasons, up to 24 weeks, but rare after 16th week (1% of all abortions).	a. up to 12 weeks, for medical or socio/economic reasons, in case of rape or foetal abnormality. b. up to 20 weeks, if woman is minor, or for special reasons, eg. mental condition. c. up to 24 weeks, on medical grounds.	Up to 10th week if the pregnancy places the woman "in a state of distress".
Conditions	On request, must be at least 6 months from previous abortion, unless woman over 35, has given birth twice, or pregnancy results from rape.	Abortions only in state hospitals.	In case of a. above, medical permission needed. In cases b. and c. above, permission of National Board of Health necessary.	Consultation with doctor and social worker/counseller, plus week of reflection, but final decision is that of woman.
Incidence of abortion	High by Western European standards, but not as high as some former Communist states. Abortion as usual method of family planning.	21,000 p.a. High in comparison with other Nordic countries.	11,000 p.a. and falling. Second lowest rate in Nordic countries.	165,000 p.a.
Cost	Free in first 6 weeks (80% of all abortions) or if medical indication.			Free.
Current politics	Anti-abortion groups now active. Independent pro-choice groups not strong yet. Slovaks likely to be less pro-choice than Czechs.	Widespread support for current law. No political parties support major change. Anti-abortion groups active, but strong pro-choice lobby.	No strong opposition to current law. Religious fundamentalists have little policy influence. Only debate about how to encourage earlier abortions.	Anti-abortion groups involved in public action, including violence. But limited influence on public opinion.
Future	Moves to restrict liberal law and practice in both republics. Slovaks more likely to introduce restrictions, but law will remain relatively liberal. Charge likely to be introduced.	Abortion seen by all as last resort. Hence increasing emphasis on contraception. Legal change unlikely.	Major legal change unlikely. Efforts to reduce number of abortions.	

Table 2 (*continued*)

Country	Germany	Hungary	Ireland	Netherlands
Year of current law	1993	1993	1861	1984
Grounds for abortion	Abortion illegal (except on medical indication), but not punishable by law if occurs in first 12 weeks of gestation and after compulsory counselling. Abortions in state hospitals no longer possible.	a. up to 12 weeks, if risk to woman's health or severe stress. b. up to 18 weeks, if woman unable to act independently or pregnancy has exceeded time limit due to clerical delay or diagnostic failure. c. up to 20 weeks (24 if diagnostic delay), if risk of foetal abnormality is 50%. d. no limit if woman's life in danger or foetal abnormality incompatible with post-natal life.	North: in practice, a small number of abortions take place for therapeutic reasons. South: no abortions legal, even for therapeutic reasons, as result of 1983 referendum and subsequent amendment to Constitution.	Abortion on request if woman is 'in situation of emergency'. 'Menstrual regulation', up to 16 days from missed period (20% of all abortions). Abortion allowed to viability, in practice 30% before 8th week, 1% after 15th week.
Conditions	Compulsory counselling favouring protection of foetus, plus three days waiting period.	Agreement of gynaecologist and Family Welfare Services nurse necessary.		Consultation with doctor followed by five day waiting period.
Incidence of abortion	Previously 120,000 p.a. in West. Problems of accessibility, especially in East, likely as result of recent legislation.	60,000 p.a.	North: estimated 200 p.a. South: probably none. Estimated 3,000 p.a. from North and 6,000 from South travel to Britain.	Very low rate: half of English rate, one-fifth of U.S. rate. Great reliance on contraception.
Cost	Abortions considered 'wrongful', therefore can no longer be paid from state health service.	Fee can be reduced or waived in exceptional circumstances.		Free.
Current politics	Unification of country led to liberal law. Challenged by parliamentary Right. Federal Constitutional Court ruled transitional arrangements as above pending reformulated law.	Anti-abortion groups active; challenged law in Constitutional Court (1991) on grounds that policies result from ministerial decree rather than democratic law. New law resulted.	Powerful fundamentalist lobbies: in North, oppose extension of British 1967 Act; in South, active in constitutional change and legal injunctions against pro-choice and other groups.	Majority of population support current law. Abortion seen as measure of last resort.
Future	Parliament must reformulate law in line with judgement of Constitutional Court.		North: prohibition of abortion likely to remain. South: legislation on abortion necessary as result of 1992 referendum. Will ensure abortion on narrow range of therapeutic reasons only.	Change in current law and practice highly unlikely

Country	Norway	Poland	Portugal	Spain
Year of current law	1978	1993	1984	1985
Grounds for abortion	a. up to 12th week, on request. b. after 12th week, medical, socio-medical, eugenic and ethical indications. No abortion after 18th week if chance that foetus is viable.	If threat to life or health of woman, if evidence of serious incurable deformity of foetus, in cases of rape and incest.	If danger to health of woman, foetal abnormality or rape. Normally up to 12 weeks, 16 weeks in case of foetal abnormality. No socio-economic indication.	If danger to physical or mental health of woman, rape (12 week limit), or foetal abnormality (22 week limit).
Conditions	In case of a. above, no obligatory counselling, only medical advice. In case of b. above, two doctors must agree.			Doctor's approval needed. In case of b. above, rape must be reported before abortion is sought.
Incidence of abortion	Rate not particularly high in comparison with other Nordic countries. Liberalisation led to decrease in abortion.	60,000 - 300,000 p.a. Rate of illegal abortions on increase since introduction of stricter law.	Very few legal abortions (400) between 1984 and 1992). Surveys show 1 in 10 women having 5 or more abortions. Abortion as method of family planning.	100,000 p.a., 70% of which illegal. Latter proportion would be higher if less liberal interpretation of mental health indication in private clinics where 98% of legal abortions occur.
Cost	Free.	Free if legal. Illegal abortions performed by private doctors are costly.	Free or low cost if legal.	Free if in state hospital (only 2% of legal abortions, less than 1% of all abortions).
Current politics	Majority of population, including political parties and state church, more or less support current law.	Public opinion more liberal than current law which has been initiated by Catholic church and Christian fundamentalists.	Strong political, medical and religious opposition to more liberal law. But also beginning of debate because of prosecutions of women.	Right attacks private clinics through court action. 80% of population favour current law. But many favour further liberalisation.
Future	Moves to restrict large proportion of late abortions. Legal change highly unlikely.	Women's groups now organised and urging laws which reflect public opinion, better and more widely available contraception, and sex education for young people.	Revision of Penal Code current. Legal change possible.	Reform of Penal Code imminent. May lead to 4th indication - socio-economic - or abortion on request within time limit. Likely no more free abortions.

Table 2 (*continued*)

Country	Sweden	Switzerland	USSR
Year of current law	1975	1942	1987
Grounds for abortion	a. up to 18th week, on request. b. after 18th week, if serious medical, psychological or social problem.	Abortion prohibited except on medical grounds. Otherwise, imprecision, leaving interpretation of 'medical' wide open. Implementation left to each canton, resulting in liberal interpretation in some, not in others.	a. mini-abortions, up to 20 days after missed period. b. up to 28 weeks, on request on medical, eugenic, ethical, or socio-economic grounds. Abortion as main form of family planning.
Conditions	Between 12th and 18th week, counselling necessary. After 18th week, permission of National Board of Health necessary; given in 50% of all cases (100 p.a.). No agreement if foetus deemed viable or after 22nd week.	Consultation with doctor, plus written agreement of second doctor. Otherwise, no conditions - no time limit, no permission of parents in case of minor, no counselling or waiting period.	None.
Incidence of abortion	No rise in abortion rate after liberalisation.	13,000 p.a., 83% of which are in six liberal cantons.	Officially 6 - 7 million p.a., unofficially 10 - 11 million. 20 - 25% of world total.
Cost	Minimal.		
Current politics	Vast majority of population support current law. Some politicians want to make counselling compulsory or reduce time limit for abortion on request to 12 weeks.	Numerous attempts to clarify legal imprecision from both pro- and anti-choice positions. Pro-choice dissatisfied that liberal abortion practice is not underwritten by liberal abortion law.	Politics determined in past by economic doctrine and ideology. Early days for independent democratic groups active on issue, whether pro- or anti-choice.
Future	All, pro- and anti-choice, see lowering of number of abortions as priority. Change in current law unlikely.	Liberal practice unlikely to change, but liberal abortion law as in many other Western European states also unlikely.	Contraceptive revolution necessary to curtail reliance on abortion, but unlikely in near future.

Other people helped us in this task of detection: Jacqueline Bernat de Celis (Paris, France), Dilys Cossey (London, England), Henry David (Bethesda, Maryland, U.S.), Zdenek Dytrych (Prague, Czech Republic), Luz Muñoz González (San Sebastian, Spain), Ilona Görgenyi (Miskolc, Hungary), Nila Kapor-Stanlovic (Copenhagen, Denmark), Ida Koch (Gentofte, Denmark), Zdenek Matejcek (Prague, Czech Republic), Beppe Mosconi (Padova, Italy), Daniel Pierotti (Copenhagen, Denmark), Arno Pilgrim (Vienna, Austria), Monika Platek (Warsaw, Poland), Wendy Savage (London, England), Angelika Schafft (Oslo, Norway), Jan Stepan (Lausanne, Switzerland), and Rita Taskinen (Helsinki, Finland). It is customary to thank such people as a matter of form. We would like to go further and state that without their help, we could never have found the authors to write the chapters that follow.

CONCLUSION

Given the extent of current and potential changes in relation to abortion law and practice in various European countries, this book is in some ways outdated already. For all the historical information presented by each author, the book in many ways portrays a picture of abortion in Europe at a fixed moment in time. But it is crucial that that picture exist. The trends for future changes on abortion are in many cases currently in existence. No matter what the future holds in relation to abortion in Europe, it is important to have the contemporary picture, not only to know retrospectively how we got there but also to prepare for what is ahead.

Towards the beginning of this introduction we asked if the end of the millennium would see the decriminalisation of abortion in Europe or its recriminalisation. On the basis of the information in these chapters it is impossible to answer that question simply. There are some trends towards liberalisation. On the other hand, the heyday of liberalisation of abortion law was in the 1970s and is past. There are trends towards increasing restriction in many countries. Even though these do not of themselves lead to a recriminalisation of abortion, there is every reason to believe that abortion law reform, once achieved, is not guaranteed in perpetuity without continuing political struggle.

REFERENCES

Cook, Rebecca. "International Protection of Women's Reproductive Rights." *New York University Journal of International Law and Politics* 24 (1992): 645–727.

David, Henry. "Romania Ends Compulsory Childbearing." *Entre Nous* nos. 14–15 (June 1990): 9–10.

Eser, A., and H. G. Koch. *Schwangerschaftaabbruch im internationalen Vergleich*. Baden-Baden: Nomos Verlag, 1988.

Gottlieb, Anthony. "Sex, Science and Silliness." In Dudley Fishburn (ed.), *The World in 1990*. London: The Economist Publications, 1989: 157–59.

IPPF Europe Region. *Late Abortion in Europe: Report of a Colloquium*. London: IPPF, 1989.

Jacobson, Jodi. *The Global Politics of Abortion*, Worldwatch Paper 97. Washington, D.C.: Worldwatch Institute, 1990.

Ketting, E., and P. Van Praag. *Schwangerschaftaabbruch: Gesetz und Praxis im internationalen Vergleich*. Tübingen: DGVT Verlag, 1985.

Lovenduski, J., and J. Outshoorn. *The New Politics of Abortion*. London, Sage, 1986.

Popov, A. A. "Sky-high Abortion Rates Reflect Dire Lack of Choice." *Entre Nous* 16 (September 1990): 5–7.

Tietze, C., and S. Henshaw. *Induced Abortion: A World View*. New York, The Alan Guttmacher Institute, 1986.

ABORTION IN THE
NEW EUROPE

AUSTRIA

Oskar Lehner

THE HISTORY OF ABORTION LAW

Abortion in the Penal Code

Although in ancient Greek and Roman law abortion was legal or punished only minimally, the influence of Christianity on medieval Austrian law resulted in abortion being treated as a major crime. Deriving its position from Aristotle, canon law distinguished between the *foetus inanimatus* (during the first 40 days after conception) and the *foetus animatus*.[1] Using an incorrect translation of the Bible (Exodus 2:22–23), canon law specified the death penalty for procuring abortion to a *foetus animatus*. In Austrian medieval criminal law, persons found guilty of abortion were executed by impalement or were drowned in a sack together with a dog, a rooster, a cat, and a snake.

In the 17th century, the Austrian legislature (Landesgerichtsordnung für das Land ob und unter der Enns 1656) was influenced by Saxon law. Punishment by death was laid down by law only for abortions performed in the second half of pregnancy. The Constitutio Criminalis Theresiana (1768) categorised abortion as manslaughter; the woman and any person having assisted the woman were to be beheaded by sword.

Criminal law under Joseph II (1787) was the first to break with the tradition of the death sentence. Influenced by the Enlightment, it mitigated the legislative sanction to indefinite imprisonment. Married women should receive a more severe sentence. There was no distinction regarding at what stage the abortion took place. The penal codes of 1803 (StG Para. 128–132) and 1852 (StG Para. 144–148), valid until 1974, sanctioned abortion with imprisonment of between one and five years.

In the late 19th century and during the first three decades of the 20th century, several commissions of the Secretary of Justice recommended—without any results—a reduction of the legislative sanction and the introduction of a medical indication. After the Austrian courts acknowledged medical indication as a reason for exemption from punishment in 1937, an amendment of the penal code was passed into law allowing abortion within a narrow medical indication on the basis of the opinion of a special commission consisting of three physicians (BGBl. Nos. 202 and 203).

Parliament and Abortion Law Reform

After World War I, the women's organisation of the Social Democrats fought for a liberalisation of the abortion law. At the party convention of 1926, women achieved a majority of their demands on total impunity of abortion. Nevertheless, in the following years, the Social Democrat party introduced a bill in the Austrian parliament demanding only a lowering of the sanction and an indication, medical, ethical, eugenic, and social (Lehner 1989).

During the period of Nazi occupation, Austrian laws concerning abortion were replaced with the rigorous German laws (1943), which were part of a general programme aimed at increasing the population. Women who consented to an abortion faced imprisonment on the basis of a law that had no upper limit on the duration of the imprisonment. According to this law, third persons who performed an abortion were to be executed when "they continually impair the life power of the German people."

After World War II, Austria re-established its rules on abortion with one exception: the commission competent to give opinions on medical indications was abolished (Rittler 1962, 20 f.). In the 1950s and 1960s, several proposals for reform were discussed but not passed by the parliament. The most important suggestion was presented by the commission of the Secretary of Justice in 1962: abortion in general should be punishable (maximum sanction one year), but within a wider-ranging medical indication (including abortion after rape), abortion should go unpunished. Resistance to this reform programme was launched, especially by the Catholic Church and the conservative ÖVP, which, until 1970, was the leading party in Austria.

In 1970 and 1971, the political landscape of Austria changed completely. For the first time, the Social Democrat party (SPÖ), which during most of the years since 1945 had been the junior partner in a coalition with the ÖVP, won an absolute majority. The SPÖ, with the exception of constitutional law, was able to pass laws against the will of the other parties in the parliament. In 1971, the Social Democratic government presented a bill for total reform of Austria's criminal law. This draft bill suggested a very moderate indication solution based on the 1962 proposal, including medical, eugenic, and social indications.

This government bill provoked opposition on both sides. On the one hand, the ÖVP, the FPÖ (Liberal party), and the churches fought the proposal, which in their eyes would have gone too far. With the help of the Catholic Church, Aktion Leben (Action Life) was founded to mobilize resistance to every kind of reform that went further than a strict medical indication. On the other hand, the women's and the youth organization of the SPÖ and the Committee to Abolish Para. 144 pressured the government for a far-reaching liberalisation of abortion. At the SPÖ Party Congress of April 1972, these organizations—against the will of some of the party leaders—gained an overwhelming majority for their demand for a term solution. Because of this pressure from its members and the impossibility of reaching a compromise with the opposition and the church in 1973, the SPÖ tabled a bill in the parliament combining a three months' term solution with an indication model.

Needless to say, the opposition parties and the churches were not willing to accept this proposal. The ÖVP proposed its own bill in which abortion would be free from punishment in two cases: when the pregnant woman faced an extraordinary affliction that was not avoidable by any other means; or when the abortion was performed to prevent the woman from facing severe danger to her life or severe damage to her health, which could in no other way be avoided. In the latter case, the expert opinion of two physicians would be necessary before the abortion. The FPÖ proposed an indication solution, including social indication.

After an intense and controversial public discussion that caused a severe conflict between the SPÖ and the Catholic Church, the term solution was passed by the Austrian parliament and became effective on January 1, 1975. Ninety-two members of the parliament voted for the bill, 89 against.

As expected, the opponents of liberalisation tried to hinder the establishment of the term solution (but not the indication solution) by appealing to the Supreme Constitutional Court. As mentioned above, in 1974 the court found the term solution compatible with Austrian constitutional law.

With the support of the Catholic Church, Aktion Leben initiated a popular initiative in 1975 against the term solution and for an indication solution that was very similar to the suggestions of the ÖVP. This initiative was signed by nearly 900,000 citizens (about 17.9 percent of eligible voters). In the ÖVP-dominated federal states and in rural areas, support was significantly higher than in the federal states dominated by the SPÖ and in the cities. Despite this, the parliament decided in 1976 not to change the legal position. It declined the draft bill of Aktion Leben by 103 votes to 75, signifying that some of the ÖVP and FPÖ deputies voted against the bill.

ABORTION: CURRENT LAW AND PRACTICE

The Law of 1975

Para. 96–98 StGB 1975 deals with abortion. These provisions distinguish between whether the abortion is carried out with or without the consent of the pregnant woman. With consent, abortion is legal during the first three months of pregnancy (term solution). The pregnancy is deemed to begin at the time of implantation. Moreover, abortion is free from punishment from the beginning of the fourth month of pregnancy to the birth if the mother is an under-age minor (under-age indication) or if the abortion is performed for medical or eugenic purposes.

The law provides for different punishments for an illegal abortion depending on whether the defendant is the mother, a licensed physician, or a nonmedical person. There is no interdependency in the punitive process between the acts of the mother, the physician, and the nonmedical person. This means that the rules concerning complicity or joint perpetration of crime are not applicable; each person has to be punished under the regulations applicable to him or her.

Technically, the legislature stated that abortion is illegal and should be punished, but it created several exceptions to this rule, exempting abortion from punishment if certain criteria are met.[2] Fundamentally, legislators weighed the competing interests of the mother (self-determination, health risks), the right of the embryo to life, the interests of the father, and the interests of the state (development of the population, taboo against killing). The father's interests and population-policy concerns were not reflected in Para. 96–98, but the Austrian legislature gave careful consideration to the interests of the mother and the unborn child. Human life was seen as an evolutionary process in which the conception, the implantation of the fertilized egg in the uterus, the completion of the third month after the implantation, and the beginning of birth are legally relevant dates. As the pregnancy progresses, the right of the foetus to life acquires more and more weight while the mother's right to self-determination recedes.

Negligent abortion is not punished. Punishment occurs only when the abortion is committed with intent (Kienapfel 1990, §96, RN 14; Leukauf and Steininger 1979, §96, RN 9 and 11; Dearing 1988, 1097).

Para. 96 and 97 require the explicit or implied consent of the pregnant woman (Kienapfel 1990, §96, RN 9). The consent is seen as a strictly personal act of the expectant mother, except in the case of some minors. While there is some question in the commentary, the predominant view is that an under-age woman (younger than 14 years) must have the consent of her legal representative (normally her parents). On the other hand, a minor aged between 14 and 19 years is able to consent by herself (even against the will of her parents) if she possesses the necessary capacity to understand the situation.

The criminal law distinguishes three different phases (Kienapfel 1990, introduction to §96 RN 4; Dearing 1988, 1100).

1. *Early phase:* This phase extends from the point of conception to the implantation of the fertilized egg in the uterus on the 13th day. In other words, it includes the first four weeks after the last menstruation. The removal of the fertilized but not yet implanted egg does not count as an abortion. From the Austrian legal point of view, pregnancy begins with implantation.

2. *Initial phase:* This period includes the first three months of pregnancy that follow implantation. During this time, the term solution applies. An abortion can be legally performed if the following criteria are satisfied:

- Consent of the expectant mother
- Observance of the three-month time limit
- Medical consultation prior to abortion
- Performance of the abortion by a physician

The medical consultation can be carried out by the same physician performing the abortion and must include a personal conversation with the pregnant mother about the circumstances and the physical consequences of the abortion, but need not include a discussion of its social impact (Kienapfel 1990, §97 RN 5; Zipf 1984, §97 RN 8). As a general principle, every physician (even a dental surgeon) in the possession of an Austrian or foreign licence is allowed to satisfy the consultation requirement and perform the abortion. It is not necessary for the abortion to be done in a hospital.

3. *Main phase:* From the beginning of the fourth month after the implantation until the commencement of birth (start of labour pains), abortion is exempt from punishment only if it occurs with the consent of the pregnant woman and one of the following three indications exists:

- Medical indication—if the abortion is necessary to prevent a severe danger to the life of the mother that cannot be averted by other means or to avoid grave damage to the physical or psychological health of the woman
- Eugenic indication—when a severe danger exists that the child would be severely damaged physically or mentally
- Under-age indication—when the pregnant woman at the time of conception was under 14 years of age

If the medical indications are met and the regulations above fulfilled, even a person who is not a physician will be exempt from punishment for carrying out an abortion. This is so even without the consent of the woman if there is no other way to save her life and professional medical help cannot be obtained in time.

In relation to legislative sanctions, it makes a difference whether the actor is the pregnant woman, a physician, or a person who is not a physician. If an expectant mother carries out the abortion by herself, or allows somebody else to, and it is not a case in which the abortion is legal, she can be imprisoned for up to one year. A physician who performs an illegal abortion with the consent of the woman can be imprisoned for up to one year. If the physician is in the abortion business, she or he can be imprisoned for up to three years. If the immediate actor is not a licensed physician, the punitive sanction goes up to three years of imprisonment. In aggravated cases, such as the death of the woman or where the defendent is in the abortion business, the legislative sanction requires a minimum sentence of six months, but not longer than five years. By performing an abortion without the consent of the woman, the actor (physician or otherwise) may be sentenced to up to three years in prison. If the operation results in the death of the woman, there is a minimum sentence of six months but not longer than five years.

Neither a physician nor the medical staff is obliged to perform an abortion or cooperate in it. Only one exception exists: when the abortion is necessary without any delay to save the woman from an immediate, nonpreventable danger to her life. In this case, the medical person who refuses on grounds of conscience could be prosecuted for failure to render assistance, or even eventually some other offence—for example, negligent homicide. The law also stipulates that, within these conditions, neither the person who performs a legal abortion nor the person who refuses to participate in an abortion can be discriminated against in his or her professional career.

The Austrian legal system contains a hierachy of laws, with constitutional law at the top. According to Article 140 of the Austrian Constitution (Bundes-Verfassungsgesetz), the Supreme Constitutional Court (Verfassungsgerichtshof) has to review the compatibility of statutes with the Constitution.

In 1974, the federal government of Salzburg appealed to the Supreme Constitutional Court on the question of whether or not the term solution is unconstitutional. In the complaint the government stated that the term solution would contradict several constitutional norms—for example, the European Convention on Human Rights, or ECHR (which has constitutional status in Austria); the Treaty of St. Germain 1919; the Basic Law of the State concerning the General Rights of the Citizens (Staatsgrundgesetz über die allgemeinen Rechte der Staatsbürger 1867); and the principle of equality.

In the judgment, dating from October 11, 1974, the Supreme Constitutional Court stated that the term solution is compatible with Austrian constitutional law (VfSlg 7400/1974 - JB1 1975, 310 - EuGRZ 1975, 74). The court took the view that Article 2, section 1 ECHR, which protects "everyone's right to life," does not contradict the term solution because Article 2 does not lay down any rule about when life begins. After noting the controversial discussion in the international literature, the court stated that Article 2 seen as a whole only applies to persons after birth. The court based its opinion on the argument that the exhaustively enumerated exceptions of Article 2 (death penalty, self-defence, seizure and arrest, prevention of escape, repression of insurrection or rebellion) apply only to post-natal life. Moreover, if Article 2 included pre-natal life too, it would be a protection without any exceptions, with the result that even a medical indication would be prohibited. Pre-natal life would therefore be preserved better than post-natal life.

Next, the court referred to Article 8 ECHR, which guarantees everyone the respect of private and family life. The federal government had argued that the term solution violated this principle of equality because the decision of abortion is left with the mother and excludes the father. The Constitutional Court responded that Article 8 does not require a government to adopt statutes to criminally punish persons who interfere with a right to respect of private and family life. For the same reason, the court found no contradiction between the new abortion law and Article 12 ECHR, which gives the right to men and women to set up a family.

While the Basic Law of the State 1867 does not explicitly protect the right to life, that right is implied from those guaranteed rights which are explicitly stated. The Basic Law, however, is seen as a vehicle to protect the individual against the acts of the state. Consequently, the Constitutional Court found that it did not protect against acts of third persons. The term solution is not an interference by the state in the right to life, but rather prevents punishment for abortion within the first three months.

Finally, the court examined whether the term solution violates the principle of equality, which is repeatedly embodied in the Austrian Constitution,[3] in that the protection of unborn life is different before and after the third month of pregnancy. The court took the view that human life evolves from fertilisation via viability to birth. The foetus at the time of implantation is not the same as the foetus at later stages of its development, and therefore the Constitution does not require equal treatment.

Of course, the judgement of the Supreme Constitutional Court on the term solution was widely discussed in Austria. Most of the juridical publications criticised the court, stating that the term solution should have been regarded as unconstitutional.[4]

Abortion in Practice

Abortion practice in Austria is an area in which very little research work exists. One reason is that, in spite of legal liberalisation, abortion still is a taboo subject, and further investigation on this subject might bar career opportunities at certain institutions. The other reason is the total lack of statistics. The few publications on the subject deal with the motivations of women who have decided for or against an abortion and with the opportunities for public or private consultations. Generally one can find a surprising contrast between the rather liberal legal situation and the practice on abortion. In fact, there are some federal states in which there is no or nearly no possibility for a woman to have an abortion performed.

One source exists, dating from 1982 (Wimmer-Puchinger 1983), which investigated the motivations of women who decided to have an abortion. The survey—questionnaire and interviews—was conducted in hospitals with women who had had an abortion for the first time (the average age being around 22 years). The women were interviewed about four or five days before the abortion was performed. The results of these interviews were compared to interviews of pregnant women who were determined to have the baby. In total, the situations of about 800 women were analysed.

The study showed that position in life for the two groups of women differed fundamentally. In general, women who decide to have an abortion are in a less stable position. The following circumstances contributed to their decision to have an abortion: lack of a partner, unsatisfactory relationship with the partner, or short duration of the relationship; negative attitude towards sexuality; being a student; positive career opportunities; bad housing conditions; low income in relation to the number of persons to support; feelings of depression; negative attitude towards marriage; strong family or religious rules; positive attitude towards equality of the sexes in professional life; or an unsatisfactory relationship with parents.

Nearly all women in satisfactory relationships with their partners arrived at their decision in consensus with the partner. Of the group waiting for an abortion, 89 percent supported a general decriminalisation of abortion, 5 percent in the case of a social indication, and 2 percent when only a health risk exists; 1 percent rejected decriminalisation in any circumstance. Among the group of pregnant women who were determined to have the baby, the figures were: 56 percent, 12 percent, 23 percent, and 2 percent, respectively. It is therefore not surprising that punishment would fail to prevent women from deciding to have an abortion. Of the women waiting for the abortion, 64 percent would have made the same choice even if the abortion had been illegal.

In Austria, only the performance of an abortion in a hospital has to be registered. Since the vast majority of abortions are performed in outpatient clinics or by private physicians, and hospital statistics do not distinguish between abortions and miscarriages, official statistics are unreliable.[5] Some estimates indicate that there are between 30,000 and 40,000 abortions per annum, while others assume 70,000 to 100,000. This would mean that there is one abortion for every birth.[6] Unanimity exists that, in relation to the international average, the rate of pregnancies that end with an abortion is rather high in Austria. In general the standard of contraception in Austria is

Table 1
Sentences for Abortion in Austria, 1955–1990 (under § § 144, 146 StG, § 96 StGB)

Year	Persons Convicted			Imprisonment		
	Total	Female	For- eigner	Immediate Sentence	With Suspension of Sentence	Other (Fine)
1955	710	505	27	109	595	6
1958	324	206	12	56	262	6
1961	257	167	10	49	205	3
1964	172	108	3	30	141	1
1966	378	321	2	16	361	1
1968	306	196	0	28	275	3
1970	192	119	11	15	176	1
1972	120	71	11	8	109	3
1974	56	36	10	2	53	1
1975	21	13	10	2	11	8
1976	23	19	6	2	11	10
1977	23	21	18	2	17	4
1978	24	20	16	2	14	8
1979	15	9	3	3	10	2
1980	9	7	4	1	7	1
1981	7	6	4	0	5	2
1982	7	6	5	0	5	2
1983	8	4	1	1	6	1
1984	0	0	0	0	0	0
1985	3	3	3	0	0	3
1986	5	4	1	1	2	2
1987	0	0	0	0	0	0
1988	2	2	2	0	2	0
1989	2	0	1	0	1	1
1990	0	0	0	0	0	0

Source: Judicial Statistics on Crime 1955 - 1990.

rather low; on average only every second Austrian woman uses contraceptives. No data are available on the use of prophylactics by Austrian men.

Of course, there are no statistics available on the extent of illegal abortions in Austria, but as shown below, illegal abortions do occur. Between 1975 and 1990, more than 40 persons classified as unqualified physicians were sentenced for performing an abortion.

There are, in addition, figures available on how many persons were sentenced for illegal abortions in recent years (see Table 1). There has been a general decrease of convictions since 1955. The fluctuating trend in the 1960s runs parallel to the political affiliation of the Ministry of Justice—for example, if it was dominated by the SPÖ (until 1966) or the ÖVP (until 1970). During the early 1970s, when the liberalisation of abortion was under discussion, the conviction rate declined to a very low level. In 1974 (the last year of total punishability), 56 persons were sentenced; in 1975 (the first year of the term solution), 21 persons. Proceeding on the assumption that the number of abortions performed has not reduced dramatically between 1970 and 1974, one can conclude that the courts had already anticipated the introduction of the term solution.

Between 1975 and 1990, 149 persons were sentenced for illegal abortions. Among them were 114 women, seven of them under the age of 18 years. Of the persons convicted, 77 were Austrians and 69 came from Yugoslavia. The conviction rate was always under 10 persons per year, and in 1984, 1987, and 1990, nobody was sentenced for abortion.

From the introduction of the term solution in 1975 until the end of 1990, 80 women have been sentenced for performing an illegal abortion by themselves or consenting to it. In the same period, 25 physicians and 44 unlicenced practitioners have been convicted. Among the types of penalty one can find a tendency toward imprisonment: 105 persons (14 of whom were sentenced immediately) had to face a prison sentence. In only 44 cases was a pecuniary penalty or other measure imposed. Women who were sentenced under Para. 96, sec. 3, were penalized with an immediate sentence of a fine or an imprisonment with suspension of sentence (Dearing 1988, 1145).

While the legal situation in Austria is rather liberal, the actual availability of abortion is not guaranteed. One can say that in Austria, as a whole, a woman opting to have an abortion will succeed in having one. But in several of the nine Austrian federal states, actual availability is restricted or entirely absent. No additional restrictions in relation to class, ethnic origin, or religious group exist.

In Vienna and Upper Austria there are sufficient opportunities for an abortion. In Tirol, Styria, Lower Austria, Salzburg, and Carinthia, the situation is not so satisfactory. Vorarlberg and Burgenland are the two federal states in which a woman has no possibility of having an abortion except in the case of medical indication. This situation has created a sort of "inland tourism," in which women travel to Vienna or Upper Austria for an abortion. A small number of expectant mothers even go abroad, especially to the Netherlands, Great Britain, or Hungary. On the other hand, it is said that a number of women come from Germany to Austria for an abortion.

The majority of the abortions occur in the private practices of physicians. Only in Vienna is there an outpatient clinic specializing in abortions. There are several reasons for these restrictions on the availability of abortion. A considerable number of Austrian hospitals are run by confessional owners—for example, Catholic orders. Because the churches oppose abortion with a vehemence, it is forbidden to perform abortions there. The same situation can be found in most of the hospitals owned by the federal states. With the exception of Vienna (ruled by the Social Democrats), whether the federal state is ruled by Conservatives or Social Democrats does not play as decisive a role as other factors, such as the general political climate in the region. Among physicians, especially gynaecologists (most of whom are of a conservative nature), only a small group supports the term solution. Performing an abortion can hinder one's professional career in hospitals or at the university. In the 1980s, physicians—especially in smaller towns—who were known to perform abortions were the target of demonstrations and campaigns carried out by radical opponents of abortion.

The suction method (sometimes combined with scraping) is the sole means of abortion used by physicians. The woman is required to stay overnight only in some hospitals. Women's organisations are especially critical of the lack of institutions for after-care.

As abortion in Austria is still taboo, women—especially in the rural regions—who have had abortions usually tend not to talk much about their experience to acquaintances. In an opinion poll among women determined to have an abortion performed within the next few days, 15 percent feared disapproval within their social environment and 42 percent were afraid that people would talk about them behind their backs. On the other hand, 61 percent expected that people would understand the decision (Wimmer-Puchinger 1983, 55).

Until liberalisation in 1975, the prices for abortions were very high. Currently, the cost of an abortion (without an overnight stay) runs between 4,000 and 8,000 Austrian Schillings (about US$380 to $750).[7] Only a few private physicians use staggered prices adapted to the economic situation of the woman. Health insurance does not pay for an abortion, except in the case of a medical indication. In some federal states, public welfare bears the costs when the woman is disabled, an under-age minor, or in serious financial hardship.

The Politics of Abortion

The attitude of the Austrian population towards the decriminalisation of abortion in the first three months has changed significally since liberalization in 1975. The results of public opinion research show that the impunity of abortion in the first three months has gained more and more acceptance among the Austrian people.

In 1974, directly before liberalisation, IMAS (Institut für Markt-und Sozialanalysen) conducted an opinion poll that revealed that 36 percent supported the term solution, 49 percent favored a medical or social indication, and 10 percent preferred total punishability as laid down in the old Para. 144 StG. Among voters for the Social Democrat party, there was a majority for the term solution (51 percent, 42 percent, and 4 percent, respectively), while a large section of Conservative party (ÖVP) supporters were in favour of the indication solution (17 percent, 63 percent, and 18 percent, respectively).

Nine years later, in 1983, IFES conducted another opinion poll indicating that 58 percent of the population were for the retention of the term solution, 15 percent supported a restriction, and 18 percent favored the extension of punishability. Remarkably, 41 percent of Conservative party voters and 59 percent of Liberal party voters wanted to maintain the term solution. In 1990, FESSEL+GFK asked in an opinion poll "whether a woman should be allowed to have an abortion, independent of what reasons she has." The results showed that 47 percent indicated that this should be permitted (with 37 percent disagreeing and 16 percent undecided).[8] All surveys show one remarkable result: more men than women support the impunity of abortion in the first three months.

Because the law binds the impunity of an abortion to its performance by a physician, the attitude of these people is of special interest for the realisation of the term solution. In 1971 the powerful Austrian Medical Society stated in relation to the first reform bill (indication solution) that it would reject any reform that moved further than a medical indication. As far as physicians themselves engaged in the public controversy about impunity, the majority were on the side of the opposition. An opinion poll among 331 Austrian gynaecologists in the early 1970s indicated a 77 percent majority against the term solution (Edlinger 1981, 111).

In the 1970s, the term solution was a source of severe conflict between the SPÖ on one side and the Catholic Church and ÖVP on the other side. It seemed that the maintenance of punishability within the first three months would be a cornerstone of conservative policy in Austria. Today, 16 years after the entry into force of the term solution, the situation has changed completely. To date, each party is of the opinion that "abortion is neither a socially desirable nor a medically recommendable method of birth control or family planning,"[9] but currently none of the parties holding seats in the Austrian parliament demands the reintroduction of punishment. This is noteworthy, since the SPÖ lost its absolute majority in 1983 and theoretically the conservative parties have enough representatives in the national assembly to change the law.

The SPÖ, since 1986 in a coalition with the ÖVP, views itself as a protector of the maintenance of the term solution but makes only a few attempts to guarantee fuller implementation. Sections of the SPÖ, especially the women's and youth organizations, demand improvements of abortion in practice—for example, foundation of public outpatient clinics for abortion in every federal state, with the cost covered by health insurance.

In the 1980s, the ÖVP modified its position and no longer demanded the reintroduction of punishment. In August 1990, the Conservative party leader declared that "a return to the punishment of women would be unthinkable and has to be rejected." Currently the ÖVP is aiming at restriction of the practical availability of abortion—for example, closing clinics that cater only to abortion seekers.

The FPÖ does not want a return to the criminalisation of women. The current party programme explicitly expresses women's right of choice. In contrast to the ÖVP, the FPÖ does not support the plan that the physician conducting the medical consultation and the physician who performs the abortion be two different persons.

The two ecological parties existing in Austria support the exemption of punishment of abortion within the first three months.

In the 1970s, the Austrian Catholic Church with its lay organizations was one of the main powers fighting the term solution and demanding maintainance of punishability in nearly every case (Österreichische Bischofskonferenz 1974). Although this subject was of fundamental importance to the church, it did not escalate the conflict beyond a certain point. Today some sections of the Catholic Church—for example, the Catholic Family Federation[10]—no longer concentrate their work on the re-establishment of punitive sanctions. On the other hand, owing to newly appointed bishops, the Austrian Catholic church—at least in the upper ranks—is approaching a more fundamentalist and conservative position. It is expected that within the next few years, on subjects such as sexuality, contraception, and abortion, the Austrian Catholic Church will fall into line with the views of the Pope.

The Austrian Protestant Church has always held a less rigorous view. One section, the Helvetic Confession, has even supported decriminalisation. Currently, a majority of Protestant churches still rejects the term solution; however, a minority regard it as an adequate legislative concept.

Among the activists supporting the term solution or further liberalisation is the Autonomous Women's Movement and the Women's Organisation of the Social Democrat Party. Their demands specifically aim at improving the practical availability of abortion.

Opponents have been organised by the Catholic lay organizations and in groups dedicated specifically to this subject—for example, Action Life and Born for Unborn. The latter developed from the youth organisation of Action Life and follows a more restrictive line. Between 1982 and 1986, during the last big campaigns, Action Life, the most powerful of these groups, distributed about 1 million booklets, 2.5 million information papers, and 3 million leaflets.[11] These organisations have ideological and organisational support from the Catholic Church. While some members still uphold the demand that abortion be liable to prosecution within the first three months, Action Life has officially dropped this demand. The organisation concentrates its efforts on making the public aware of the situation and consulting expectant mothers. Furthermore, it demands social, financial, and legal provisions so that abortion would no longer be necessary and exerts pressure for modifications on the term solution that would render abortion more difficult in practice.

THE FUTURE

The issue of impunity versus punishability does not represent a major problem in domestic Austrian politics currently. Nevertheless, the issue does get raised periodically in the run-up to elections. In 1990, for example, the parties disagreed on the registration of RU 486, a drug which can be taken orally to induce abortion.

The conflict over abortion currently does not concentrate on the question of impunity versus punishability. Both parties are now trying to change the practical availability of abortion. The women's movements demand the opportunity to have an abortion performed in every public hospital with the costs covered by health insurance. On the contrary, the opponents of abortion insist that only certain physicians be allowed to perform abortions. They further demand that consultation and abortion be done by two different persons and that there be an obligatory time for reflection in between.

NOTES

Abbreviations

BGBl	Bundesgesetzblatt
BT	Besonderer Teil
ECHR	European Convention on Human Rights
EuGRZ	Europäische Grundrechtezeitschrift
FPÖ	Freiheitliche Partei Österreichs
JBl	Juristische Blätter
ÖVP	Österreichische Volkspartei
SPÖ	Sozialdemokratische Partei Österreichs
ÖJZ	Österreichische Juristen-Zeitung
RN	Randnummer
StG	Strafgesetz
StGB	Strafgesetzbuch 1975
VfGH	Verfassungsgerichtshof
VfSlg	Sammlung der Erkenntnisse und wichtigsten Beschlüsse des VFGH

1. This distinction was valid until 1745.

2. According to majority opinion, these exceptions of punishment constitute a defence to an illegal act (Kienapfel 1990, § 97 RN 1; Leukauf and Steininger 1979,

§ 97 RN 2; Foregger and Serini, Strafgesetzbuch, § 97 I). The minority position (Zipf 1984, § 97 RN 3) is that these exceptions alter the elements of the offence.

3. For example, Art. 7 sec. 1: "All citizens are equal before the law. Privileges of birth, sex, rank, class and confession are precluded."

4. K. Marschall, "Grundsatzfragen der Schwangerschaftsunterbrechung im Hinblick auf die verfassungsrechtlich gewährleisteten Rechte auf Leben," *JBI* 1972, 497; D. Grimm, "Die Fristenlösungsurteile in Österreich und Deutschland und die Grundrechtstheorie," *JBI* 1976, 74; R. Nowak, "Das Fristenlösungs-Erkenntnis des österreichischen Verfassungsgerichtshofes," *EuGRZ* 1975, 197; R. Machacek, "Das Recht auf Leben in Österreich," *EuGRZ* 1983, 453; W. Groiss, G. Schantl, and M. Welan, "Der verfassungsrechtliche Schutz des menschlichen Lebens," *ÖJZ* 1978, 1; H. Spanner, "Lebendiges Verfassungsrecht," *JBI* 1977, 20. However, the following authors denied a contravention of the Constitution: Dearing 1987, 154; W. Rosenzweig, "Drei Verfassungsgerichte zur Fristenlösung," in FS Broda 1976, 231.

5. Since the establishment of the term solution in 1975, the argument between the pro and anti factions centres on the issue of compulsory registration. While the opponents of impunity demand statistical recording of all abortions, many of the supporters of the term solution are against it. They cite the desire of the women to remain anonymous and the fear that these data could be misused. In addition, they are afraid of the possibility that a high rate of abortion might be used as another argument by their opponents. Furthermore, it is implied that there is some resistance by physicians to registration for fiscal reasons.

6. Edlinger, *Studien zur Reform des österreichischen Strafgesetzes*, 131 ff; Rainer Münz, "Zur Zahl der Abtreibungen in Österreich," in Benedikt and Potz (Eds.) 1986, 165 ff. Alfred Rockenschaub, one of Austria's leading gynaecologists, alleges that in his experience, because of the low standard of contraception, an Austrian woman who has borne two children in her life has also had two abortions and two miscarriages.

7. In 1989 in Austria, 50 percent of female workers earned less than 7,830 and 50 percent of male employees less than 10,390 Austrian Schillings (Mikrozensus, June 1989).

8. The Austrian newspaper *Der Standard* (27.9.90, Pg. 8) published other opinion polls from FESSEL that indicated growing approval in the Austrian population of the term solution: 53 percent (1976), 56 percent (1983), 63 percent (1990). On the other hand, the opposition to impunity decreased: 40 percent (1976), 35 percent (1983), 27 percent (1990).

9. Resolution passed by the Austrian parliament on November 11, 1973, the same day the term solution was adopted.

10. For example, on September 7, 1990, this organization published a press release stating: "The Catholic Family Federation still stands up emphatically for the full protection of human life from conception to death, without aiming at a persecution of women by criminal law."

11. Information brochure *Dem Leben eine Chance* (2/87) of this organisation.

REFERENCES

Benedikt, Michael, and Richard Potz, (eds.). *Zygote-Fötus-Mensch: Zur Anthropologie des werdenden Lebens* (Zygote-Foetus-Man: Anthropology to the Becoming of Life). Vienna: Jugend und Volk, 1986.

Broda F.S., *Festschrift für Christian Broda zum 60. Geburtstag* (Publication in Honour of the 60th birthday of Christian Broda). Vienna: Europa Verlag, 1976.

Dearing, Albin. "Landesbericht Österreich" (Austrian Report). In Eser, Albin, and Hans-Georg Koch (eds.). *Schwangerschaftsabbruch im internationalen Vergleich* (Abortion in International Comparison). Baden-Baden: Nomos Verlang, 1988.

Dearing, Albin. "Austria." In Frankowski, Stanislaw J. and George F. Cole (eds.). *Abortion and Protection of the Human Fetus: Legal Problems in a Cross-Cultural Perspective.* Dordrecht-Boston-Lancaster: Martinus Nijhoff, 1987.

Edlinger, Gertrude. *Dokumentation der politischen Geschichte zur Reform des §144 StG* (Documentation of the Political History of the Reform of Para. 144 StG.). Vienna, 1981.

Flossmann, Ursula (ed.). *Frau im Recht: Geschichte-Praxis-Politik* (Woman in Law: History-Practice-Politics). Linz: Universitätsverlag Rudolf Travner, 1988.

Foregger E., and E. Serini. *Strafgesetzbuch Penal Code*, Wien: Manz.

Gründel, Johannes. *Abtreibung pro und contra* (Abortion Pros and Cons). Innsbruck: Tyrolia-Echter Verlag, 1971.

Ketting, Evert, and Philip van Praag. *Schwangerschaftsabbruch: Gesetz und Praxis im internationalen Vergleich* (Abortion: Legal Situation and Practice in International Comparison). Tübingen: Deutsche Gesellschaft für Verhaltens Therapie, 1985.

Kienapfel, Diethelm. *Grundriss des österreichischen Strafrechts Besonderer Teil 13* (Compendium on the Austrian Criminal Law, Special Part 13). Vienna: Manz Verlag, 1990.

Lehner, Karin. *Verpöonte Eingriffe: Sozialdemokratische Reformbestrebungen zu den Abtreibungsbestimmungen in der Zwischenkriegszeit* (Illegal Abortion: Social Democratic Reform Attempts to the Law of Abortion Between the Two World Wars). Vienna: Picus Verlag, 1989.

Leukauf, Otto, and Herbert Steininger. *Kommentar zum Strafgesetzbuch 2* (Commentary to the Penal Code 2). Eisenstadt: Prugg Verlag, 1979.

Münz, Rainer, and Jürgen M. Pelikan. *Geburt oder Abtreibung: Eine soziologische Analyse von Schwangerschaftskarrieren* (Birth or Abortion). Vienna: Jugend and Volk, 1978.

Österreichische, Bischofskonferenz (ed.). *Worte der österreichischen Bischöfe zum Schutz menschlichen Lebens* (Statements of Austrian Bishops to the Protection of Human Life). Vienna, 1974.

Rittler, Theodor. *Lehrbuch des österreichischen Strafrechts II* (Manual on the Austrian Criminal Law, II). Vienna: Springer Verlag, 1962.

Sagmeister, Reimund. *Fristenlösung: Wie kam es dazu?* (Term solution: How did it come about?). Salzburg-Munich: Verlag Anton Pustet, 1981.

Sozialwissenschaftliche Arbeitsgemeinschaft: *Vom Volksbegehren zum Schutz des menschlichen Lebens* (From Popular Initiative to the Protection of Human Life).

Wimmer-Puchinger, Beate. *Empirische Untersuchung der Motive zum Schwangerschaftsabbruch: Soziale und psychische Situation der Frau* (Empirical Investigation on the Motivation of Abortion: Social and Psychological Situation of the Woman). Vienna: Bundesministeriun für Umwelt, Jugend und Familie, 1983.

Wimmer-Puchinger, Beate, Michael Kundi, and Gertrud Bronneberg. *Frauen im Schwangerschaftskonflikt: Beratungsangebote* (Women in the Conflict of Abortion: Possibilities of Consultation). Vienna: Bundesministeriun für Umwelt, Jugend und Familie, 1988.

Zipf, Heinz. "§§ 96–98 StGB." In Foregger, Egmont, and Friedrich Nowakovsky (Eds.), *Wiener Kommentar zum Strafgesetzbuch, 25. Lieferung* (Viennese Commentary to the Penal Code, 25th Delivery). Vienna: Manz Verlag, 1984.

BELGIUM

Vicky Claeys

THE HISTORY OF ABORTION LAW

The Emergence of a Political Debate

For centuries Belgium was under occupation and therefore subject to the laws of other countries. It was once part of the Kingdom of the Low Lands, which in turn was annexed by France. In France, justice was defined by the penal code of Napoleon.

In 1830, Belgium became a sovereign country, but it was 1867 before it got its own penal code. The articles concerning abortion, however, were an exact copy of Napoleon's. Abortion was forbidden in all circumstances. The woman was liable to punishment and the abortionist, if a midwife, nurse, or medical doctor, was subject to even more severe punishment. In addition, information and advice about the sale of abortifacients was punishable. In short, nothing was legal and lots of women suffered or died from clandestine abortions performed by nonmedical people.

The debate on abortion originated in a number of different organisations. The Belgian Family Planning Association (FCGSO), established in 1955, was the first to talk openly about abortion. The goal of this organisation was merely to provide contraceptives, but from the beginning its members stood at the barricades to change the abortion law.

The second important group to contribute to the debate was the Socialist Women's Movement (SVV). Their opinion was very important and influential for the official stance of the Socialist party. They pointed out that abortion was also a matter of class difference. Illegal abortion was dangerous, but it was much more dangerous for poor women because rich women could always find a solution by paying a private doctor or going to another country where abortion was legal. Therefore, SVV demanded the right to medical help for every woman and was the first organisation to stress the woman's autonomy, given that she was the one to get pregnant and to have the abortion.

The Free University of Brussels (ULB-VUB) took an early part in the discussions by organising seminars about the subject. The freethinkers added new ideological dimensions to the debate. They stipulated the right of the human being to control nature. Respect for the quality of life was a value of global concern. Humanist morality stressed the importance of individual responsibility and personal decision making. State intervention in the private lives of human beings was not to be tolerated. A pluralist society allowed for a difference in ideas rather than that one opinion be dictated to everyone.

Subsequently, debate also began among people who were confronted with abortion in reality, such as lawyers, medical doctors, and gynaecologists. The lawyers were witnesses to the harsh legal procedures against women, and the doctors experienced how bad illegal and nonmedical abortions were for the health of women.

Points of view formulated at international conferences and the statements of the World Health Organisation (WHO) on the concept of health made clear to doctors that they were in any case obliged to help. Only the most radical among them were convinced that the wish of the woman to have an abortion was sufficient. Others were afraid to be reduced to the position of technicians and wanted to judge for themselves—to have the possibility to refuse. Whatever the category to which they belonged, that doctors spoke out about abortion was an important element in breaking the taboo. Only a few of them openly told the press that they had performed abortions. One of these was Dr. Peers, who was imprisoned in 1973. This was the action that served to put the issue firmly in the political arena.

Another important voice in this matter was that of CEFA (Centre d'Education à la Famille et à l'Amour), led by Canon De Locht. They talked about the difference between ethics and justice. The Catholic Church, they said, stands for the absolute principle of the right to life. CEFA acknowledges this to be a fundamental fact but not an unquestionable one. For CEFA, it was only the woman (or the couple) who could decide if the pregnancy was feasible. Contrary to the church's position, CEFA stressed that the life of the foetus is of no more value than that of the woman. The foetus only acquires human value when the mother (or the couple) assumes responsibility. In the same period, Pro Vita published their *Manifesto for the Protection and Development of Human Life*. Catholic women's and youth organisations have a different approach. They support a partial change in the law but not complete legalisation.

By 1972 the abortion issue was attracting the attention of all politicians. Feminists, communists, and socialists shared the platform with freethinkers, while moderate liberals tried to link up with progressive Christians. All of them had problems with those who clung to the traditional ideas of Catholicism.

The new openness about sexuality and the fact that several groups formulated their wish to change the abortion law forced political parties to consider their position on abortion. In the 1970s different parties approached the issue in different ways.

The Communist party (KP) had no problem at all. Their contacts with Eastern Europe, where abortion was legal, made it clear to them that it should be made legal in Belgium too. They introduced a proposal to make abortion legal up to 12 weeks of pregnancy if performed in a hospital by a specialist doctor. They stressed that abortion should be reimbursed out of social security and the final decision was to be the woman's.

The day after Dr. Peers was arrested, the Congress of the Socialist party (SP) declared solidarity with Dr. Peers and demanded a change in the law. At the same time they declared their willingness to enter into government (previously they were in opposition). But it was W. Calewaert, a Socialist minister, who introduced for the first time a proposal in the parliament to change the abortion law—more a personal initiative than one from the party. That said, until about 1978 the party agreed on its content. Calewaert's point was that abortion should be legal until 15 weeks of pregnancy and should be performed by a gynaecologist. If it was an abortion on medical grounds, the woman had to consult two doctors. If it was on social grounds, she had to see a commission of three doctors, one of whom needed to be a neuropsychiatrist and another a gynaecologist. The proposal highlighted the need for such a consultation to allow the doctor performing the abortion to have the possibility of persuading the woman to change her mind. Calewaert was against too liberal a law because he feared this would detract attention from planned parenthood and the use of contraceptives. His proposal was not accepted by the Socialist women's groups because it was too restrictive. It was never discussed at the political level.

The Christian Democrats (CVP), of course, did not agree with Calewaert's proposal because, as far as they were concerned, it made abortion on demand possible. In February 1973 they issued a statement wherein they agreed to legalise the selling of and information and advice about the use of contraceptives and agreed on nonprosecution of therapeutic abortion. This statement was clearly an evolution, making it possible to change Article 383. This happened on July 3, 1973, when the law was changed as part of a political deal for ending debate on the abortion issue.

The most positive aspect of legal changes allowing contraception was that the Family Planning Association (FPA) and its local centres got recognition and government funding.

The difference between the CVP position and the stance of the Catholic Church is remarkable. Following *Humanae Vitae*, the church was and is against any change in the law. In 1972, the Liberal party (PVV) supported abortion only if the life of the woman was in danger, if the child was likely to be handicapped, or if the pregnancy was the result of rape or incest. The Nationalist party (Volksunie-VU) stated that abortion was a personal decision but could only be taken in very severe situations.

This brief summary of the views of the political parties at that time shows the overall conservative position on moral matters in Belgian society. Only the small and noninfluential Communists had a progressive point of view, but the sources of that view lay in Eastern Europe where the reasons for providing legal abortions were (and are) very different from ours.

Parliamentary Activity

Although in the 1950s and 1960s several medical doctors had been imprisoned in Flanders, it was not until 1973, with the imprisonment of Dr. Peers, that a general public reaction emerged. The time was right to begin actions and demonstrations. All the above-mentioned political groups condemned his imprisonment, more so because the abortion was performed on a 15-year-old handicapped girl.

Within three weeks, about 250,000 signatures were collected, and 200 doctors and 800 women confirmed their active participation in performing or undergoing an abortion.

The case also sharpened the views of the opposition. The bishops reacted. De Locht was dismissed as chaplain and representative of his own organisation, CEFA. These events got a lot of press coverage, which increased public interest. A public opinion poll in February 1973 showed that a large majority of the people questioned were in favour of a change in the law. The abortion issue was a political hot potato. The question was: How long could they wait until it was not hot anymore?

A coalition of Christian Democrats and Liberals announced in their government's *Declaration of Policy* (1974) the establishment of a State Commission on Ethical Problems. This commission had to prepare and advise the government on issues of contraception and abortion in order to enable the government to take a position in parliamentary debates. The government also requested a parliamentary "armistice" on the abortion debate while the commission was at work. The armistice was extended when the Minister of Justice also made an agreement with the Central Court to stop prosecutions. The activists also suspended their activities until 1978.

The succeeding coalitions did not find a solution and returned the matter again and again to parliament. In the meantime, there occurred so many (much more important) political problems that no political party dared to endanger the continuity of government.

The results of the commission's study were very important because they came out with both minority and majority proposals (1974) and reinforced the government's unwillingness to handle the problem. But they had also collected lots of information and data that proved valuable in the ongoing discussion. It was also clear that every member of the commission was convinced that the law needed to be changed, although they did not agree on the form.

Between 1973 and 1983 there was a lot of parliamentary activity on the issue. No fewer than 39 proposals to change the law were submitted, including proposals to stop the prosecutions. For the most part this activity involved two political parties. The Liberals continued their strategy of looking for compromises and gathering as many parliamentarians as possible behind their proposals. Within the Liberal party people were divided, but one representative, Ms. Lucienne Herman-Michielsens, worked consistently on the issue and became a real specialist. It is she who finally succeeded in bringing about legislative change.

The Socialists became more radical. They wanted abortion taken completely out of the penal code. In this party it was also a woman, Léona Detiège, who was most prominent. Both Detiège and Herman-Michielsens were Flemish. In the Francophone part of the country the lawyer Roger Lallemand took the initiative from the moment he became a Socialist senator. He became an expert on the abortion issue as a solicitor in many court cases, and eventually made an "abortion coalition" with Lucienne Herman-Michielsens to introduce the law that was finally voted in.

By 1978 there were many organisations, both big and small, active on abortion, but there was no coordination among them. It was the right moment for the Committee for the Suspension of Prosecutions to start their activities. Two feminist women began this initiative. They were involved in family planning, socialist movements, the universities of Brussels, the freethinkers' organisations, and government departments. They were thus very well placed to get most of the organisations and persons involved around the table. The meetings were national (both languages) and included the prosecuted doctors, their lawyers, parliamentarians, women's organisations, representatives of abortion centres and family planning organisations, and Freemasons.[1] This committee tried to reach a common position and to organise the necessary lobbying of parliament. They succeeded to the extent that we can say that the law finally passed was prepared in their midst.

The Rise of Abortion Centres

What was happening in real life was at least as thrilling as what was happening on the political level. With the introduction of easier methods of abortion at the beginning of the 1970s, a whole network of abortion centres was established in the Netherlands. This was the start of the important phenomenon of "abortion tourism." In 1975 about 12,000 abortions were performed in the Netherlands on Belgian women. Some of the centres on the Dutch border worked almost exclusively for Belgian clients. Abortions performed in another country were never punishable in Belgium.

In the mid-1970s the first abortion centres in Belgium were established. They were separate from the hospitals and most of them performed abortions only in combination with contraceptive advice. There were differences in practice between the Francophone and Flemish-speaking regions. While the abortion centres are part of the FPA in Francophone Belgium, this is not the case in Flanders. For political reasons (Flanders is far more Catholic), the FPA did not risk starting abortion services and endangering their family planning work. It was not until 1980 that the first Flemish abortion centre opened its doors. Legally it is a separate organisation.

Up until 1981 matters were fairly quiet in relation to prosecutions. But then the attorney general of Brussels decided that he had given parliament enough time to clarify legal matters. Because they had not succeeded, he concluded, the former law was still applicable and justice had to be done. From that moment on hard times were in store for women undergoing abortions as well as for the medical staff of hospitals and abortion centres. Many cases were brought to court, but fortunately they always ended with the lowest possible punishment for the medical staff and no punishment at all for the women. Even so, it was a very stressful time. It provided a reason to organise demonstrations and to work on public and political opinion.

In mid-1991 there were five centres operating in Flanders, and about 23 in Francophone Belgium. Next to these centres there are, of course, the hospitals. It depends on their internal policy whether or not they perform abortions. The Catholic hospitals were instructed not to organise a counseling service, so in fact they cannot perform legal abortions.

Reliable statistics are elusive; legal abortion is recent and there are no reliable figures from the previous period when abortion was illegal. Specialists conclude, however, that there are 15,000 to 20,000 abortions annually. Since the start of the abortion centres, the figures for abortions for Belgian women in the Netherlands dropped except in periods of prosecutions. The annual report of Stimezo for 1987 through 1988, reveals that there were 4,652 abortions on Belgian women in 1986, 4,833 in 1987, and 4,430 in 1988.

ABORTION: CURRENT LAW AND PRACTICE

The Law of 1990

A new abortion law passed the House of Commons on March 20, 1990, and has been operative since April 3, 1990. Abortion still remains in the penal code, but it is no longer punishable in certain cases. A prerequisite is the "untenable situation" of the woman, whether physical, psychological, or social. It is the woman and only she who decides that she is in this position. Nobody, including the doctor, is allowed to debate this point. When the woman is in an untenable situation she can have a legal abortion up to the 12th week of pregnancy (14 weeks of amenorrhoea). The abortion must be performed by a medical doctor in a health centre. The woman must be fully informed beforehand about her rights and alternatives to abortion by an information service in the (abortion) clinic. After six days, and after signing a paper whereby she declares that she is fully convinced about having the abortion, the abortion can be performed.

After 12 weeks' pregnancy, an abortion can be legally performed only when the life of the woman is in danger or when the foetus is severely handicapped and is likely not to survive.

The doctor must fill out a registration form that has to be sent to the Evaluation Commission. This commission was set up in March 1991. Official guidelines are published about the structure and tasks of the commission, but discussions at the political level about who is "acceptable" as a member of the commission have taken a very long time. The structure provides for 16 members. Nine of them are women. The background of these people is also specified. Eight members have to be doctors, four have to be doctors of medicine, and four need to be lawyers. Four people must be working in the field. This committee is supposed to be the watchdog in the application of the abortion law.

As mentioned, abortion is still in the penal code. There are different degrees of punishment, depending on the circumstances in which the abortion takes place.

1. If the woman has an abortion that cannot be seen as falling under the circumstances described in the law, she can be punished with one month to one year of imprisonment and a fine of between 50 and 200 Belgian francs.

2. When the abortion method causes the death of the woman or when the woman agreed to have the abortion but it was performed outside legal stipulations, the one who performed the abortion will go to prison (no time specified).

3. If the abortion is performed illegally and without the woman's consent, the abortionist will get 10 to 15 years of forced labour.

Abortion in Practice

In 1990, the Family Planning Association tried to inform the general public about the steps to take in case of an unwanted pregnancy. In its opinion there are three possibilities.

1. *The abortion centre:* As abortion is legal and the addresses of the centres are available, the woman can choose to go straight to the centre. There she will have a medical examination and counselling to see if her decision is

clear. Six days later she can get an appointment for the abortion. Afterwards she can go for a postabortion medical examination to her own doctor or a family planning association.

2. *The family doctor:* If this contact is good, she can have her medical examination there and get the address of an abortion centre. When she makes contact with the centre the same procedure described under (1) starts.

3. *The family planning centre:* These centres used to be the first contact for women who wanted an abortion. That image still remains. If the woman is not sure about her decision and/or has other problems in her relationship, the family planning centre is a more neutral place to discuss this and to obtain multidisciplinary help. If the decision is clear, the procedure as under (1) starts.

The cost of an abortion in a centre is approximately 6,000 Bfr. About 2,500 Bfr. is repaid by social security for the curettage element in the abortion. Discussions are going on currently on this point, since it may be necessary to reclassify abortion under a special social security code in order to get financial reimbursement. Social security will not agree to pay for the cost of the whole abortion operation under the title of "curettage."

As was explained earlier, the current abortion law makes abortion legal until the 12th week of pregnancy. Although there are no other limitations, there can be some difficulty for very young women. The question is whether the parents need to be informed or not. In practice the medical staff inform the parents only when the girl is under 12 or 13 years of age. For older girls it is important to have very good counselling to make sure the decision is really theirs. As there are no obligations concerning a written consent from parents or partner, there also is no obligation to inform them.

The article in the law that obliges the woman to have a preliminary visit to the abortion centre (with medical and psychological services) and the abortion six days later can cause problems if the pregnancy is advanced. The problem is even greater if she first visits her doctor or a family planning centre. This is the main negative aspect we have experienced in relation to the quality of the services provided.

We can presume that from the mid-1970s on illegal abortions (i.e., nonmedical) have been scarce. The only information we have is that in the big hospitals there were fewer women appearing with serious health problems because of a badly performed abortion.

The fact that the law is very recent makes it difficult to assess the current situation. The FPA still gets women in consultation who are badly informed and who are not even aware of the existence of the law. There is much more work needed to provide information to the public in general and to women particularly, but the press is no longer cooperative on this issue. Having spent the previous year covering the political debate, they are now really fed up with it.

In addition, medical doctors are, generally speaking, not well informed, either. Not all of them know where to refer the woman; some are unwilling to do so. In the latter case the woman should be aware that the doctor is obliged to say immediately that she or he is not willing to help her on moral grounds. In this case the law leaves the doctor the possibility to refuse, but on the other hand it is clear that the doctor should provide an address where the woman can find help (e.g., a family planning centre).

One of the big advantages of the law is that abortion is no longer secret. In the past we had to explain to women not to tell anybody about their abortion. We had to do so because all the prosecutions started with a charge from someone close to the victim (parents, husband, boyfriend). We knew that hardly anyone was to be trusted and certainly not in the case of problematic relationships. In spite of all our counseling, this constraint clearly was not positive in helping the woman come to terms with the emotions an abortion can cause.

The Politics of Abortion

Belgium has always had a majority of Roman Catholics, especially in Flanders. The Christian Democratic party has been the major party for at least the last 40 years. There is also a Catholic royal family. At the time the new abortion law was passed in parliament, the king refused to sign it and failed to respect the democratic decision because of his own moral beliefs.[2] In addition, the Catholic Church has an important influence. Sometimes it is difficult to see precisely how powerful it is, but on abortion it is surely a counterforce.

With this in mind it is no surprise that the general attitude towards matters of sexual morality is complex and often turns out to be a conflict between Catholics and freethinkers. As a matter of fact, this is exactly the split between pro and anti-abortionists. On the pro side are the Socialists and Liberals with their socio-cultural and women's organisations. The growing pluralistic movement is also pro.[3] All of them respect the right of the woman to choose.

On the other side, we find the church and the Catholic organisations, with Pro Vita in the lead, and the extreme right-wing political party, Vlaams Blok. Currently some people in the Catholic welfare organisations are developing alternative structures to avoid abortion. A woman with an unwanted pregnancy will be helped through her pregnancy. After delivery, she will be helped either to keep the baby or give it up for adoption. Nothing is wrong with this, if the choice of the woman is respected.

Pro Vita is active in Catholic schools, showing their videos and convincing young people what horrible people the "pro-abortionists" are. They have a monthly publication wherein they attack "the godless" and give a list of the schools they visited.

A positive development recently has been that the majority of people, even politicians, agree on the necessity of sex education but with a focus on relationships. At the time the law was passed, three Christian Democrat ministers (education, welfare, and health) began initiatives to prevent unwanted pregnancies. They got additional funds (approximately 180 million BFr.). Most of the services of these three departments were assigned special tasks in this field, with additional personnel and funds. The family planning centres were recognized as the major organisation with which to collaborate, and got most of the money. In addition to providing intensive personal counselling services, especially for women having an unwanted pregnancy, the family planning centres also organised information and educational activities on the subject. The branches that were members of the Belgian Federation CGSO (and of IPPF, or International Planned Parenthood Federation) had had a policy on information and educational activities for years, but they did this on a voluntary and almost unpaid base.

So the positive result is twofold. On the one hand, there is a change in attitude on the part of the government, which finally recognizes the need to talk about sex (they prefer to say relationships); at the same time, the family planning organisations got more people and money to do what some of them had been doing for many years. Of course, such a sudden change also has negative aspects. The government has some naïve ideas about who is capable of providing information and education. Many people (teachers, doctors, etc.) do not like to do it and do not feel comfortable. We can only hope that they will look for collaboration with trained and experienced people.

THE FUTURE

As has already been pointed out, there was a slow but steady change of opinion towards abortion, which made it possible to change the law. However, this legal change is so recent that we cannot foresee what the practical outcome will be. What is certain is that the law must be followed very strictly to avoid prosecutions starting again. If this should happen, punishments would be severe and public opinion could swing from apathy to a negative reaction to abortion services, and by extension to the law itself. The slightest mistake will be taken up by the church, the Christian Democrats, and Pro Vita in order to abandon the law.

In 1991, a survey was conducted to ascertain general public opinion concerning the law. Recently some of the results were revealed to the press. Men and women aged 21 to 40 were asked under what circumstances they would accept that a woman could have an abortion. Most respondents, men and women, agreed with abortion when the woman's health is at risk. Two-thirds agreed in the case of the risk of a handicapped child. The same proportion agreed to abortion when the woman was in an "untenable situation." Not being married or simply not wanting the pregnancy is not regarded as valid reason for an abortion by the majority of those questioned. In short, 67 percent of the respondents were in favour of the abortion law as voted in 1990.

The above figures do not mean that the general public is fully aware of the exact content of the law. Apart from the 5 percent who don't know, about 10 percent of respondents think that abortion is allowed in all circumstances. Only 3 out of 10 refer to the exact phrase "untenable situation."

The situation is even worse when we look at the level of knowledge concerning the abortion services available. More than one year after implementation of the law, more than half the population reveals that they do not know where to obtain an abortion. Figures show a relevant difference in knowledge according to general educational level.

The major challenge in the future will be dealing with the activities of the Evaluation Commission mentioned earlier. The existence of such a commission is due to pressure from the Christian Democrats. It resulted from a political deal ensuring that a commission would assess the law and its effects. Within two years the commission has to report on the quantity, content, and social circumstances of the abortions performed and of the unwanted pregnancies that did not end in an abortion. This report must be submitted to parliament as a basis for reopening discussions and changing the law again, whether positively or negatively. It is clear that the commission's report will be of enormous importance for the future of the law and the help that can be given to women. The members of the commission have very different backgrounds and we cannot at this moment foresee the balance between those for and those against the law.

People working in the abortion centres, family planning centres, and other resources in the field already experience the limits of the law and will probably try to present this message to the commission. The most important constraint is the time limit on abortion (up to 12 weeks), which presents an obstacle to women who do not succeed in finding help within this time. We are still obliged to send these women over the border. A second major constraint is the reflection time of six days, which can be too long in some circumstances. A third problem is the obligation to make two visits to the abortion centre, which can be unnecessary if the woman has had a worthwhile first consultation with her doctor or in a family planning centre. This rule forces her to tell too many people about the most personal matters in her life. Laws exist to provide rules, which are necessary in any organised society. But there are always exceptions to the rules—extraordinary circumstances in people's lives. At this moment women in these difficult situations have no recourse and the law is too recent to show what exceptions will be accepted by the courts.

In general—and this is not only the case for Belgium—the evolution of abortion laws in other countries will be of major influence. What happens in the United States is always used as an example in Europe, in spite of the different social and cultural backgrounds. The attempts to change the laws in Poland and Bulgaria, and the revival of the Catholic Church in Eastern Europe in general, are also rather frightening.

To end this story of Belgium positively, we hope and are convinced that it is almost unthinkable that this law can be changed regressively. Once something is implemented and accepted by the public, it is almost impossible to go back to the past. We have had this experience as regards contraceptives, which are acceptable despite the Catholic Church's admonition to Catholics not to use them. Belgium has a high rate of pill use, and many users say they are Catholic. On issues of sexuality and family planning, there is a growing gap between the rules of the church and people's own lives. Let's hope people will never allow the church or the politicians to deprive them of the rights for which they have fought.

NOTES

1. In Belgium there is a group of freethinking Freemasons who have taken progressive stances on a number of social issues, including abortion.

2. The Belgian royal family has close relations with the Catholic Church. The queen is Spanish. She and her husband have remained childless and have never made a secret of their support for "the rights of the unborn." The king's failure to sign the abortion law caused political embarrassment. In an apparent paradox, it also led to a decline in the political influence of the Christian Democratic party.

3. Previously it was difficult to survive politically independent of the major political parties in Belgium. CGSO has managed to do so, often against the odds. Recently there has been a much greater tendency of other organisations to break any links with formal political parties and to work, like CGSO, independently.

REFERENCES

Belgisch Strafwetboek, art. Titel VII, hoofdstuk 1, vruchtafdrijving.
Claeys, V.. *Het Belgische Abortusverhaal.* Brussels: Federatie CGSO, 1985.
Press conference, Centre for Population and Family Studies, Brussels, May 5, 1992.
Witte, E. "Twintig Jaar Politieke Strijd Rond de Abortuswetgeving in België (1970–
        1990)," *Res Publica* 32, no. 4 (1990).

BRITAIN

Madeleine Simms

THE HISTORY OF ABORTION LAW

Between the Wars

The cause of abortion law reform has a comparatively long history in England. The Abortion Law Reform Association was founded in 1936 by a group of women, most of whom had been involved in other progressive causes of the period. Some had campaigned for votes for women 25 years earlier, some had been active in the birth-control cause, some had been involved in the work of the Labour party, and several were active freethinkers. They were aware that there had been a striking improvement in public health since the First World War.

In his annual report for 1933, the chief medical officer of the Ministry of Health had observed that mortality from tuberculosis had been halved during the previous 20 years, a reduction comparable with the decline in infant mortality. This provided a striking contrast with maternal mortality: "For twenty years that rate has remained static at or about four deaths per 1,000 births" (HMSO 1934, 259). He said that one reason for this was: "A substantial increase in abortion, and in the habit of abortion . . . which is now materially affecting maternal mortality" (261).

In 1933, 463 women died as a direct result of abortion. Another 97 women died for reasons "associated with abortion." These were the official figures. The chief medical officer recognised that these figures were incomplete and that additional deaths took place from abortion that were ascribed to other more respectable causes. The social stigma then attached to the subject ensured its systematic underreporting.

Whereas birth control had always been legal, abortion was illegal in England and Wales under the Offences Against the Person Act of 1861. However, a small but increasing number of abortions were performed in public hospitals when the woman's life was in danger. At the same time, middle-class women bought abortions privately from expensive doctors, while working-class women bought them more cheaply and more dangerously from illegal abortionists who, although unqualified, were often quite experienced. By contrast to England and Wales, in Scotland it had long been possible for a doctor to carry out an abortion if it was necessary in his clinical judgement. A doctor could not be charged with illegal abortion unless a specific complaint had been brought against him and there was evidence that he had not acted in good faith. In practice, however, abortions were probably carried out on much the same grounds as in England, though there were variations within Scotland according to local religious tradition.

Nobody knew how many illegal abortions took place each year. Estimates varied from about 50,000 to 250,000 a year. Meanwhile, without benefit of modern contraception, birth rates fell relentlessly. In 1933, the birth rate in England and Wales fell to 14 per 1,000, the lowest figure ever recorded until that time. This too caused public and professional anxiety. The medical profession and the government set up committees to investigate the abortion problem.

The British Medical Association published its *Report on the Medical Aspects of Abortion* in 1936. It recommended that abortion should be legal where it was necessary to preserve the physical or mental health of the woman, where sexual assault had taken place or where the baby would be likely to be born abnormal. It aroused much controversy by also suggesting that the community as a whole should consider whether abortion should be legalised "for social and economic reasons."

In 1937, the government appointed a committee under Mr. Norman Birkett, a senior barrister, later a High Court judge, to inquire into abortion. The committee was dominated by a group of eminent and conservative doctors and its conclusions were correspondingly cautious. It confined itself to recommending that abortion should be legalised where this was necessary to preserve the life or health of the woman. However, one member of the Birkett Committee, Dorothy Thurtle, a Labour party politician, went further. She recognised, even then, that early, medically induced abortion was at least as safe as childbirth itself. Recent experience in the Soviet Union had demonstrated this. She therefore recommended that abortion also be made legal in cases of sexual assault, where the baby might be born abnormal, and where the women had already had four pregnancies.

While this committee was sitting, a notable trial took place that was to have a great impact on public opinion. A 14-year-old girl had been assaulted and raped by two soldiers. A courageous gynaecologist, Mr. Alec Bourne, agreed to carry out an abortion, and informed the police of his action because he did not wish to be accused of acting illegally. He was arrested amid much publicity. After a long trial he was acquitted on the grounds that the original 1861 act referred to instances when abortion was "unlawful" and therefore it followed that it must sometimes also be lawful. An obvious instance was when the woman's life was at stake. However, it was not possible to distinguish between danger to life and danger to health. Thus, the judge concluded, abortion must be lawful if the pregnancy would otherwise severely damage a woman's physical or mental health. The Bourne judgement greatly liberalised English abortion law, even though it was only a single case and did not go to the Appeal Court. There still remained some doubts that a higher court might reverse this judgement, though as time went by and the Bourne judgement was reinforced by further legal cases, these fears lessened.

This case caused many people who had not thought very much about the issue before to declare their public support for abortion-law reform in the face of religious and conventional opinion.

Parliamentary Activity

During the Second World War, all abortion-law reform activities ceased. In 1951, however, the abortion issue was sharply revived when the Pope, in a speech delivered to Italian midwives, repeated the Catholic Church's traditional objection to birth control, adding that abortion was never justified, not even to save the life of the woman. This announcement was very badly received, even by leading members of the Church of England, in the more radical postwar atmosphere that prevailed in Britain. The following year, 1952, Mr. Joseph Reeves, a Labour MP, introduced the first of what were to be six parliamentary bills that attempted to reform the antiquated abortion laws. All abortion bills in Britain have been introduced into Parliament by individual Members of Parliament and not by governments, which do not wish to get actively involved in such controversial matters. Since little parliamentary time is available for such private legislation, Members of Parliament enter a ballot once a year, and only those who are fortunate enough to come out near the top of the list (usually the first six or eight names) can hope to obtain enough parliamentary time not only to introduce a measure in the House of Commons but also to guide it through all the necessary stages until it becomes law. Mr. Reeve's bill failed, and was succeeded in 1961 by another attempt, by Mr. Kenneth Robinson, MP, who was to become Labour Minister of Health a few years later. Roman Catholic MPs of all parties combined to defeat this measure, but now against a rising tide of public opinion that the Abortion Law Reform Association was helping to organise outside Parliament by publicity and political lobbying.

It was at this point that the thalidomide tragedy occurred. Pregnant women had taken drugs prescribed by their doctors to combat nausea in pregnancy, and now they learned that these drugs sometimes caused severe deformities in babies. When some pregnant women who had taken this drug requested legal abortions they were informed that, although the prescription they had been given was legal, the proposed remedy—abortion—was illegal. This argument immediately swept the abortion issue into the arena of public health, and it ceased to be associated solely with criminal and surreptitious activities. It also swept a new and energetic generation into the Abortion Law Reform Association, determined to bring about a more liberal and humane law. On July 25, 1962, a London national newspaper, the *Daily Mail*, published a startling public opinion poll showing that 73 percent of the public was in favour of abortion where a child might be born deformed. The thalidomide tragedy educated a new generation into the realities of the abortion situation. Many new and useful drugs were coming onto the market that might nonetheless be found subsequently to produce unexpected and dreadful side effects. Abortion needed to be made widely available at least on health grounds to take account of these developments. Many couples in the child-bearing groups felt concerned about this. Two further parliamentary bills were introduced into the House of Commons, one by a Labour MP, Mrs. Renée Short, and another by a Conservative MP, Mr. Simon Wingfield Digby. Again they were defeated by the Catholic MPs of all parties, who spoke so long in the debate that allotted parliamentary time ran out. But these parliamentary tactics were now openly criticised by people in all political parties.

When Lord Silkin introduced the first abortion bill into the House of Lords in 1965, he was surprised at the good progress it made in the now altered state of public opinion. A general election intervened that brought his bill to an end, but he successfully re-introduced it in the new session of Parliament. In 1966, however, Mr. David Steel, a young Scottish Liberal MP, who in later years was to become leader of the Liberal party, drew third place in the Private Members' ballot and agreed to introduce a bill in the House of Commons to liberalise the abortion law, thus convincing Lord Silkin to withdraw his own bill in the House of Lords in favour of Mr. Steel's. The bill was opposed by the more right-wing Conservative MPs and by Roman Catholic MPs of all parties, as was now the established pattern of opposition to abortion-law reform. At the same time the bill was supported by a large number of non-Catholic Labour MPs, by a small number of more progressive Conservative MPs, as well as by many of the small number of Liberal MPs. The struggle to bring the bill to a successful conclusion was a long and arduous one. The by now very experienced Lord Silkin guided Mr. Steel's bill through its various stages in the House of Lords. So bitter was the opposition that the bill nearly ran out of time but the Labour government, which was on the whole sympathetic to abortion law reform, agreed to allow some additional government time to permit the debate to finish and the necessary votes to be taken. The bill finally passed into law on October 27, 1967, and came into operation on April 27, 1968.

Social and Economic Factors Underlying Reform

It is always difficult to pinpoint why a particular piece of reform legislation comes about in one decade rather than another. The Second World War had unleashed radical forces in British domestic politics. The urge towards greater social equality and justice for all sections of society was partly embodied in the programme of the first postwar Labour government with its emphasis on public ownership, social security, and the establishment of the National Health Service, legal aid, and the children's services. The social legislation of the 1960s was probably the final manifestation of the aspirations and optimism of this postwar era. This was an era of unprecedented prosperity for Britain. Despite a series of economic crises, there was full employment, a rapidly rising standard of living, and confidence in the future—a strikingly different world from that of the 1990s. Social confidence allows compassion, generosity, and innovation to flourish. It creates an ambience that is sympathetic to social reform.

Another feature of the 1960s that is not often remarked upon is that it contained the first substantial generation of women graduates. Many of these educated women were now sitting at home with young children, wondering what to do with their lives. In that period, middle-class women with very young children did not often go out to work. A considerable number of these young, house-bound, graduate married women, many with young children, formed the core of the revitalised Abortion Law Reform Association, and many other similar reforming groups, that became such formidable campaign organisations in the 1960s. These women were feminists, but not by present-day standards very liberated. Their spare-time activities were subsidised by their husbands' earnings, not their own. The women's movement—the third wave of modern feminism—was in its early days and the abortion-law reform movement owed nothing to it as yet.

With the advent of the contraceptive pill, birth control was almost universally practiced by married couples, and increasingly by the unmarried also. The Brook Advisory Centres were established during this period to cater to the contraceptive needs of young women in their late teens and early twenties.

Religious practice had become a minority preoccupation and the Roman Catholic Church was in growing disarray over its social morality. Catholics were now openly using birth control by methods forbidden by their church, and this was causing heated public debate.

The reform of abortion laws was increasingly seen as a logical extension of other methods of fertility control. National Opinion Polls carried out a national abortion survey in 1965, which showed that 75 percent of Anglicans, 68 percent of nonconformists, 65 percent of Presbyterians, and even 60 percent of Roman Catholics favoured a measure of abortion-law reform. Doctors' opinions, too, were changing rapidly. The majority of general practitioners were known to favour a liberal abortion law, though this grass-roots view had not yet penetrated the rarefied atmosphere of the Royal Colleges, the associations of specialists and consultants which dominate the medical profession in Britain. But then it was the family doctors, not the specialists, who were on the front line and had to face the patients who were desperate for terminations.

Finally, and perhaps most important of all, was the composition of the Labour back benches after the 1966 general election. This brought 363 Labour MPs into the House of Commons, the highest number since 1945, of whom more than half were university graduates and nearly 100 were teachers, university lecturers, writers, or journalists. Moreover, nearly 100 were in their twenties or thirties. They wanted to see action. Abortion was one of a number of obvious social reforms where the state of the law was absurdly antiquated and widely ignored. Additionally, it was an inexpensive reform. Indeed, it was one that, properly considered, would actually save large sums of public money in the long run by reducing the number of septic abortions requiring hospital treatment. Here, surely was a reform whose time had come, and the Labour intake of the mid-1960s was composed of a high proportion of liberal-minded intellectuals who would be eager to take advantage of this fact.

ABORTION: CURRENT LAW AND PRACTICE

The Law of 1967

How did the Abortion Act change the situation? It confirmed that abortion was legal where it was necessary to preserve the physical or mental health of the woman. This ground had already been established by the 1938 Bourne judgement, but now it was strengthened by being turned into statute law. Legal abortion was also extended to avoid the birth of a seriously handicapped child. There were two important innovations. In the first place, a medico-social clause was introduced. The effect of the pregnancy on the health of the existing children of the family could be taken into account by doctors. In the early years of the abortion-law reform campaign, the argument had centred mainly on health issues. But social issues became increasingly important in the later stages of the debate. The extreme difficulty in distinguishing medical from social grounds in the context of both birth control and abortion became recognised, and found expression in this wording of the act. The second innovation came about as a result of intervention by the Lord Chief Justice, who wanted a clear criterion for judges when trying

Table 1
Abortions in Great Britain, 1970–1990

Year	Residents				Foreign and Irish	Grand Total
	England and Wales		Scotland			
	Nos.	Rates	Nos.	Rates	Nos	Grand Total
1970	76,000	7.0	5,000	5.0	11,000	92,000
1980	129,000	11.0	8,000	7.0	32,000	169,000
1990	173,000	16.0	10,000	9.0	13,000	196,000

Source: Abortion Statistics 1990, London, HMSO 1991, p. 6.

abortion cases in the courts. Abortion was held to be legal if it was safer for the woman than continuing with the pregnancy. Opponents of legal abortion allowed this principle to be incorporated into the act because they genuinely believed abortion to be an extremely dangerous operation. As early abortion carried out by qualified doctors in medical settings became increasingly safer than childbirth, the importance of this aspect of the Abortion Act grew.

The Abortion Act also contained three constraints that were new to the abortion situation in Britain. All abortions had to be notified to the chief medical officer at the Department of Health. Not one, but now two doctors had to agree to the abortion and sign the necessary documents. The abortion had to be carried out in a National Health Service hospital or a private clinic approved by the minister. This meant that the private clinics had to be licensed and inspected by government officials.

These regulations were not welcomed by all abortion reformers, for they hedged the abortion operation with rules that did not apply to other much more dangerous surgical procedures. The regulations were restrictive in intention and thus strongly supported by the act's opponents, who argued that this degree of medical and civil service supervision would reduce the likelihood of abortion "abuses" occurring. The reformers, who saw quite clearly the intentions that lay behind these regulations, regarded them as part of a necessary price to be paid for obtaining some reform of the law. It was a compromise, but a worthwhile one, given the benefits to women that the Abortion Act brought in its wake.

Abortion in Practice

The Abortion Act legalised abortion in Great Britain in 1967, but not in Northern Ireland. From that date onwards, as Table 1 shows, the numbers of legal abortions carried out in Great Britain rose rapidly to a peak of nearly 200,000 in 1990, when the abortion rate per 1,000 women in the childbearing ages was 16 in England and Wales and 9 in Scotland. Thereafter the figures started to decline, though it is too early to say whether this decline will prove permanent.

As Table 2 shows, the largest number of abortions in England and Wales is carried out on women in their early twenties, where the abortion rate is 28 per 1,000. Less than half of all abortions are carried out by or paid for by the National Health Service, though this could alter with current changes in the organisation of the National Health Service. Nearly 90 percent of all abortions are carried out in the first trimester of pregnancy and only 2 percent, less than 4,000, are carried out at or after 20 weeks gestation.

Nearly all early abortions are at present carried out by vacuum or menstrual aspiration, and many of the later ones by prostaglandins, alone or with other procedures. Nearly all legal abortions are carried out on the grounds that continuance of the pregnancy would involve risk of injury to the physical or mental health of the pregnant woman. Less than 20,000 are carried out for medico-social reasons of risk to the health of existing children in the family. Between 1,000 and 2,000 each year are carried out on grounds of serious handicap to the child if born. About half of all abortions are now carried out as day cases.

Some abortions were carried out on foreign women who came to Britain for this purpose from countries, mostly in Europe, where abortion was illegal or otherwise hard to obtain. The number of such abortions rose to a peak of 50,000 in the early 1970s, and then declined rapidly as abortion was legalised throughout most of the developed world. However, 4,000 women come to Britain each year from the Republic of Ireland for legal abortions denied them in their own country, and many more are thought to provide English addresses and thus entered under the English statistics. The same applies to Northern Ireland, which is not covered by the 1967 Abortion Act. About 2,000 women come each year officially, but the real figure is thought to be much larger.

Before abortion laws were reformed abroad, 20,000 Spanish women came to London for abortions in one year, in addition to 15,000 French women, 4,000 West German women, and even close to 2,000 American women. Now, very few women from these countries need come any longer to England for legal and safe abortions they can obtain at home, or, in the case of some German abortions, much nearer home in the Netherlands. In 1990, only 6,000 foreign women from Europe and the United States had abortions in Britain.

The Politics of Abortion

Attacks on the Abortion Act started almost as soon as it had passed into law. Opponents seemed to fear that unless the act could be destroyed

Table 2
Aspects of Legal Abortion in England and Wales, 1990

	All ages	Under 15	15	16-19	20-24	25-29	30-34	35-39	40-44	45 and over	Not stated
All legal abortions	186,912	933	2,689	37,950	59,799	41,555	23,988	14,002	5,538	446	12
Statutory grounds+											
1 (with any other)	437	6	12	87	115	84	62	467	21	3	-
2 (alone)	167,641	924	2,662	36,993	55,379	36,171	19,668	11,119	4,366	348	11
3 (with or without 2)	17,223	3	11	742	3,988	4,848	3,964	2,608	987	71	1
4 (alone)	1,175	-	2	89	242	364	225	170	74	9	-
4 (with any other except 1, excluding 4 alone)	431	-	2	38	73	87	68	58	90	15	-
5 or 6	5	-	-	1	2	1	1	-	-	-	-
Gestation weeks											
Under 9	65,638	230	611	10,207	20,441	16,177	9,799	5,757	2,235	175	6
9-12	94,462	442	1,423	20,179	30,342	20,558	11,768	6,850	2,697	197	6
13-19	23,027	210	515	6,454	7,725	4,246	2,098	1,200	520	59	-
20 and over	3,780	51	139	1,109	1,288	574	323	195	86	15	-
Not stated	5	-	1	1	3	-	-	-	-	-	-
Procedure											
Hysterotomy (only)	74	-	1	5	17	21	16	10	4	-	-
Hysterectomy (only)	38	-	-	-	1	8	12	10	6	1	-
Vacuum aspiration (only)	134,989	643	1,908	27,192	42,487	30,129	17,681	10,448	4,168	324	9
Vacuum aspiration with D & C or D & E	35,339	88	278	5,930	11,918	8,574	4,844	2,653	976	75	3
D & C or D & E (including menstrual aspiration)	6,046	55	143	1,602	2,129	1,062	558	336	144	17	-
Other surgical	55	-	5	15	19	10	3	2	1	-	-
Prostaglandins (only)	4,372	67	147	1,244	1,330	783	405	264	113	19	-
Prostaglandins with other agents	2,911	41	104	1,014	932	440	206	112	55	7	-
Other medical	111	1	1	11	37	29	16	13	3	-	-
Other and combined methods	2,977	·38	102	937	929	499	247	154	68	3	-

+ 1. risk to life of pregnant woman
  2. risk to health of pregnant woman
  3. risk to health of existing children in the family
  4. risk of serious foetal handicap
5 & 6. life or health in emergency

quickly, it might remain on the statute books forever. Attacks came from three main sources: from Roman Catholic MPs, from other MPs representing heavily Catholic constituencies, and from MPs on the far right of the Conservative party. Twenty attempts to amend, limit, or destroy the Abortion Act were made between 1969 and 1989. Some sought to limit the grounds for abortion, some to destroy the link between the referral agencies and the nonprofit abortion clinics, some to reduce gestation limits, some to alter the conscience clause or other aspects of the act. All possible parliamentary procedures and stratagems were resorted to, including repeated demands on the part of Roman Catholic MPs that a government committee of enquiry be set up to investigate the working of the Abortion Act. Eventually the Secretary of State for Health acceded and appointed a committee under a High Court judge, the Hon. Mrs. Justice Lane. The Lane Committee sat for two-and-a-half years and published a 700-page report in three volumes in April 1974. The Catholic lobby was not pleased when the main conclusion reached by the committee was published: "By facilitating a greatly increased number of abortions the Act has relieved a vast amount of individual suffering. . . . We have no doubt that the gains facilitated by the Act have much outweighed any disadvantages for which it has been criticised."

The immense publicity these interventions generated educated the public in the realities of the abortion issue, and, paradoxically, steadily increased the proportion of citizens supporting reform, which the frequent public opinion surveys mapped.

In 1990, however, a bill was passed that slightly affected existing abortion legislation, although that was not its primary purpose. The Human Fertilisation and Embryology Act permitted abortions to be carried out legally without any time limit where the life and health of the woman were at risk or where there was risk of serious foetal handicap. (This had always been the law in Scotland, where a time limit had never operated.) Other abortions were restricted to a 24-week gestation time limit. Since very few abortions on other grounds had ever been carried out after 24 weeks, this amendment to the 1967 Abortion Act had negligible effects. It also brought selective reduction in multiple pregnancies from treatments for infertility under the terms of the Abortion Act, in cases where a foetus in a multiple pregnancy was at risk of handicap or if too many embryos had been implanted. Thus Clause 37 of the Human Fertilisation and Embryology Act could be said to have updated the Abortion Act in the light of advances in medical technology without altering the basis of access to abortion.

THE FUTURE

The 1967 Abortion Act was an early and pioneering attempt at comprehensive reform of the abortion laws. The act proved serviceable but far from perfect. Some women who need abortions are still denied them, particularly the young, the poor, and the badly educated. Many other women who need abortions find they are unable to obtain them free under the National Health Service, and have to pay for them privately, which they can often ill afford. Moreover, it is much more difficult to obtain an abortion in some regions of the country than in others. Much still depends on the personal predilections of the doctors in charge.

On the other hand, more than 4 million abortions have been obtained legally and safely since 1967, making the Abortion Act one of the most important public health measures for British women since the end of World War II. Deaths from abortion have been virtually eliminated, as has illegal abortion. The criminal abortionist is now a figure only in folklore. In a 1991 paper "Vital Statistics of Birth" in the *British Medical Journal*, the distinguished gynaecologist Professor Geoffrey Chamberlain observed: "It must give satisfaction to those who fought for the Abortion Act 1967 to find that in the last two triennia reported by the confidential enquiry committee (1982–4 and 1985–7) there was not a single death from illegal abortion in England and Wales."

More than 40,000 women have been spared the despair of giving birth to a severely handicapped child requiring, in some cases, a lifetime's care. Many thousand women from other parts of the world have been able to obtain safe abortions in safe conditions and taken back with them to their own countries the message that legal abortion is worth fighting for. Throughout the 1970s American and Western European abortion laws were transformed, and Britain's example was often influential.

Ideally, of course, no specific abortion law is required, any more than we have specific laws dealing with other much more difficult and serious operations. Sound medical practice should be enforced for abortion as for all other medical or surgical procedures. Women who need abortions should be encouraged to come early. Abortion on request by self-referral in the first trimester, in licensed specialist abortion clinics, would cut out delay and ensure safety and high-quality care, including, most importantly, birth control instruction and abortion counselling if these are required. The nonprofit pregnancy advisory services, which were established soon after the Abortion Act was passed to cope with the demand for abortion which the NHS was unable to meet, already embody good practice in this field and demonstrate the virtues of specialisation. Under the latest changes in the administration of the National Health Service, it may become increasingly possible for Directors of Public Health to purchase services on what is called "an agency basis" from these strongly consumer-orientated organisations for pregnant women in their health districts who need abortions.

In 1991, the Minister of State for Health pointed out in the House of Commons (June 7 and July 3) that the average cost of an NHS abortion in England and Wales was £250, whereas the average hospital cost of having a baby was £1,170. It is now widely accepted that no good comes of compelling a woman to continue with an unwanted pregnancy, least of all one that costs the taxpayer more than four times as much as an urgently needed abortion. Moreover, research suggests that unwanted children are more likely to require continuing social support for many years.

Attempts will no doubt continue to be made by some sectarian extremists and antifeminists to reduce the scope of legal abortion. But now most people of childbearing age have grown up in an era of legal and safe abortion. So have a generation of young doctors, lawyers, and Members of Parliament. The forces of intolerance cannot expect any more easy victories such as they enjoyed between 1950 and 1965, when they consistently blocked all efforts for reform, thus causing the unnecessary deaths from illegal abortion of many pregnant women.

Methods of carrying out abortions are becoming simpler, cheaper, and safer all the time. Ethics, health economics, and medical technology have converged in the 1990s. All point toward the motto of the Abortion Law Reform Association: "Every Child a Wanted Child." This is the goal that all abortion-law reformers and family planners have always aimed at, and the 1967 Abortion Act made a giant stride towards this goal.

REFERENCES

Birkett Report. *Report of the Inter-Departmental Committee on Abortion.* Ministry of Health and Home Office. London: HMSO, 1939.

Chief Medical Officer. *On the State of the Public Health: Annual Report 1933.* London: HMSO, 1934.

Hindell, K., and M. Simms. *Abortion Law Reformed.* London: Peter Owen, 1971.

Lane Report. *Report of the Committee on the Working of the Abortion Act.* London: HMSO, 1974.

Marsh, D., and J. Chambers. *Abortion Politics.* London: Junction Books, 1981.

Office of Population Censuses and Surveys. *Abortion Statistics.* Statistics Series AB. London: HMSO, 1990.

Simms, M. *Abortion in Britain before the Abortion Act.* London: Birth Control Trust, 1980.

———. "The Compulsory Pregnancy Lobby—Then and Now." The Marie Stopes Memorial Lecture 1975. *Journal of the Royal College of General Practitioners* 25, no. 159 (1975): 709–19.

———. "Abortion: The Myth of the Golden Age." In Hutter, B. and Williams, G. (eds.), *Controlling Women.* London: Croom Helm, 1981.

Williams, Glanville. *The Sanctity of Life and the Criminal Law.* London: Faber and Faber, 1958.

BULGARIA

Dimiter Vassilev

THE HISTORY OF ABORTION LAW

Abortion on Demand

Artificial interruption of pregnancy on grounds of medical indication was introduced in Bulgaria for the first time in 1932. At that time the most frequent indication for the procedure was the presence of tuberculosis. After the Second World War, following the example of the Soviet Union, China, and Czechoslovakia, the Bulgarian parliament passed an amendment to the existing penal code (Paragraph 135), cancelling the punishment of abortionists and women having abortions, provided the interruption of pregnancy took place in a medical institution. As an addition to the law, a further special decree was issued in 1956 by the Ministry of Public Health and Social Welfare. As a result, abortion on demand was allowed in practice.

The social and demographic policy of Bulgaria during the last four and a half decades was strongly influenced by the fact that the ruling power was the Bulgarian Communist party and the state accepted the principles of socialism. Both the Communist party and the state oriented their policy toward the pro-natalist goals of extensive population development. The aim of demographic policy was two or three children per family. Families themselves were on average two children families.

The government followed a dual policy. On one hand, unable to support families with an intensive housing programme, incentives, and a higher living standard, the government was forced to accept, approve, and practice abortion policy. The lack of contraceptives made abortion the only birth control measure. At the same time, the government tried to suspend women's right to abortion at every level.

Thus a strange situation resulted whereby officials were pronouncing the liberal stance that women had the right to an abortion as one of the advantages of the "socialist revolution," with the Soviet Union as its example, and at the same time were punishing women who had abortions as having done something against society and state policy (deprivation of sick leave, humiliation through the lack of confidentiality, psychological attack, and accusations of irresponsibility and selfishness).

Restricting Abortion

The birth rate in Bulgaria decreased significantly in the 1960s. The rate of natural increase of the population has also dropped. This reduction in birth rate was used by the government to explain the country's economic crises and its government's failures. Hence a strongly pro-natalist atmosphere emerged that influenced newer abortion policy. The rulers decided that restricting abortions was an essential element of social and demographic policy, and the right of women to abortion on demand was slowly and gradually suspended.

At the end of 1967, a special decree was published (Decree of the Council of Ministers and the Central Committee of the Bulgarian Communist Party #69) that sought to encourage births. The point of the decree was to limit a woman's right to abortion, and so some serious restrictions were set up. Abortion was forbidden for all married women having no children or having only one child. Bureaucratic barriers were placed in the way of other abortions. Candidates for abortion were obliged to apply before a special commission at outpatients' clinics. Women were categorized on the basis of marital status, social status, and so on. The pro-natalists limited the right of abortion to women who had "fulfilled their patriotic obligation" to deliver at least one child (1969) or two children (1984). That was the beginning of a long period of violence in the field of family planning, during which pregnant women seeking abortions were humiliated.

The situation got worse in 1973, when the ruling pro-natalists increased in power. New limitations on the right to abortion were introduced; for example, abortion became impossible for all unmarried women. Public reaction was negative, since the new amendments to the legislation went against concepts and practices that had been accepted for decades. After several months in which some groups fought to have the restrictions eliminated, the Ministry of Public Health was forced to liberalise the decree. During this time there were several maternal deaths owing to illegal abortions. In the following year (1974), as a result of public pressure, some relaxation of rules was introduced, relating mainly to unmarried pregnant women.

New restrictions were introduced in 1984, when it became clear that previous measures to increase the birth rate had not been effective. Pressed by some political forces of a conservative pro-natalist nature, the Ministry of Public Health set up a new type of committee that included neighbourhood representatives who were nonmedical persons. The principle of confidentiality, which had been respected for more than 30 years, was now abandoned, and the right of women to abort was discussed openly.

The fight against a more liberal abortion law continued up to the beginning of 1990, when new democratic changes took effect. It is significant that the present decree on freer access to abortion was signed by the former minister on the night before he was discharged. The changing atmosphere in the country did not allow the pro-natalists to react to the new legislation, and it became fact.

The Bulgarian experience has shown that the emergence and survival of liberal abortion legislation is a result of an ongoing struggle in which involvement by the media, social organisations, and the Family Planning Association were of significant importance. Because of the antidemocratic, totalitarian character of the communist system, these groups were effective in expressing public opinion in support of the liberalisation of abortion law.

ABORTION: CURRENT LAW AND PRACTICE

The Law since 1990

A woman's right to legal abortion in Bulgaria is defined by a special decree of the Ministry of Health and Social Welfare.[1] According to this decree, an abortion can be performed on request or for medical indications on Bulgarian citizens, foreign citizens, and women without citizenship who are allowed to live in Bulgaria. In practice, the law guarantees interruption of an unwanted pregnancy without discrimination based on marital or family status, citizenship, age, and so on. Women with severe mental disabilities can have an abortion only if their legal representatives or guardians agree.

Although medical care in Bulgaria is free for all citizens, women must pay a fee to have an abortion. This is determined by their income; the maximum fee payable equals US$5. This fee is regarded as a tax, not as the price for the operation, since it does not cover the real cost of the medical care involved.

Abortion is performed free if it is medically indicated, if the pregnancy is a result of rape, or if the pregnant woman is under the age of 18. This last exemption is made in order to treat teenagers when they have the problem and are in danger of delay owing to financial difficulties.

All hospitals and medical institutions authorised to perform abortions must admit the pregnant woman within three days of her request or of the medical decision about contra-indication being taken. Women have the right to select the place of operation in order to keep the abortion confidential.

Two main reasons for performing an abortion are acknowledged: on request, and because of some medical indications. Abortion on request can be done if the pregnancy is not more than 12 gestational weeks and the pregnant woman suffers from an illness that might be aggravated by the pregnancy and delivery, thus endangering her health or life.[2]

The procedure that the candidate for an abortion has to follow includes diagnosis of pregnancy at the local (regional) women's consultation office, laboratory examinations, and final decision. All of this has to be done within a period of 10 days, or shorter if the pregnancy is closer to the term of 12 weeks. The local regional obstetrician is obliged to direct and refer the pregnant woman to the hospital she has chosen as a preferred place for the operation. In the presence of medical contra-indications to abortion, the local gynaecologist has to treat the patient before sending her to the appropriate medical institution.

Artificial interruption of pregnancy can be carried out only in specialised obstetrical hospitals or in the obstetrical wards of general hospitals. The logic is that the pregnant woman has to be ensured the most qualified medical care—in the hospital environment, operated on by a specialist doctor, under anaesthesia, and so on. Termination of a pregnancy on an outpatient basis is considered an illegal procedure. Local or general anaesthesia is obligatory, although the evidence is that many abortions are done without or with insufficient anaesthesia.

Medically indicated abortions have to be performed on request too; that is, when the pregnant woman is suffering from a proven illness endangering her health or life (at the moment or in the future), or when risks to the offspring are shown beyond any doubt to exist. Medically indicated abortion can be done up to 20 gestational weeks if the illness indicated is one included in the addendum to the decree. If the condition or the illness is not listed in the addendum, the abortion is allowed as an exception.

Termination of a pregnancy of more than 20 gestational weeks is allowed only if the woman's life is in danger or in the case of severe morphological changes of the foetus, as well as if the foetus is severely genetically harmed ("genetic abortion").

Candidates for medical abortions are assessed by specially appointed medical committees authorised to give the appropriate permission. For the safety of the patient, all problems connected with the interruption of a pregnancy of more than 20 gestational weeks are decided by special commissions established at the University Obstetrical and Gynaecological Clinics and bigger obstetrical hospitals. Logically speaking, throughout the decision making and operation, a corresponding specialist competent to the specific illness indicating the abortion must be present.

If the commission decides that no abortion should be performed, this decision can be appealed within seven days before a special committee appointed by the Ministry of Health. The committee has to investigate the case and make a decision within seven days. The decision is final and cannot be appealed.

For the safety of the patient, the operation in a medically indicated abortion is done in a specialised hospital, engaging not only the gynaecologist but also a specialist in the disease indicating the operation. The abortion can be carried out in the nearest medical institution by the same specialist if it is an emergency or if there are medical reasons against transporting the woman.

It must be emphasised that the list of medical indications is wide, including some obstetrical and gynaecological indications. For example, a woman who has previously had a caesarian section followed by complications is allowed to decide, in the case of a later pregnancy, whether to continue with the pregnancy or have an abortion at an early stage. The same goes for any pregnancy likely to end in caesarian section.

Genetically motivated abortion is the second big group of medically indicated abortions. This group includes a huge majority of pregnant women over 35 years of age. The concept behind the legislation has been to protect the offspring from some genetically determined damage caused by the age of the mother. At the opposite extreme, abortions for teenagers below the age of 16 are regarded as medically indicated. A new medical indication for abortion is if one or both parents has AIDS or is HIV positive.

In conclusion, the current abortion legislation of Bulgaria could be classified as among the most liberal. The law not only protects the woman's right to abortion but allows her to make choices and guarantees confidentiality, quality medical care, and quality of life for the offspring. The legislation opens the door to medically indicated abortion based on modern concepts.

The Incidence of Abortion

The legalisation of abortion in Bulgaria was followed by a sharp increase in the number of registered terminations of pregnancy. The rise was almost linear. The specific character of abortion in Bulgaria was such that, once the rate of abortion rose, it stayed at a high level for several decades. In other European countries that legalised abortion at the same time, the level of abortions remained high for no longer than 10 years. The first signs of a reduction in abortion rate in Bulgaria have been seen only in the last few years, and the decrease does not exceed 10 percent.

Table 1
Abortions per 1,000 Females, 15–49 Years of Age (Selected Eastern
European Countries with Liberal Abortion Laws)

Country	Abortions
USSR	118.0
Romania	98.2
Bulgaria	61.9
Hungary	37.1
Czechoslovakia	34.5
GDR	26.6

Source: Ketting 1989.

The higher abortion rate and the relatively constant level of absolute number of abortions were a natural result of the role that abortion played in the dynamics of population increase. It was obvious that abortion was a birth-control and family-planning instrument, broadly practiced and accepted by people who had no other alternative than primitive traditional contraception, which by itself was creating abortions because of its huge number of failures. In short, spouses were forced to terminate unwanted pregnancies.

Approximately 30 years after legalisation, the abortion rate and the absolute number of abortions in Bulgaria has remained relatively high compared to other European countries with legalised abortion. Coming after the Soviet Union and Romania, with their huge number of abortions, Bulgaria has occupied third or fourth place in the league table of abortion rates (see Table 1). Approximately half of all registered pregnancies still end in abortion. Although the abortion rate has been decreasing since 1987, the abortion-to-birth ratio remains unchanged (see Table 2).

In 1990–91, the abortion-to-birth ratio increased dramatically owing to a sharp drop in the birth rate; the latter reached a level never before registered in Bulgaria except during the First World War. The main reason for this was the severe economic and political crisis arising in the transition from totalitarianism to democracy.

Some specific features of the occurrence of abortion in Bulgaria are:

• The relative safety of the operation, which is performed in hospitals by skilled medical specialists, has made abortion a birth regulating instrument.
• Abortions are performed free or for a low fee.
• The wider list of medical indications has transformed abortion on demand into a medically indicated procedure.
• There are no other effective alternative methods of birth control.
• There are no social, religious, psychological, or ethical constraints on women in reaching a decision; having an abortion does not lower a woman's status or reputation in the family or society.

Table 2
Births and Abortions per 1,000 Females, 15–49 Years of Age, 1980–89

Year	Births	Artificial Abortion
1980	60.4	65.5
1981	58.6	64.0
1982	58.8	62.5
1983	58.4	56.5
1984	58.1	55.3
1985	56.6	55.8
1986	57.1	57.3
1987	55.4	56.6
1988	55.6	56.8
1989	52.2	55.7

- Defeat of the hard-line pro-natalists was a victory for supporters of liberal abortion.

- Unlike in a number of other European and non-European countries, younger women and teenagers make up a minority of those having abortions (see Table 3).

Research has shown that when teenagers or younger women get pregnant, they usually marry. Thus, in 1989, when there were 114 abortions performed on girls below 15 years of age, 890 births to girls in the same age group were registered (see Table 4). Figures from recent years demonstrate that women below the age of 19 having abortions represent around 8 percent of all those having abortions, although their share is gradually increasing. The same is true of unmarried and childless women having abortions.

The fact that abortion is typical for women of 30 years or more shows that it is serving as a method of birth control after the marriage and delivery of the first child. The issue of repeated abortions remains unstudied. There is some indication, however, that its role is slowly decreasing.

A comparison of fertility rates and abortion rates by age shows that abortion is practiced mainly during the intergenetic interval—that is, between the delivery of the first and second child in the family—and less often as a preventive of the delivery of the third child.

More than half of all abortions are performed at the most specialised hospitals—obstetrical hospitals, university clinics, and district hospitals. Pregnant women prefer medical institutions where there are enough facilities. They do not like to risk their health and life. Usually they find their way to the hospital where they believe they will obtain adequate medical care.

The operative technique used is vacuum aspiration (80–85 percent), followed by dilatation and curettage (D & C). Vacuum aspiration was introduced in Bulgaria in 1963. There are several studies demonstrating that the well-performed operation (by an experienced operator, with adequate pre-

Table 3
Age-Related Abortion Rate, 1989

Age Group	No. of Registered Abortions	Percentage Distribution of women having abortions
Less than 15	114	0.01
15-19	9,301	8.80
20-24	25,562	23.11
25-29	29,250	27.25
30-34	25,822	23.25
35-39	14,534	13.25
40-44	4,831	4.40
45-49	452	0.41

Source: Public Health Statistics Annual, Bulgaria, 1989, p. 46.

vention of complications, by the less traumatic technique), is not harmful, as is sometimes feared. In principle, an abortion performed in a specialised hospital has to be a safe procedure. Pregnancies that are advanced—over 20 gestational weeks—are usually terminated by instillation. More than half the women having abortions leave the hospital the same day after having spent some hours under observation by medical staff, but maternal mortality owing to abortion is relatively high (see Table 5).

Illegal Abortions

The absolute number of illegal abortions, and indeed the ratio of illegal abortions, is not high. Annually, about 200 to 220 cases are registered, mainly as a result of medical treatment required because of complications (see Table 6). In the case of an abortion begun or completed outside a medical institution, the law requires careful registration of the data in the presence of witnesses such as a second doctor or nurse. The data are then signed off by the patient or the witness.

If there is suspicion that an illegal abortion has been performed, the doctor must inform the hospital administration, the nearest prosecutor, and the police within 24 hours. In practice, medical staff try to avoid this long procedure (except when the evidence is obvious or there are life-threatening complications). The prosecutor's office and the police must decide if an investigation is necessary or not. The doctor who treated the woman who had the abortion is obliged to preserve all evidence: histological specimens, results of tests, foetus, parts of the egg, and so on.

Table 4
Probability to Abort or Deliver as a Ratio by Age, 1989

Age Group	Probability Abortion/Delivery
Less than 15	0.125
15-19	0.435
20-24	0.666
25-29	1.428
30-34	2.500
35-39	5.000
40-49	10.000

Source: Vassilev 1982.

The number of illegal abortions strongly correlates with legislative changes; a restrictive regime is always tied to some increase in the number and ratio. This phenomenon was observed very clearly in 1973–74, when limits on abortion rights was most severe.

The penal code requires a prison sentence of up to three years for the illegal abortionist, or up to eight years in the case of fatal complications. In practice, the court never uses the maximum sentence, probably because of the generally accepted concept that abortion outside a medical institution is not always unsafe and life threatening. Usually abortionists are medically qualified gynaecologists or midwives.

The woman who has had an illegal abortion is excused by the law. The logic is that if she is not regarded as guilty, she will not wait when complications start to manifest themselves, nor will she have any motivation to keep the operation secret.

The medical profession has accepted abortion as a reality. Among doctors and midwives, there was no strong opposition to it. In fact, the legalisation of abortion brought a drop in the number of illegal abortions and a dramatic reduction in their fatal complications and consequences.

The data on illegal abortions show how closely linked are medically indicated abortions, miscarriages, and registered illegal abortions. From 1984 to 1990, restrictions on abortions for mothers of only one child led to a rise in medically indicated abortions, but not in illegal abortions. Obviously the medical profession was helping women who were deprived of their rights. Some of the medical indications were in fact pseudo-medical.

THE FUTURE

Bulgaria entered its demographic transition at the beginning of the second decade of the twentieth century (1912). At that time, the fertility rate was

Table 5
Deaths from Abortion Complications per 100,000 Women Ages 15–49, by Country, 1977

Country	Deaths registered
Romania	9.8
USSR	1.0
Bulgaria	0.9
Denmark	0.1
Finland	0.1
Holland	0.1
Poland	0.1
Switzerland	0.1

Source: WHO/MCH/90,4: 115

high; in the ensuing eight decades, the fertility rate dropped to a third, and the two-child model of a family has become the preferred one. During this time, and especially after the Second World War, abortion played an important role in reducing the fertility rate. Unfortunately, families are still planning their size by means of artificial interruption of pregnancy when other methods of family planning have failed or have been exhausted.

A high abortion rate correlates with a high rate of classical contraception, leading to a high percentage of failures. The shortage of modern, effective, and safe contraceptives is one of the basic reasons for Bulgaria's excessively high rate of unwanted pregnancies—more than half of all registered pregnancies. It is obvious that during the next decade, family planning in Bulgaria has to introduce modern contraception methods in an effort to replace abortion.

Surgical contraception in Bulgaria does not exist. It is traditionally regarded as a Nazi eugenic method, unacceptable to both the public and the medical profession.

Also, in recent years, Bulgaria has been practically isolated from the latest advances in reproductive medicine and biology. There is no experience in some modern methods of family planning, such as antiprogestins, new barrier methods, subdermal implants, and new hormonal formulae. This gap has to be closed in order to help the transition from abortion to contraception.

Unfortunately, the severe economic crisis has blocked the normal supply of medical preparations, including contraceptives. If the supply does not improve, no significant results can be expected in combating abortion use. Several studies have shown that the contraceptive technology used by the Bulgarian population is out of date, but future improvements depend on the general development of the country and its social and medical care delivery

Table 6
Registered Abortions in Bulgaria by Type, 1980–89

Type of abortion	Absolute number by year		
	1980	1985	1989
Total abortions	156,056	162,266	132,021
medically indicated	3,830	5,586	7,134
miscarriage	15,787	14,242	13,627
illegal, clandestine	180	228	218
on demand	136,259	112,210	111,042

systems. In addition, it is not clear yet how reorganization of the health insurance system will affect abortion coverage.

An increase in "genetic abortion" is expected; this is abortion medically indicated to prevent defective offspring. The concept is still not very popular, although the first step has been taken: 1,000 genetic abortions were performed in the last few years.

When explained properly to them, spouses have proved receptive to the idea of interrupting a pregnancy that is likely to lead to the birth of a genetically disabled baby. This is substantiated by the fact that only 1 percent of parents in such cases have refused a medico-genetic abortion. As a rule, those refusing were parents with low educational level and insufficient information. It must be clear that the increase in genetic abortions in the future will lead to medico-psychological problems. It is not easy for a couple to agree to terminate a planned pregnancy, especially when there is no child in the family yet.

For the first time, in 1991 Bulgaria experienced the pronouncements of informal pro-life groups against the legal status of abortion. It is not known what will effect democraticisation will have on the concept of free choice. Although not popular, pro-life groups could find support not only among "old" pro-natalists but also among the new ruling party members.

From the time of legalisation up until now, Bulgaria has gained experience in relation to abortion. Between 1956 and 1991, more than 3.5 million pregnancies were interrupted. The medical profession has been deeply involved in this phenomenon. Rhetorically, the profession has accepted the desirability of contraception over abortion. But in practice, the abortion ratio and abortion rate remain relatively unchanged. That is why abortion still continues to present a serious problem for public health and demographic policy. Research has shown that about half (47 percent) of the practical activities of the outpatient obstetrical and gynaecological services are engaged in care connected with abortion: reference of the patient, examinations, preparations for the operation, postoperative follow-up, treatment of consequences and complications.

The forthcoming transition in the political and economic system, and the expected restructuring of the public health system, will probably be a difficult period for combating abortion. The problem has its ideological, political, psychological, and economic aspects.

At the same time, it has to be emphasised that Bulgaria has long experience in legal abortion practice. The process of liberalisation in the presence of a strong and powerful anti-abortion lobby could be instructive for some countries in Europe. Lots of aspects of abortion have been studied in detail: incidence, factors and determinants, motivation, psychological controversies created by the interruption of pregnancy, organization of abortion services, abortion counseling, influence of different technologies and their correlation with the rate of complication, late consequences, etc. The failure of family planning and contraception to combat abortion has its causes, mechanisms, sources, and determinants, and Bulgaria's experience could be of use in countries that are having or expect to have similar experiences.

NOTES

1. Decree #2, February 1990, Concerning the Conditions and Order for Pregnancy Termination, Ministry of Health. Bulgaria occupies the central part of the Balkan Peninsula, covering 119,000 square kilometres, with a population of 8.99 million (1989). Life expectancy is 71.19 years, some 6.27 years longer for females. The educational level is relatively high. The public health system is financed by the state budget and is free for the population.

2. The contra-indications to abortion are clarified in the addendum to the decree and include acute or subacute inflammatory diseases of the genitalia and pelvic organs, presence of some septic focuses, or acute general infections when they themselves are not the cause for seeking the pregnancy termination.

REFERENCES

Ketting, E. "Induced Abortion in Europe: An Overview." *Planned Parenthood in Europe* 18 (1989): pp. 2–4.
Public Health Statistics Annual. Bulgaria, 1989, p. 46.
Vassilev, D. "Obstetrical Aspects of the Parental Function of the Family." Doctoral thesis, Sofia, 1982.

CZECH AND SLOVAK REPUBLICS

Radim Uzel

THE HISTORY OF ABORTION LAW

Abortion in the Communist Era

Before Czechoslovakia came into being, in 1910–1914, the number of illegal abortions performed in the territory was estimated at about 100,000 per year. This is despite the fact that there was a penal code since 1852 that inflicted strict and long-term punishment not only on the woman and the father of the child but also on persons who carried out the operation. The number of abortions was more or less the same after the Czechoslovak state came into being, between the two world wars and even later, until a new penal code took up a more liberal position on "foetus killing."

The law that was passed in 1957 was a real turning point in abortion legislation. In addition to health reasons, the law conceded some other situations considered "worthy of special regard," such as housing problems, social reasons, large number of children, and "the hard position of a single woman." A woman who wanted to undergo the operation had only to have approval by a special board. Thus Czechoslovakia was among the first European countries that liberalised their abortion laws.

Most of the once-illegal abortions were now taking place in common hospitals and gynaecological wards, where they were carried out by trained physicians. This situation led to a reduction in female mortality. The duty to inform health authorities of these operations also facilitated research on abortion, making data more accurate. Since that time, the Ministry of Health issued accurate abortion statistics annually.

The period between 1958 and 1986 can be divided into five stages.

1. 1958–1962. The possibility of abortion gradually came into women's minds, and the annual abortion rate increased from 61,480 to 89,815. This increase reflected the easy availability of the operation. It was free of charge and unlimited, as long as an application was submitted. Obviously, economic factors and the lack of safe contraceptive methods contributed to this increase.

2. 1963–1964. A quick drop in the annual abortion rate (70,546 and 70,698) was a result of a new restrictive edict that bound the applicant to her place of residence and introduced a charge of up to 800 crowns for abortions for all but health reasons. This edict also stressed the responsibility of abortion boards. There were now lay women on the boards, usually mothers of several children.

3. 1965–1969. The annual abortion rate increased again, from 79,591 to its maximum of 102,797 in 1969. The abortion-to-birth index at that time was 57.7.

4. 1970–1975. There was a quick rise in the birth rate in Czechoslovakia during this time. The activity of the abortion boards became more strict again, and this cut down on the number of abortions (99,766–81,641).

5. 1976–1986. The period saw an increase in the number of abortions (84,589–124,188). Those in favour of restricting abortion lost ground as Czechoslovakia was affected by an energy crisis and the economic situation worsened.

The legal position in the Czech and Slovak Republics involved further liberalisation of abortion operations. The abortion boards were abolished and abortions up to the eighth week of pregnancy were declared free of charge. The main argument against the abortion boards was the delays they caused, whereby a woman got to her doctor for the operation at least one to two weeks later than if the boards had not existed. Activity by these abortion boards was liberal during their final years; they agreed with about 96 percent of all applications. It is little wonder that the boards were found to be useless.

The new legal position, valid since January 1, 1987, also introduced the question of contraceptives. Free pills and IUDs had been provided to all women since 1987. Unfortunately, the previous assumption that this would decrease the number of abortions has not proved true. The use of birth-control pills and IUDs has remained the same (about 5 percent for pills and about 15 percent for the IUD) for women between the ages of 15 and 44 years and the abortion rate has increased by 26 percent (by one-third in the Czech Republic and one-fifth in the Slovak Republic).

The "Velvet Revolution"

The so-called Velvet Revolution occurred in November 1989, and the first free elections were held in June 1990, marking the end of the 40-year totalitarian communist dictatorship. It was the victory of democratic forces once concentrated in dissent circles, mostly around the Charter 77 movement. One would have expected that the democratic forces that fought for human rights under the communist regime would not object to a fairly liberal abortion law. But the political forces that won the free elections as the Civic Forum party involved many, rather different elements.

There are many opponents of the democratic approach to family planning, and these forces are mostly representatives of the Roman Catholic Church. Religion was suppressed for 40 years, so during the revolution it was received as a welcome ally of the democratic dissident movement. However, after communism was defeated, differences of opinion in the Civic Forum became more and more evident. New political groups and organizations were formed, and some of these organizations will fight "to protect unborn life." They are against abortions, even against all methods of modern contraception except so-called natural methods—that is, periodic sexual abstention.

The differences of opinion are intensified by the various levels of religious belief in different regions of the republics. The number of believers is much lower in the Czech Republic, excluding some parts of southern Moravia. The Slovak Republic, on the other hand, is a traditionally Roman Catholic state—in some parts, quite similar to that in orthodox Catholic Poland.

Until complete separation, there were three governments and three parliaments in the Check and Slovak Federal Republics (CSFR). There was the Czech government and parliament in the Czech Republic (about 10 million inhabitants) and the Slovak government and parliament in the Slovak Republic (about 5 million inhabitants). There was also the federal government whose task became an increasingly difficult one as the tendency to complete separation between the Czech Republic and Slovakia increased.

As with arguments over economics, debates on family planning revealed the different views of people in the two republics and led to political instability. The pro-life pressure groups were more aggressive in the Slovak Republic and were well represented in both government and the parliament.

There were more and more intensive efforts to restrain the abortion law. The pro-choice position was represented as a legacy of communist ideology, the abortion law as a product of the totalitarian regime, and termination of pregnancy as a result of 40 years of devastation of moral values. To some extent, these arguments played into the hands of ideological opponents of the fairly liberal abortion law. Followers of a liberal position were often said to be secret agents, sad leftovers of the previous communist regime.

Some important posts in the media and the Ministry of Health were occupied by people who openly supported the ideology of religion. Thus, just prior to separation, the movement for restriction of abortion was gaining strength, with amendments to the legislation prepared by the Czech and Slovak parliaments. We shall mention them in detail later.

ABORTION: CURRENT LAW AND PRACTICE

The Law of 1987

The law dealing with pregnancy termination in the Czech and Slovak Federal Republic was valid since January 1, 1987, some three years before the November 1989 revolution. The law allowed for termination of pregnancy to protect a woman's life and health, and in favour of planned and responsible parenthood.[1]

According to this law, every woman can undergo termination of pregnancy if she submits a written application, she has been pregnant for no more than 12 weeks, and there are no health complications. In addition, pregnancy can be terminated for health reasons with a woman's agreement if either her life or health or the development of the foetus is in danger, or if there is an evident genetic defect of the foetus. A woman under 16 can undergo termination of pregnancy only with the agreement of her parents or legal guardian. Between the ages of 16 and 18, this operation is available without parental agreement; however, according to the law the gynaecologist who carried out the operation must inform the parents or legal guardian of the abortion.

In practice the procedure is as follows: a woman submits a written application to a gynaecologist according to the place of her permanent residence, workplace, or school. This gynaecologist confirms the woman's application and sends her to a hospital where she undergoes the operation. Though it is not compulsory for a woman to go to her local hospital, most women have no other choice because the other hospitals usually refuse nonresident women patients.

Permission for abortion will not be granted if there are disorders that would be worsened by abortion, or if it has been less than six months since her previous abortion. This latter restrictive step was included in the law after long discussion. It does not apply in the case of women who have given birth at least twice, or are over 35 years of age, or who have become pregnant as a consequence of a criminal offence (rape).

In the CSFR, women paid 500 crowns for the termination of their pregnancy (i.e., one-fifth or one-sixth of an average month's income). See Note 1 for more recent costs.

To reduce health complications, there is a special precaution dealing with so-called mini-abortions (*miniinterrupce* in Czech)—that is, terminations at early stages of pregnancy. Such an operation is free of charge, limited only by the length of pregnancy—45 days for women who have not borne children yet, and 55 days for those who have, counting from the first day of the last menstruation. The result of this financial motivation is that nearly 80 percent of all abortions are carried out at the early stages of pregnancy. Although the operation is carried out in a hospital ward, the woman need not be hospitalized; she can go home after several hours.

This fairly liberal law is the reason why there were hardly any illegal abortions carried out in the CSFR. Termination of pregnancy was readily available to every woman. There might have been a few exceptions of women who did not fulfill the obligatory six-month limit or who attempted to exceed the "ration" of two abortions per year. But these women usually could find an acceptable solution in terms of health indications. Very often they made use of the psychiatric indication clause.

Nevertheless, illegal abortion is mentioned in the republics' penal codes. A person who helps a pregnant woman to abort or encourages her to terminate her pregnancy by herself, or to ask or give permission to someone else to perform the abortion contrary to the law on termination of pregnancy, is to be punished by a custodial sentence of up to one year in length; in the case of causing serious damage to the health of the pregnant women, it is up to five years. There are even more strict punishments set for abortionists. The maximum sentence is five years' imprisonment if a profit is made or damage is caused to the woman's health; acting without a woman's agreement can bring an eight-year sentence; and 15 years is the sentence if the abortion causes a woman's death. A woman who terminates her pregnancy by herself or asks someone else to do it, or allows someone to do it, is not punishable at all. Considering the liberal abortion law, no one has been punished according to this article of the law.

Abortion in Practice

The international conference From Abortion to Contraception, held in Tbilisi, Georgia, in 1990, suggested that the CSFR, together with the former German Democratic Republic, belonged among the states with the best and most accurate abortion statistics. In fact, no abortion could miss statistical registration in the Czech and Slovak Republics.

Paradoxically, such accuracy in abortion statistics makes comparison with international statistics difficult. Early pregnancy termination data and "menstruation regulations" are not included in the statistics of many other countries. In the CSFR, there were some efforts to legalize menstruation regulations which is often used as a code for mini-abortions. Unfortunately, the efforts were not successful. Every termination of pregnancy, even if done at the earliest stage of gestation, was statistically recorded.

Tables 1 to 3 shows both absolute and relative numbers of abortions during the last five years; we can notice a slight increase in 1987 (as mentioned above) as a consequence of liberalization of the abortion law. In recent years,

Table 1
Number of Abortions, Czech and Slovak Republics, 1986–1990

Year	Number of Abortions		
	Total	Czech Republic	Slovak Republic
1986	124,188	83,564	40,624
1987	156,542	107,717	48,825
1988	160,241	110,394	49,847
1989	157,912	109,815	48,097
1990	157,262	109,361	47,901

Source: Ministry of Health, *Statistical Yearbook*, Prague, 1991.

the number of children born in the CSFR was slightly exceeded by the number of abortions in some parts of the country, particularly in the capitals of the two republics, Prague and Bratislava.

The data on age of applicants for pregnancy termination is interesting, too. Unlike in Western European countries, the number of young women under 18 is quite small. Women between 20 and 30, who usually already have one or two children, form the largest category. Some unwanted pregnancies do occur in the teenage category, too. However, more than half of those pregnancies are solved by early marriage. More than 50 percent of first-born children to married women are conceived before the wedding. Unmarried women's confinements are very rare.

In comparison to Western European countries, the number of abortions in the CSFR was very high, although not as high as in other formerly communist countries, with the exception of Catholic Poland. Today's opponents of liberal abortion policy often suggest that such high numbers of abortions are caused by nothing other than the liberal law. They even exaggerate the numbers of abortions in their arguments. The media have repeated the data given by a press officer from the Ministry of Health (a person of Catholic orientation), who introduced the number of 180,000 abortions per year—a purposefully distorted figure obtained by the addition of 23,000 spontaneous abortions. Besides this, opponents say that the number of children born is exceeded by the number of abortions, which is also false.

In practice, abortion is quite easily available in the republics. However, the fact that the woman must ask for the operation in the place of her permanent residence may be rather disadvantageous, especially in small

Table 2
Number of Abortions per 1,000 Women Ages 15–44, 1986–1990

Year	Number of Abortions		
	Total (%)	Czech Republic (%)	Slovak Republic (%)
1986	37.1	37.9	34.6
1987	46.7	48.7	42.7
1988	47.4	49.7	43.1
1989	46.3	49.1	41.1
1990	45.7	48.4	40.5

Source: Ministry of Health, *Statistical Yearbook*, Prague, 1991.

towns and villages where people know each other well. Nevertheless, this operation is readily available to all in the population, no matter their social position. Only Gypsies constitute a rather unusual group. There are an estimated half million or more Gypsies in the republics. For them, fertility is one of the basic values of life, and thus they refuse contraception and abortion. Propagation of family planning methods does not generally meet with any notable success in this population group.

The charge for women pregnant more than eight weeks is not an obstruction to abortion. These operations account for only 20 percent of the total number of abortions. Sometimes it is difficult to ascertain the accurate length of pregnancy because ultrasonic diagnostic apparatus is rarely available in many hospitals and information on the last menstruation is often inaccurate. The operation is free for women who must undergo the operation for health reasons.

The amount of money collected for abortions in the republics overall is not higher than 10 million crowns per year, and it goes to health service budgets in general, not only to the family planning service. The abortion charge is paid through a mail payment slip on health institution credit.

Abortions are always carried out by vacuum aspiration with a brand new cannula, followed by the curette examination. Mini-abortions are carried out under local or light complete anaesthesia; abortions between the eighth and twelfth weeks are under complete anaesthesia. During the period the CSFR abortion law was valid, only two cases of complications from this operation resulted in death. Other complications are not followed statistically. The

Table 3
Number of Abortions per 100 Births, 1986–1990

Year	Number of abortions		
	Total	Czech Republic	Slovak Republic
1986	56.0	62.4	46.4
1987	72.5	81.9	57.8
1988	73.9	82.9	59.6
1989	75.4	85.2	59.8
1990	74.4	83.4	59.6

Source: Ministry of Health, *Statistical Yearbook*, Prague, 1991.

frequency of applications submitted by individual women shows no harmful influence on further fertility.

As for the willingness of medical practitioners to carry out abortions, one must take into account the health service system. All the doctors and medical practitioners in the republics are civil servants (employed by the state) and carry out abortions within the framework of their service duties. All the operations are performed in hospital wards. The operation is so usual and widespread that the ability to carry out an abortion is specified as one of the requirements for obtaining a speciality in gynaecology and obstetrics in the first degree (three years after finishing medical studies).

There is no special money given to medical practitioners for carrying out the operation. They get a regular month's salary, which for doctors is often lower than the average salary of a qualified worker. Considering these circumstances, medical practitioners are used to accepting abortions as "a necessary evil" and there have been no cases of refusal to carry out an abortion. Doctors and other medical practitioners who do not want to participate or carry out abortions for moral or religious reasons usually chose other medical fields or work outside of hospitals.

There is only one case of administrative force to carry out abortion recorded during the time of the communist regime. But the necessity of carrying out such operations did not cause the emigration of gynaecologists abroad. The reasons for emigration were political and economic.

Most Czech or Slovak women consider abortion a usual method of family planning. This attitude may derive from specific factors. There were no modern contraception devices (pills and IUDs) at their disposal during the first liberalization of the abortion law in 1957, and women got used to solving the problem of unwanted pregnancy by abortion. In contrast, liberalisation of abortions in Western European countries came later, and by that time women had access to modern and safe contraceptive methods.

Czech and Slovak women are not ashamed of abortion. They openly talk about their abortions, not only with their friends and neighbours but even in the media. But this relates mainly to the largest group of women undergoing abortions: married women between 20 and 30. Younger women and unmarried women usually keep the operation secret, even from their own parents.

The Politics of Abortion

According to the current law, termination of pregnancy is widely accepted and a woman's right to choose freely is fully respected, with the exception of the necessary six-month time limit between abortions and the duty to ask for the operation according to place of residence. Some of the pro-life pressure groups, especially those of Roman Catholic orientation, have recently attacked the politics of abortion, sometimes in an aggressive and intolerant way. Through leaflet campaigns and newspaper articles they try to suggest that abortion, even when done at an early stage of pregnancy, is murder of a human being. They exaggerate the negative consequences of abortion and try to influence public opinion emotionally by distribution of a film and video cassette called *The Silent Cry*, in which an intrauterine camera recorded limb crushing and the destruction of an embryo during abortion. In meetings held by religious activists one can see slides that in multiple enlargement show torn limbs and mashed heads of embryos at later stages of pregnancy.

These militant groups are centred in bigger towns as organisations called For Unborn Life Protection. Besides antiabortion propaganda, they are concerned with exaggerating the negative effects of contraception methods, and they often fight against pre-marital sexual activity and open sex education, both in schools and at home. They consider sexual education as a source of bad mores for society, and call for the prohibition of information on all questions connected with sexual life. It is interesting that even some official representatives of cultural, scientific, and political institutions tend toward these restrictive opinions. Their position was further strengthened by the Pope's visit in April 1990.

The Roman Catholic Church is the strongest religious element in the republics; at a guess, more than 50 percent of the population belong to this church, though not all of its members live according to its religious teachings. The other, smaller churches are much more tolerant towards abortion and family planning, including contraception.

A counter-balance to these groups can be seen in the organisation The Association for Family Planning and Sex Education (Společnost Pro Plánováni Rodiny a Sexuálui Výchovu—SPRSV). This association was a former department of the Czech Sexologist Association, but in February 1991 was organised as family planning associations (FPAs) in both the Czech and Slovak Republics. The memoranda of both associations have their origin in the International Planned Parenthood Federation (IPPF) memorandum. For more than 20 years, Czechoslovakia tried to become a full member of this international organization, however it was not possible because of disagreements between the governing Communist party and the Ministry of Interior Affairs. During this time, Czechoslovak representatives were only observers. Now there are no political barriers and both FPAs are trying to reach full membership in IPPF.

It was rather difficult, however, to establish friendly contact with groups of MPs, the Ministry of Health, and the President of the Republic's Office. On January 9, 1991, the federal parliament accepted the Bill of Human Rights. The controversial matter of free access to abortion involved a long discussion, and the parliament, under the influence of religious groups, finally accepted a formulation that rather ambiguously guaranteed a woman the right to decide freely and responsibly about the number of her children, a position appropriate to the international pacts that Czechoslovakia had signed. The parliament finally accepted a compromise formulation stating that "human life is worthy of protection even before birth."

In 1991, the parliament was writing new constitutions. Political parties and citizen's action groups were expressing their opinions on drafts of the constitutions for the Czech Republic, the Slovak Republic, and the Federal Republic. In this context, the SPRSV (Společnost Pro Plánováni Rodiny a Sexuálni Výchova) already sent several petitions stressing the "pro-choice" position to the parliamentary committee and the President of the Republic. Unfortunately, most of these letters were not answered, and the right to family planning was not included in the draft of the new federal constitution.

Support for a woman's free choice suffers from the absence of a feminist movement in both the Czech and Slovak Republics. Close cooperation with the Communist party of Czechoslovakia had brought a monopolistic women's organization—the Czechoslovak Women's Union—into discredit. New women's organizations are not very numerous and lack political influence. In fact, there is not feminist movement in the countries—that is, there is no movement that represents a powerful political force and a "pro-choice" pressure group, such as exists in many western countries. This political passivity of women may be a result of the high employment rate (more than 90 percent) of women of reproductive age, by the low level of services, and by worries of shopping for everyday necessities. Women, after finishing their normal work shift, start another one connected with household duties at home. They suffer from an absolute lack of free time, something which is so important for public activities. Control of the government, parliament, and political parties is, in fact, in the hands of men.

A public opinion poll, conducted in March 1991 by the Federal Public Opinion Research Institute, found that 61 percent of people questioned agreed that a woman should have the right to choose for or against abortion (the Czech Republic 63 percent, the Slovak Republic 56 percent); 23 percent said that termination should be carried out only with regard to health and social conditions; 11 percent felt that it should be allowed only in cases where a woman's life is endangered; and 4 percent supported an absolute ban. The greatest support for an absolute ban was in Bratislava, the capital of the Slovak Republic (13 percent). Of those questioned, 41 percent in the Slovak Republic stated that the partner's agreement should be necessary for the operation, while the same opinion was very rare in the Czech Republic.

There was another difference of opinion that affected the professional gynaecology-obstetrics associations in the CSFR. While the Czech Association unanimously occupied the pro-choice position, there was controversy among Slovak gynaecologists at the National Conference in February 1991. The leaders of the association—mostly older doctors and representatives of attitudes restricting the possibility of abortion—stood against the younger generation of gynaecologists who supported their Czech colleagues. After an open vote it was clear that the liberal attitude of the younger opposition won; however, leadership of the Slovak Gynaecologists Association is still in the hands of the minority that supports restrictive measures. Such differentiation between pro-life and pro-choice attitudes is going to increasingly reflect a generational conflict in the republic, not only within professional associations. Representatives of the older generation still occupy influential posts in many institutions.

THE FUTURE

Public opinion polls have suggested that in the CSFR there was hardly any challenge to a woman's free access to abortion and free choice about the number of children to have. Nevertheless, there were supporters of legislative change who had been intervening in the parliaments. In addition, the parliament of the Slovak Republic drafted amendments to the abortion law that were very restrictive.

The draft amendment of the abortion law prepared by the Ministry of Health of the Czech Republic mentioned in its introduction some critical opinions of experts and laymen. Some of them suggested restricting the existing law, with the greatest opposition voiced by 700 doctors from Bohemia and Moravia, the Bishops' Conference of the CSFR, the Unborn Life Protection Association, and the Czech Family Association. On the other hand, there was support for maximum liberalisation of abortions, establishment of an institution of menstruation regulation, and the possibility of carrying it out in private surgeries (the attitude of the Czech Gynaecologist Association).

This proposed new amendment seemed to be a compromise between these extreme demands. Most of all, it changed the name of the operation. Instead of calling abortion "pregnancy interruption," it spoke about "pregnancy termination." A woman who asks for an abortion would be allowed to terminate her pregnancy up until the end of the twelfth week of pregnancy. She could ask for this operation in writing, and choose a doctor by herself. The doctor would inform the woman of possible consequences of the operation and of its possible impact on her emotional and mental health and future pregnancies. The doctor must also inform the woman of alternative ways and possibilities of help (especially the possibility of adoption). The operation could be carried out only in the hospital wards of the common health service net. The woman's selection of a doctor and hospital would not be limited by her place of permanent residence.

Pregnancy termination for health reasons was to be free of charge, but payment would be necessary in other situations. The sum a woman would pay had not been set, and it was not clear whether the sum was to be differentiated according to pregnancy stages (see Note 1). Pregnancy termination would be available to teenagers under 18 only after agreement by the parents or legal guardians.

There were more restrictive changes involved in the draft suggested by the Ministry of Health in the Slovak Republic. Their title of the law was On Human Life Protection and, apart from abortion, it dealt with the ban on euthanasia. From the moment of conception, the foetus was given a so-called foetal right. Nevertheless, the law accepted five indications that allowed an abortion, as follows:

1. Direct and irreversible danger to the mother's life or detriment to her state of health

2. A serious abnormality of the foetus, causing serious effects on the woman's psychosomatic development or an abnormality incompatible with life

3. Danger to the foetus's life

4. Pregnancy as a consequence of a criminal offence

5. A serious social and economic exigency that cannot be averted by any other way and that is so serious that one cannot ask a woman to bring her pregnancy to its natural conclusion

Women under 18 would have to have their parents' agreement. The father of the child could express his opinion if asked for it. Conditions for pregnancy termination had to be supported by a written acknowledgment, and every application was to be judged by the Ethical Council nominated by the director of a hospital. Appeals would be judged by the Ethical Council of the Ministry of Health in the Slovak Republic. The operations in cases 1 and 3 above would be free of charge; those in cases 2 and 5 would be paid by the woman; the operation in case 4 would be paid by the offender. The sum had not been set (see Note 1).

If most of the gynaecology-obstetrics wards in Slovak hospitals refused to carry out these operations, the Ministry of Health would provide at least three wards equipped for these operations for the whole of Slovakia.

The draft suggested by the Ministry of Health claimed in its introductory article that pregnancy termination is not a method of family planning and any operation carried out other than according to this law would be prosecuted.

The differencies between these two drafts were so great that, were they both to become law, there would have been an immediate flourishing of abortion tourism between the Czech and Slovak Republics. Besides this, the Slovak draft of the law was rather unrealistic. Above all, it did not mention the planned parenthood pact (Teheran Declaration) signed by the CSFR. Delegating the final decision to a special Ethical Council and the restricting indications for abortion would mean a serious infringement of human rights. Acceptance of this new law would shift the situation back to what it was before 1957. Besides that, the draft mentioned the unfortunate six-month time limit between two abortions, which would introduce a strict control according to place of residence, rather than the suggested free choice of a doctor. Abolition of these territorial-administrative limitations would have been the greatest change in the health service since the revolution of 1989. In the interests of the efficient operation of pregnancy termination in Czechoslovakia, it was surely advisable for both parts of the federation to have, if not the same laws, then at least very similar laws on the matter.

This was a touchy sphere, where the interests of the pro-life and pro-choice groups would meet in conflict again and again. Nevertheless, changes in the existing law could not affect the real number of abortions. At most, a too restrictive law would affect the number of illegal abortions, with all the sad consequences to the health and lives of Czech and Slovak women. As a warning, we need only look at the example of what happened in Romania a short time ago.

NOTE

1. The Czech and Slovak federation split into two separate republics—the Czech Republic and Slovakia—on January 1, 1993. After the split, the federal law described in this article continued to pertain in both republics. The only difference is that abortions are no longer free, except on medical indication, in the Czech Republic. They now cost between 2,000 and 3,000 crowns (about US$70–100). In Slovakia, abortion is still free.

REFERENCES

Buresova, A. "Czechoslovakia 1991: Abortion and Contraception." *Planned Parenthood in Europe* 20, no 2 (1991): 6–7.

Havranek, F. *Interruptio Graviditatis*. Prague: Avicenum, 1982.

Henshaw, S. K. "Induced Abortion: A World Review 1990." *International Family Planning Perspectives* 16 (1990).

Uzel, R., E. Ketting, A. Visser, and P. Lehert. *Contraceptive Practices and Attitudes of Czech and Slovak Women*. Brussels: International Health Foundation, 1992.

Visser, A., R. Uzel, E. Ketting, and N. Bruyniks. *Attitudes of Czech and Slovak Gynaecologists on Family Planning*. Brussels: International Health Foundation, 1993.

DENMARK

Nell Rasmussen

THE HISTORY OF ABORTION LAW

Limited Abortion Rights

Having for several hundred years been regarded and punished as foeticide, induced termination of pregnancy gradually came to be permitted under particular circumstances in Denmark. In the 1920s and 1930s a public debate on contraception and abortion started within the context of demands for equal rights for women and as a quest for an abortion law. In the 1866 penal code, still in force, termination of pregnancy was punishable by up to eight years of forced labour, the sole exception being where the pregnancy constituted a severe threat to the woman's health. The penal code of 1930 made no provision for cases in which abortion was not punishable, however the conditions of the 1866 penal code were applied in practice.

Termination of pregnancy was criminalised until 1937, when the first act on Termination of Pregnancy (still the legal term) was passed.[1] The act came into effect in 1939, and made provision for access to abortion on medical, ethical, and eugenic grounds. A majority of 18 of the 19 members on the preparatory commission on the law also proposed access to abortion on social grounds. However, this was not included in the law proposed in parliament. Instead, Mothers' Aid, a government-supported private organisation, which since 1939 acted as an advisory agency on abortion and provided additional financial support for pregnant women, set up local branches all over the country to expand the social aid for single pregnant women and mothers.

The act was due for revision 10 years later. In 1950, a new commission on abortion was set up, which completed its work in 1954. The proposals of the commission were accepted by parliament in 1956.[2] In this act, the medical reason for abortion was extended to a socio-medical indication; the ethical and eugenic indications were largely unchanged. A woman's inability to take care of a child owing to physical and psychological defects or other medically stated conditions was accepted as a fourth condition. During the debate it became clear that Mothers' Aid had in reality already expanded the medical indication to include "social-medical-humanitarian" reasons. The penalty for illegal abortion was minimised by the law. A woman who willfully terminated her pregnancy illegally could be sentenced for up to three months of deprivation of liberty. A doctor performing an abortion outside the conditions stipulated could normally be sentenced to up to two years of imprisonment. If he or she did so for personal gain, the sentence could be up to four years.

The Fight for Free Abortion

The fight for free abortion really started in the 1960s. One event more than any other triggered the debate on liberalisation of the abortion law. In January 1967 the youth group of the Danish Women's Society—the oldest women's organisation—announced that it was going to establish an office in which women who had not been able to obtain permission for a legal abortion could get an itinerary and names and addresses of clinics in Eastern Europe where the abortion could be performed (Bregnsbo, 1971). In February the Socialist People's party proposed abortion on request for all women up to the end of the 12th week of pregnancy. Later in 1967 the minister of justice appointed a new pregnancy commission that finished its work in 1969. The commission concluded that the rising number of women applying for abortion was because the widespread media coverage and public debate had led more women to consider applying to have an abortion. It also concluded that the declining birthrate was due to the widespread use of contraception. A majority of the commission proposed substantial liberalisation of access to abortion, while the minority proposed free abortion. Finally the commission proposed the decriminalisation of abortion for any woman. No such decriminalisation was proposed in the case of a doctor or other person actually performing the abortion. The Socialist People's party proposed its bill on free abortion in five consecutive sessions in the parliament, but was not successful.

The demand for liberalisation of abortion legislation and practice and for the introduction of free abortion must be viewed in the light of the fact that illegal abortions involving a risk to the woman's health and a risk of punishment were a rampant social problem in the 1960s. The commission estimated that 15,000 to 16,000 illegal abortions were performed each year.

Consequently in 1970, the minister of justice proposed and had adopted a law that extended access to abortion on social grounds, including young age and immaturity.[3] In addition, a woman would be allowed without special permission to have abortion if she had turned 38 years old by the end of the 12th week of pregnancy, or if she had four children below 18 years who were living with her. These indications were added to the existing indications for abortion. The act had a short life.

The major opponent of the new act was the Christian People's party, which came into existence as part of a protest movement against the 1970 abortion act. During the 1970s the party regularly proposed changing the law back to the situation in 1956, but without any penalty for the woman. The opponents of the abortion act in the late 1970s formed the organisation Respect for Human Life, which belongs to the international anti-choice movement. Since 1979 the organisation has published a small journal.

ABORTION: CURRENT LAW AND PRACTICE

The Law of 1973

In 1973, following recurrent debates in the Danish parliament on the subject, access to free abortion was embodied in Danish Act No. 350 on Termination of Pregnancy.[4] The right of every woman to have her pregnancy terminated on request up to the end of the 12th week of pregnancy (Section 1) and, under certain conditions, to have her pregnancy terminated after the end of the 12th week (Sections 2 and 3) was thus put on the statute book.

After the end of the 12th week of pregnancy, the woman's own wishes are no longer adequate grounds for having an abortion. Thereafter, it is required that one of the special indications set out in law be fulfilled, having been verified by a joint committee on abortion authorised to give permission for termination. The terms of Section 3 of the abortion act governing abortion after the 12th week of pregnancy are:

- That the pregnancy, birth, or care of the child entails a risk of deterioration of the woman's health on account of an existing or potential physical or mental illness or infirmity or as a consequence of other aspects of the conditions under which she is living (medical indication);
- That the pregnancy is due to incest, rape or other sexual assault (ethical indication);
- That there is a danger on account of a hereditary condition or injury or disease in the foetal state that the child will be affected by a serious physical or mental disorder (eugenic or genetic indication);
- That the woman is incapable of giving proper care to a child on account of her physical or mental disorder or impaired mobility;

• That the woman is currently incapable of taking care of the child properly owing to her youth or immaturity;

• That the pregnancy, birth, or care of the child can be assumed to constitute for the woman such a serious strain, which cannot in any other way be averted, that, out of consideration for the woman, the upkeep of her home or the care of the other children in her family, termination of the pregnancy must be regarded as imperative. The decision must take account of the woman's age, workload, and other personal circumstances as well as the family's residential, economic, and health conditions (psycho-social indications).

Authorization for abortion may be granted only if the grounds on which the application is based are sufficiently important to justify subjecting the woman to the increased risk to her health, which the procedure entails.

According to Section 6 of the law, a woman under 18 years of age (a legal minor) or who is incapable of managing her own affairs must have the consent of her parents or guardians to the application for abortion. However, when justified by circumstances, the committee may refrain from requiring consent. It may even authorise abortion even if consent has been refused. The decisions of the committee may be submitted to a board of appeal by the woman (Section 6, subsection 2), or the person exercising parental authority or the guardian (Section 6, subsection 3).

The act carries penal sanctions for a physician who performs an abortion without the conditions prescribed being satisfied and without authorisation having been granted. The penalty is, without prejudice to any more severe penalty imposed under the criminal code, up to two years of deprivation of liberty or imprisonment or, if there are mitigating circumstances, to a fine (Section 14). If the physician does not meet the procedural requirements of the act, the penalty is a fine.

Abortion may be performed only by a physician in a state or communal hospital or in a clinic attached to the hospital. A physician who performs an abortion in any other place shall be liable to a fine. A person performing an abortion who is not a physician is liable to up to four years of imprisonment without prejudice to any more severe penalty imposed under the criminal code. Any person providing assistance to the above-mentioned activities is liable to the same penalty (Section 14).

A chief physician of a hospital or hospital department concerned has a right to refuse to perform the procedure, even if the conditions prescribed are satisfied. However, the woman shall be referred to another hospital or hospital department where the procedure can be performed (Section 10, subsection 2). In 1989 this right to refuse to perform or assist in the performance of an abortion against personal ethical or religious beliefs was extended to doctors, midwives, and nursing aides, whereas it had previously been restricted to chief physicians, nurses, and trainee nurses.[5] This amendment caused no notable public debate.

Amendments to the act on abortion have otherwise been made only as a consequence of changes in other legislation. A major organisational change was introduced in 1975, when the Mothers' Aids Institutions were closed and their tasks transferred to the social welfare offices of the municipalities.

The Incidence of Abortion

For a number of years following the introduction of abortion on demand there was a sharp increase in the number of induced abortions. The peak occurred in 1975, when it reached 27,884. In recent years the figure has leveled off at around 21,000 abortions annually. In 1988, 21,199 abortions were performed. In 1989, there were 21,465 abortions. And in 1990, the number was 20,589. Per 100,000 women aged 15 to 49 years, the abortion ratio in 1988 was 16.4; in 1989, 16.5; and in 1990, 15.8. Both the absolute number of legally induced abortions and the incidence of abortion were roughly the same in 1989 and 1988, and only slightly higher than in preceding years (National Board of Health 1988; Knudsen and Tanska 1990).

The incidence of abortion should be seen in relation to the constantly rising birthrate.[6] In 1988, the birthrate was 59,310. For 1989, the provisional birthrate is over 60,000. Both in 1986–87 and in 1987–88, therefore, the number of induced abortions made up 26 percent of the number of births, as against 28 to 30 percent in 1985–86 and previous years. Since 1983 the birthrate has gone up by 20 percent (Knudsen and Bille 1991). The birthrate is therefore rising relative to the increase in the abortion rate (Knudsen 1989).

The breakdown of abortions by age group has changed little in recent years. They are lowest among the youngest and the oldest, with certain fluctuations in the mid-range groups. However, these fluctuations must be seen in relation to the fact that these age groups (20–34 years) together account for more than two-thirds of both induced abortions and births. There has been a marked increase in the number of women who have had an induced abortion without previously having borne a child. This shift should be viewed against the increase in the average age at which women are having their first child. The average age of women giving birth for the first time rose from 24.8 to 25.9 years between 1981 and 1987 (*Statistisk Årbog* 1989, Table 10).

The surveys show that women seeking abortion do not represent a special risk group; rather, they are in a situation where they do not wish to become pregnant at the time in question.

According to the statistics from the National Board of Health, the incidence of abortion displays large regional variations. These are—and for some time now have been—most marked for the younger age groups, where the abortion quotient is still at least twice as high in Copenhagen as in most of the counties in Jutland. The lowest total abortion quotient is found—and has been during the whole period since 1973—in Ringkøbing County (mid-west Jutland). This may be explained by much stronger religious and less liberal sexual norms in the western, rural parts of Jutland compared to Copenhagen.

The National Board of Health's statistics on recurrent abortions show that between 1985 and 1987, 4.5 to 5.4 percent of women who have had an abortion have another abortion performed within two months. The highest recurrence rate is seen among 18- to 24-year-old women. It is possible to calculate that a recurrence rate of just under 5 percent is consistent with the women's use of contraceptives with an average reliability of 95 percent.

The vast majority (97–98 percent) of induced abortions are performed before the end of the 12th week of pregnancy (first trimester). A very small proportion of abortive interventions (2–3 percent) take place after the end of the 12th week of pregnancy, although there is a somewhat higher proportion of late abortions among the very young and the oldest women (4–5 percent). After the end of the 12th week of pregnancy, there were 439 abortions in 1989, corresponding to 3 percent of all abortions. In 1990, the figure was 449, corresponding to 2 percent of all abortions.

Of the late abortions, those performed for medical, social, and genetic indications formed the largest contingent. In 1990 there were 159 abortions on medical and 137 on social indications, and 82 on genetic indication. This is the equivalent of one-fifth of late abortions.

It is a general opinion among professionals that illegal abortions hardly occur in Denmark. Abortion being free and freely available, with no practical, moral, or social restrictions to availability from the health system, the "market" for illegal abortions is virtually nonexistent. Neither the health nor the criminal statistics report any cases of illegal abortions, which, of course, does not necessarily exclude their occurrence.

The comprehensive Danish abortion statistics since 1973 are due to the fact that all abortions are performed in public hospitals. The hospitals are obliged to report statistics monthly to the National Board of Health.

The number of induced abortions in Denmark is high in comparison to other Scandinavian and northwestern European countries ("Abortsituationen i de nordiska Landerne" 1990). A number of factors may be contributory here. The more liberal sexual behaviour probably plays some role. Women's status in society, great attachment to—and a wish for permanent attachment to—the labour market, participation in education and training, and the wish for training require planning as to the timing of births and some restriction on the number of births. The upshot of this trend is that women today plan the timing of their children to a greater degree, and pregnancy no longer entails women marrying and starting a family with a man by whom they have inadvertently become pregnant. The higher average age of first-time childbearing women reflects this development, and the abortion rate must be evaluated in this light.

In 1986 the Danish Family Planning Association and the Danish Committee for Health Education (both private organizations promoting sex education and health education) summarised the most important results of various surveys and of the National Board of Health's statistics on the use of contraception and abortion (Danish Family Planning Association and the Committee on Health Education 1986). The conclusion was that the status and developmental pattern of contraceptive use generally look positive. The surveys also indicated that women who embark on an unplanned, unwanted pregnancy constitute a random selection of those who do not safeguard themselves 100 percent. Unprotected periods normally coincide with transitions between various contraceptive methods. And in a survey in 1989, the group of adolescents seeking abortion did not differ essentially from the nonpregnant women. Available surveys show that there is nothing to suggest that Danish women use abortion as a means of contraception. This still seems to be the case.

Abortion in Practice

The county health boards are responsible for ensuring that access to abortion—as well as counseling on contraception—is available. All counties in Denmark, therefore, have one or several hospitals with gynaecological and other departments performing abortions, meaning that women all over the country can have abortion in a hospital within 50 kilometers of their home.

The abortion act covers women domiciled in Denmark, meaning that foreign women cannot have an abortion performed in Denmark unless on an acute health indication. This is because the cost of abortion is covered by the national health insurance scheme. Thus abortion is free of charge at a hospital in the county in which the abortion seeker lives. If for some reason a woman is having an abortion performed in another county, she must have coverage from her own county, or she must pay herself. In practice the counties always cover the costs in these situations.

Abortion must be performed only in public state or communal hospitals at county level, by trained doctors, or in a clinic attached to a public hospital according to the act on abortion. Private clinics are not authorised to perform abortions. The first private hospital in Denmark, the Mermaid Clinic, applied in 1991 to the National Health Board for authorisation to perform abortions. The application was refused, however, according to the requirements of the law. The hospital is hoping to have the abortion act amended in order to be able to perform abortions, but so far this has not happened.

A woman living in Denmark, seeking an abortion up to the 12th week of pregnancy, can have that abortion on request. The woman's application must be presented to a general practitioner or to a county social centre (in Copenhagen and Frederiksberg, the social administration services). If the woman seeks abortion from a general practitioner (GP)—which is the most frequent course of action—the GP is obliged to offer her nondirective guidance; *inter alia*, the GP shall inform the woman that she, on application to the social authorities, is eligible for counseling on the possibilities of support for seeing the pregnancy through and support after the birth of the child. If the woman applies to a county social centre for an abortion, she must also be granted this counselling should she desire it.[7]

The woman must sign a statement that guidance has been given, and if the woman stands by her application, the GP should refer her to a hospital. No statement from a husband or cohabiter is needed. Minor girls must, as mentioned, have parental consent for abortion, whereas they can acquire all types of contraceptives without the consent of the parents. In practice, the written consent of only one of the parents is needed. The joint committee can, however, dispense with the requirement of parental consent.

The woman will go to a hospital within a week after having seen her GP, but in case of emergency she may be there within one day. At the hospital the doctor again shall ascertain that the situation complies with the conditions for performing abortion. The abortion is normally performed under general anaesthesia. Less than one-fifth of the women have abortion performed as outpatients; 41 percent stay in a hospital for less than one day (Knudsen 1990). The hospital will often persuade the woman to stay until the next day, unless she has somebody to take care of her at home.

After the 12th week of pregnancy, as mentioned, the woman must have permission for an abortion from a joint committee that verifies that one of the special indications set out in law has been fulfilled. The committee is comprised of two physicians—a specialist in gynaecology or surgery and a specialist in psychiatry or social medicine—and a lawyer or social worker from the county welfare authorities.

In 1986, 595 women applied for abortion after the 12th week of pregnancy; this corresponds to 2.6 percent of all abortions. A recent study shows that abortion was granted in 519 cases. Of these, 82 women were denied abortion, 7 of whom were later granted abortion by the board of appeal established by the minister of justice. The significant reasons for denial of abortion given in the study are the length of the pregnancy and the age of the woman, being over 25 years old and living in good social conditions (Nordentoft, Petersson, and Sidenius 1991).

The number of minors seeking dispensation from parental consent for abortion is small, but the cases are often dramatic. One reason for dispensation may be that the girl does not live with her parents and has broken off her relationship with them. Dispensation may be given if the abortion will create a serious conflict within the family. In most cases, though, the joint committee demands that the girl speak to the parents. If the parents oppose abortion, the girl can reapply, and the joint committee then can grant a dispensation from parental consent on account of familial conflict. Both the girl and the parents can appeal a decision of the joint committee to the board of appeal. In most of these cases abortion is granted by the board of appeal.

However, in recent years one group of young women seeking abortion has faced problems. According to the New Mothers' Aid (a private organization established in 1983), young women on public welfare are frequently pressured to seek abortion by the welfare authorities (Aagaard 1991). However explainable from the point of view of the social workers, this appears to be illegal with regard to both the abortion act and the social welfare act.

According to the abortion act, the woman must be informed by the physician of the nature of the procedure and its direct consequences, as well as the risks it may involve. Despite the fact that women sign a statement on having had guidance on their rights, a survey in 1989 carried out among 105 women who were referred for abortion in 1987 showed that the woman's knowledge of the nature of the intervention and possible complications was limited. Half of the women in the study reported that they had not been adequately instructed on this issue. This is attributed by some commentators to memory failure, but the conclusion of the study is that the GP's information is often insufficient. The study also showed that guidance given by GPs on the possibilities of obtaining assistance in seeing a pregnancy through was inadequate (Nielsen et al. 1988; Christiansen et al. 1988).

While doctors in general have a positive attitude, and GPs and nurses generally treat women having an abortion neutrally in order not to provoke feelings of shame, a recent study of all cases of late abortions in 1986 (519 cases) indicates that in 23 percent of the cases reported, medical errors were the cause of exceeding the 12-week limit. (Together with young age, medical errors were the main factor correlating with late abortions; Nordentoft, Petersson, and Sidenius 1991.) The authors argue that GPs, as well as women, must acknowledge subjective symptoms of pregnancy more readily. They also proposed that the abortion act be amended to include medical errors as an indication of late abortion.

The importance of adequate information concerning abortion was stressed by the National Board of Health in 1990.[8] An official communication to all doctors in the weekly *Journal for Physicians* noted that "during the years [it] had received a number of complaints from women still being pregnant in spite of the abortion intervention." The National Board of Health notes that a marginal risk of continuation of a pregnancy exists even after a correctly performed abortive intervention. Thus the board requires that information on the slight risk of a continued pregnancy after abortion be given by hospitals, in order that the patient thus informed is able to estimate and act on possible gynaecological irregularities and seek advice from the GP sooner.

Abortions can be performed up to the end of the 24th week of pregnancy; however, abortion after the 20th week is rare. In 1990, 227 women had an abortion after the 16th week of pregnancy. As a consequence of the technological possibilities of enabling extremely premature babies to survive, gynaecologists and neonatologists are having heated discussions about whether to lower the official upper limit for abortion to the 22nd week of pregnancy. No professional agreement has been reached, and practice concerning enabling extremely premature children to survive seems to differ throughout the country (Meyer 1991). Neither has any political initiative been taken to discuss the upper abortion limit.

Abortion is accepted by the population. Not just professionals but people in general are tolerant of women having an abortion. None of the existing surveys indicates a special feeling of guilt among women who have had an abortion. In my personal experience, friends and aquaintances who have had induced abortions talk of this freely, though not lightly. Several women have written books on their experiences in relation to abortion. Of course, in some Christian and other religious environments the situation is different, but such people constitute a minority of the population.

The Politics of Abortion

In 1987, an act on the formation of a council of ethics and the control of certain biomedical experiments fueled an extensive debate, partly because Section 1, subsection 3 of the act contains a turn of phrase that might at first be construed as militating against the availability of free abortion.[9] This subsection—according to which the council of ethics is to base its activities and dealings on the "assumption that human life has its origin at the instant of fertilisation"—was also debated in the parliament. A minority consisting of the Social Democrats and Social Liberals aired strong concern that the use of this phrasing might create "complications with regard to other legislation [the abortion act]." During the parliamentary discussions, however, the Democratic Liberals, the Conservative People's party, the Socialist People's party, and the Liberal Socialists also signaled that they had no desire to repeal or restrict access to free abortion. Nor did the Christian People's party indicate that this was intentional or desirable.[10]

With such statements on record, it is possible to establish that neither the government nor any political party intends to make any change in existing access to abortion. Thus, there can be no doubt as to prevailing law. Whatever reading is given to the provision, the regulations signposted by the act on a council of ethics must be compatible with access to free abortion until the end of the 12th week of pregnancy and thereafter with the permission of a joint council, providing the conditions of the act are fulfilled.

In October 1988, the organisation Respect for Human Life addressed all members of the parliament, urging them to reassess the abortion act.[11] The organisation requested that the social and economic consequences of the law be critically evaluated and that biomedical facts on the evolution of human life and ethical aspects of abortion be discussed. The address noted that the abortion act was passed without the present knowledge on the evolution of the foetus and noted, with satisfaction, that the act on a council of ethics built on the assumption that human life has its origin at the instant of fertilisation. The organisation found this inconsistent with the substance of the abortion act. It concluded that the act on abortion constitutes a "disastrous deviance" from the fundamental democratic and humane ideals of Danish society, and urged all members of the parliament to reconsider their position on abortion. The address was not debated in parliament and caused little debate in the media.

Fear that the act on the council of ethics would signal an end to free abortion led to the formation of a group of women researchers and other academics calling themselves the Women's Ethical Council. In 1989, the group published a book entitled *Life Begins at Fertilization: On the Necessity of Free Abortion* (Kjerkegard et al. 1989). The group also saw a threat to free abortion in the new methods of pre-natal diagnosis, making foetal diagnosis possible at a stage prior to the free abortion limit, thus making selective abortion on obscure reasons like sex and and normal traits possible. They recognised that since the legalisation of free abortion virtually no debate on the ethical aspects of abortion had taken place, and there had been a tendency to take the existence of abortion for granted. The group wanted to take the offensive and be prepared for a renewed debate on free abortion, seeing that this was already a hot issue in other European countries and in the United States.

The Women's Ethical Council concluded after prolonged debate that abortion is always a bad solution, but a necessary one. They stressed that it will remain so, not least because of inadequate means of contraception. They thought that abortion should always be seen as a last resort and should never be a routine matter, and argued that the tragedy today is not having an abortion but that abortion for many women is not a real choice and has become more or less forced owing to the lack of social and economic support that pregnant women have compared to, for example, 20 years ago.

The view that abortion is a necessary last report is shared by the Danish Family Planning Association and the Danish Female Medical Association. These organisations held a large conference for professionals, politicians, and members of the media in March 1990, in order to back up professionally the views expressed above. However, besides pointing to the continued need for abortion and the necessity of developing new methods of contraception, the organisations raised the question: can the abortion figures be changed? They argued that accepting abortion as a last resort implies an interest in reducing the number of abortions—not because abortion is ethically wrong per se, but because of the physical and mental strain on the woman having an induced abortion, and because the Danish abortion incidence is high compared to other (comparable) European countries.

In November 1990 a meeting was held by the Danish Women's Society and the Family Planning Association to engage larger groups of women in the debate on abortion. At the meeting and in the press feminist researchers disputed the Danish abortion incidence as too high. They argued that the incidence of induced abortions reflects the conditions of Danish women, socially and workwise. They found the argument on abortion as a last resort hypocritical and admission of abortion being ethically unacceptable. They disputed the low Dutch abortion figures as based on incomplete statistics, and claimed that the actual rate of abortion in Holland is not lower than in Denmark. In spite of differences regarding the desirability of lowering the incidence of abortion, all participants agreed on insisting on a woman's right to abortion on request.

The organisation Respect for Human Life suddenly received 200,000 krone (about £18,000) from the 1990 government budget. This should not be seen as a tribute to the objectives of the organization, however, but could be accounted for by clever negotiations by the Christian People's party, which got a great sum for private charity organisations as part of a political horse-trading deal. Respect for Human Life made the headlines for some days, but the organisation generally has played a minor role in the public debate. A pamphlet published with the financial support of the Ministry of Health in 1990, entitled *Before You Choose Abortion: An Information Pamphlet from Respect for Human Life*, has been widely criticised by doctors and other health professionals for giving incorrect information and carrying tendentious illustrations. The Ministry of Health and the National Board of Health have been requested to comment on and evaluate the contents of the pamphlet for the Parliamentary Committee on Health.[12]

In September 1990 the Council of Ethics made its mandatory report, *Foetal Diagnosis and Ethics*, to the Minister of Health (Danish Council of Ethics 1990). In it, the council also touched on the question of induced abortion. The council took the following position:

The use of foetal diagnosis still implies that the discovery of a deviation may lead to the choice of abortion. And abortion is never without its ethical problems. Fertilized ova, embryos and foetuses have, in the view of the Council, a special status; they represent various stages of the evolution towards the born child and are therefore encompassed by the notion of human worth. Consequently, freedom vis-à-vis foetuses is restricted. Induced abortion must never become routine or a matter of course. The goal must be to substitute proper treatment for abortion leading on from foetal diagnosis. (p. 58)

Though restricted in its views, the Council of Ethics has supported the ethical acceptability of induced abortion on the present legal conditions.

In the light of the public debate and the reservations expressed about the number of induced abortions, the minister of health in April 1990 circulated a memorandum on reducing the abortion rate (Ministry of Health 1990). The memorandum contains a rundown on the abortion situation and a series

of examples of initiatives to reduce the abortion rate taken by private organisations, counties, and local authorities. On the basis of some of these
attempts, the minister of health puts forward proposals for possible initiatives
in this field. It is pointed out that the abortion rate in more closely defined
groups can be lowered by a targeted information campaign. In addition to
stepping up information drives in schools—including broader use of the
counties' contraceptive clinics—possible initiatives might be support for the
pregnant woman (social, economic, and housing), if required, and closer
follow-up during "exposed periods," such as the time just after birth or
following abortion and sterilisation. The minister of health has left the initiatives to be taken by private organisations such as the Danish Family Planning Association by asking them to undertake information projects and other
projects funded by the Ministry of Health.

In January 1993 a new four-party coalition government consisting of the
Social Democrats as head of the government and, among others, the Christian People's party, took over in Denmark. In March the Progress party (a
right-wing group) introduced a bill proposing that young women between
the ages of 15 (the sexual minority age) and 18 years should no longer have
to have parental consent to abortion. The argument was that, since they are
allowed to have intercourse and are allowed to carry through the pregnancy
without parental consent, they should also be able to decide on abortion
themselves.

Three of the parties in the coalition agreed in principle to abolish parental
consent, but still the government stated that it could not support the bill.
The bill was thus abandoned without further debate.

THE FUTURE

In Denmark, the attitude and approach towards sex generally is, if not
liberal, then pragmatic rather than moralistic. Most Danes deem sexuality a
normal component of life and part of a good quality of life. An individual's
sexuality is still considered part of private life, but sexuality and contraception are discussed openly in the media and sex education is provided in the
schools.

Abortion is not a controversial topic in Denmark, and it probably will not
be to the degree in other European countries. Nevertheless, the opposition
is noticeable in local newspapers around the country. The rationale for having an abortion in the case of an unwanted pregnancy rather than giving
birth to an unwanted child, however, seems to be widely shared in the population. Likewise, knowledge and acceptance of contraception is high in the
population as such. However, the moral climate concerning abortion is
changing. Early selective abortion and other consequences of medical-
technological developments have led to renewed ethical considerations
among Danish women. Although abortion in the future may be seen more

as a last resort than previously, there is nothing to indicate that the legal right to free abortion in Denmark is endangered by the strong anti-choice movements and tendencies seen in many European countries.

NOTES

1. Act No. 163, May 18, 1937, on Provisions on Account of Pregnancy, etc.
2. Act No. 177, June 23, 1956, on Provisions on Account of Pregnancy, etc.
3. Act No. 120, March 24, 1970, on Pregnancy, etc.
4. Act No. 350, June 12, 1973, on Termination of Pregnancy.
5. Act No. 350, May 24, 1989, amending the Act on Termination of Pregnancy.
6. By January 1, 1991, there were about 1.3 million women of the fertile age between 15 and 49 years. The population of Denmark is about 5.5 million.
7. "Justitsministeriets vejledning af 24. marts 1976 om svangerskabsafbrydelse" (Instructions on termination of pregnancy of March 24, 1976).
8. "Patientklager. Fortsat graviditet trods abortus provocatusindgreb. Betydningen af tilstraekkelig information." Message in *Ugeskrift for Laeger* (weekly medical journal) 152, no. 25, June 18, 1990.
9. Act No. 535, June 3, 1987, on the Formation of a Council of Ethics and the Control of Certain Biomedical Experiments, with subsequent amendment by Act No. 315, May 16, 1990 (deferment of revision act).
10. References from the parliamentary debate.
11. Address to the members of parliament by Respect for Human Life, October 25, 1988.
12. Queries no. 182 and 183 to the Minister of Health by the parliamentary committee on health, May 17, 1991.

REFERENCES

Aagaard, A. Social adviser at the Danish Women's Medical Society and the Family Planning Association, March 1991, and article in *Berlingske Tidende* (daily newspaper), June 26, 1991.

"Abortsituationen i de nordiska Landerne," *Nordic Medicin* 105, no. 2 (1990).

Bregnsbo, H. *Aortloven 1970—en lovgirningsproces.* Copenhagen: Gyldendal, 1971.

Christiansen, T., R. Nielsen, J. Lund, O. Christensen, and J. Larsen. "Abortsogende dvinders viden om abortindgrebet," *Ugeskrift for laeger,* 150, no. 44 (1988).

Danish Council of Ethics. *Fetal Diagnosis and Ethics: A Report.* Copenhagen: Danish Council of Ethics. 1991.

Indstilling vedr. en forbedret indsats til ofrebyggelse af legale aborter. Copenhagen: Danish Family Planning Association and the Committee on Health Education. April 1986.

Kjerkegaard, E., I. Kofoed, and B. Persson (eds). *Livet begynder ved befrugtningen: Om nodvendigheden af fri abort.* Copenhagen: Tiderne Skifter, 1989.

Knudsen, L., "Det gik ikke sa galt—Abort i tal." In E. Kjerkegaard et al. (eds), *Livet begynder ved befrugtningen: Om nodvendigheden af fri abort.* Copenhagen: Tiderne Skifter, 1989.

————. "Hvad fortaeller tallene?" Contribution at a conference arranged by the Danish Female Medical Association and the Danish Family Planning Association, March 3, 1990, Kan aborttallet aendres?

Knudsen, L., and H. Bille. "Faerre kvinder vaelger abort," *Journal for Sundhedsvaesenet* (Journal for Health Services), May 2, 1991.

Knudsen, L., and I. Tanska. "Legalt provokerede aborter 1989," *Ugeskrift for Laeger*, 152, no. 34 (August 20, 1990).

Meyer, G. "Stop for de seneste aborter," *Ugeskrift for Laeger*, 153, no. 27 (July 1, 1991).

Ministry of Health. *Nedbringelse af aborttallet.* Notat, Sundhedsministeriet, April 1990.

National Board of Health. "Statistik om praevention og aborter," *Vitalstatistik,* 1, no. 25 (1989).

Nielsen, R., T. Christiansen, O. Christensen, J. Larsen, and P. Staehr. "Information af abortsøgende dvinder," *Ugeskrift for Laeger*, 150, no. 44 (1988).

Nordentoft, M., B. Petersson, and K. Sidenius. "Psykosociale aspekter hos abortsøgende efter 12. svangerskabsuge," *Ugeskrift for Laeger*, 153, no. 14 (1991).

"Patientklager. Fortsat graviditet trods abortus provocatur-indgreb.—Betyningen af tilstraekkelig information." Message in *Ugeskrift for Laeger*, 152, no. 25 (June 18, 1990).

Statistik Årbog (Statistical Yearbook). Copenhagen: Danmarks Statistik. 1989, 1990.

FINLAND

Marketta Ritamies

THE HISTORY OF ABORTION LAW

The First Abortion Law

Up until 1950, when the first abortion law came into effect, Finnish law did not recognise legal abortions at all. Punishment for performing abortions was laid down in the criminal law, and illegal abortions were rather common. It has been estimated that before the abortion law, the number of abortions would have been between 20,000 and 22,000 annually.

In 1950, Finland got its first abortion law. According to this law abortion could be granted on socio-medical and ethical grounds, as well as on medical grounds. As a result, Finland moved from category 2 to category 3 in the World Health Organization's classification (WHO 1971).

Abortion was granted on medical grounds when the pregnancy or child-birth would cause serious risk to the woman's life or health. Abortion could be induced on ethical grounds when the intercourse leading to pregnancy took place because of rape or incest, and also when the woman was under 16 years of age at the time of conception. Abortion was also possible on eugenic grounds when it could be presumed that the child would be mentally defective or that he or she could develop a serious illness or physical defect.

For an abortion on medical or ethical grounds, the agreement of two physicians was necessary, one being the physician performing the abortion and the other a physician appointed by the National Board of Health (since March 1, 1991, the National Agency for Welfare and Health). For an abortion on eugenic grounds and also when the pregnancy was over four months, permission was needed from the National Board of Health.

The Debate on Legal Reform

The 1950 abortion law was primarily intended to decrease illegal abortions and their health risks. Its purpose was also to define uniform criteria to evaluate abortions on medical grounds. However, the objectives set for the law could not be realised during the two decades it existed.

The number of illegal abortions did not decrease significantly. At the least, the research results were contradictory. According to some surveys abortions decreased to some extent; according to others no decrease was noticed. Nor, despite objectives to the contrary, was regional or social equality established. It was more difficult for those belonging to lower classes to have an abortion, as well as women living in rural and remote areas of the country. This was mostly because physicians who performed abortions were distributed unequally throughout the country. At the end of the 1960s there were about 530 physicians with a special licence to perform abortions, and they were numerous in the southern parts of Finland.

In the 1960s there was growing dissatisfaction with the abortion law. In the media, criticisms were expressed by some and the law was defended by others. Those critical of the law sought not only to reduce the number of illegal abortions but also to establish principles of a woman's freedom of choice and every child being a wanted child. Abortion was considered a measure to help individuals in the case of unwanted pregnancies. Movements dedicated to sexual equality, such as the women's liberation movement and the political left, especially Group Nine, argued for a more liberal abortion law. Furthermore, many physicians expressed their dissatisfaction with the existing law. The first group to suggest officially the liberalisation of the abortion law was the Finnish Women's Democratic Union.

Those who opposed modifying the abortion law, among whom were some physicians, emphasised ethical and Christian principles; they said in principle that a developing life should not be destroyed at any stage.

Public attitudes to abortion were revealed in attitude surveys and newspaper articles. A study carried out by Suomen Gallup (Finnish Gallup) among Finns over 21 years of age gives a picture of the attitudes regarding abortion in the late 1960s: 51 percent of those who participated in the study were in favour of easier abortion, 32 percent wanted to keep it unchanged, and 9 percent supported more restrictive abortion. Of those replying, 8 percent expressed no opinion. In 1969 it was found that 29 percent of those who participated in a survey were of the opinion that a woman should have the right to decide on abortion herself; 26 percent supported abortion for economic and social reasons; 27 percent only in cases in which the life of the mother was in danger, and 10 percent for less serious health reasons. Six percent expressed no opinion. Only 2 percent of those who participated in the survey did not accept abortion under any circumstances.

A study that analysed newspaper editorials on the issue of abortion showed that the papers generally espoused a more permissive abortion law. Left-wing papers in particular were for freer abortion. The Agrarian party news-papers were not as negative towards the new law as were their party supporters, who together with the Conservatives took a more careful attitude towards the abortion law. A more permissive abortion law was supported by 34 percent of farmers, 58 percent of factory workers, and 71 percent of those with the most education. Urban residents, men, highly educated people, and the young were more permissive towards abortion than rural people, women, less educated people, and older people. The most negative attitude towards abortion was among those belonging to revivalist movements.

In the 1960s, many different views on the abortion question were presented and the question was also discussed in the parliament. An Abortion Law Committee was set up in 1967 and concluded at the end of 1968 that the prevailing abortion grounds did not sufficiently take into consideration changes in public attitudes toward abortion. Neither did they correspond to the medical reappraisal, which was reflected in a stronger emphasis on mental health and on social and psychological elements in decisions concerning abortion. However, the committee still took a negative stand in relation to free abortion. According to the committee, abortion should still be bound to specific grounds.

The committee recommended that an abortion be allowed when the woman was under 16 or over 40 at the moment of conception. It suggested accepting socio-medical grounds and liberalised eugenic grounds. The report emphasised the necessity of increasing the use of contraceptive methods in regulating fertility. In the proposed law on birth control counseling it was suggested that fertility regulation and sex education be included in the school curriculum and medical staff should give counseling about birth control after abortion.

ABORTION: CURRENT LAW AND PRACTICE

The Law of 1970

After a long and hectic debate, the new abortion law was passed on June 1, 1970. The main difference in the new law compared to the old one was in relation to social grounds. Under the new law there are sufficient social grounds for abortion, whereas under the old they were taken into consideration only as additional factors. The new law is much broader than the previous one, but by no means does it render free abortion if the social grounds are not interpreted liberally. The law can be classified in WHO category 4.

According to the 1970 law, an abortion is granted to a woman asking for it when:

1. Pregnancy or childbirth would risk her life or health (medical grounds).
2. Childbirth and child care would be a considerable strain on her and her family economically and socially (social grounds).
3. She is made pregnant against her will (ethical grounds).
4. She was not yet 17 years of age or was over 40 or already had four children at the moment of conception (age and birth giving limitations).
5. There is reason to expect the child to be mentally defective or to have a difficult illness or physical defect (eugenic grounds).
6. Illness, disturbed psychological functioning, or a comparable factor of one or both parents seriously limits their capacity to take care of the child (limited capacity to take care of the child).

The Medical Board of Health gave detailed instructions for applying the grounds mentioned in the law. For example, in relation to social grounds, the following factors that may cause considerable strain for the woman may be considered: her civil status, family relationships, and the living conditions of the children already in the family and the effects of childbirth and care on them; the economic situation of the woman and her family; the probable effects of childbirth and care on her work and studies; the effects of childbirth and care on her significant relationships, including the marital one; the effects of childbirth and care on her future plans; her opinion of the child's father's willingness and ability to participate in child care and rearing; limitations to child care caused by her age or immaturity, or her or a family member's ill health or handicap; limitations to child care caused by her or a family member's continuous use of alcohol, criminality, or asocial way of life.

The law forbids abortion after the 16th week of pregnancy except on medical grounds, in which case there is no limitation. However, the National Board of Health has the right to give permission for a later abortion on special grounds up to and including the 20th week of pregnancy. In 1979 a restriction was included in the law according to which an abortion induced on social grounds must be performed during the first 12 weeks of pregnancy, instead of the first 16 weeks, as it was previously. Since 1985 the National Board of Health may grant permission for abortion up to the end of the 24th week when it can be presumed that the child will be mentally defective or would have a difficult illness or physical defect.

According to the prevailing law, abortion is induced by a physician on the basis of a statement given by another physician. On medical grounds, abortion may be performed in any period of gestation, and on social and ethical grounds and on grounds of limited capacity to take care of the child up to the end of the 12th week of pregnancy.

With the permission of one physician, the performing physician, abortion can be induced up to the end of the 12th week of pregnancy when the woman has been under 17 years of age, over 40, or has already four children at time of conception.

The National Board of Health may grant permission for abortion up to the end of the 24th week of pregnancy when there is reason to presume that the child would be mentally defective or that the child would have a serious illness or physical defect. It may give permission up to the end of the 20th week of pregnancy also when the woman was under 17 years of age at the time of conception or when there are other special reasons. Special reasons can be, for example, factors independent of the applicant that have caused the delay of the abortion application, such as late detection of pregnancy, difficulties in getting an appointment with a physician, or a change in the relationship of the mother and the child's father after detection of pregnancy. Special reasons may also include the woman's mental state, or her and her family's social and economic difficulties, or corresponding factors that influence the life situation of the woman.

Where the application for an abortion is rejected by the physician or physicians concerned, the woman may apply to the National Board of Health. It has to deal with the matter urgently. No appeal is allowed against the decision of the National Board of Health.

According to the present law, every authorised physician working for the state, municipality, or federation of municipalities or who is accredited by the National Board of Health may give a statement on the abortion. Abortion must be induced in a hospital accepted by the National Board of Health. Every legalised physician working for such a hospital may perform an abortion. In emergency cases, when the woman's life or health is in danger, any legalised physician may induce an abortion on medical grounds.

The National Board of Health must be informed of all abortions within a month. The tables and figures presented in this article are based on statistics compiled by the board on the basis of these returns.

In Finland, most of the abortion patients—87 percent in 1991—are treated as inpatients. This practice differs from the other Nordic countries and especially from Sweden, where over 80 percent of abortion patients are treated as outpatients. Naturally the Finnish practice means that abortions are more expensive.

The abortion patient in Finland generally stays one day at the hospital, longer if the pregnancy has lasted more than 12 weeks. In 1991 the average time for treatment in the hospital ward was 2.4 days. She pays the normal outpatient fee and bed-day fee as in cases of illness. Abortions are also performed by private physicians charging normal fees.

Figure 1
Abortions per 100 Live Births, Finland, 1969–1990

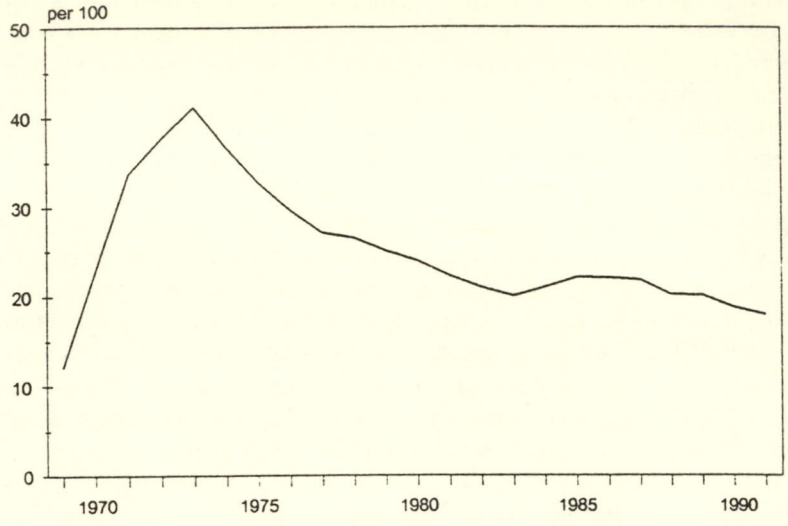

Abortion in Practice

As the new abortion law came into force in the summer of 1970 many were afraid that the number of abortions would grow significantly. In the beginning it seemed as if the fear would come true. The number of legal abortions increased rapidly and in 1973 was at a peak—23,000. However, the number of abortions started to decrease evenly year by year. In 1991 only 11,700 abortions were induced in Finland. There were 19.6 abortions per 1,000 women ages 15 to 49 in the peak year 1973, but only 9.3 in 1991. Correspondingly, the number of abortions per 100 live births went down from 41.3 to 18.0 (see Figure 1). In practice, abortion has not become a method of birth control in Finland.

It is estimated that the number of illegal abortions in the 1950s and 1960s varied between 18,000 and 25,000 annually. Under the present law they have gradually disappeared almost totally. Virtually all abortions in Finland are legal. The number of illegal abortions treated in hospitals annually is only a few dozen; there are hardly more than one or two hundred induced annually.

An indication that abortion has not become a birth control method in Finland is that the majority of abortions induced annually are first ones. In 1991, for almost 71 percent of the women having an abortion, it was their first one; for 21 percent their second, and only for 7 percent their third or more.

The low total abortion rate also indicates the small amount of repeat abortions. In Finland the total number of abortions performed during the fertile period of a woman was 0.4 in 1990; in Sweden the corresponding figure was 0.7 and in Denmark 0.6. The best standard of comparison for repeat abortions used as a birth control method has been in the former Soviet bloc countries. For example, in Romania in the early 1980s, 2.6 abortions per woman were induced. In the Soviet Union, between five and seven pregnancies were interrupted during the woman's fertile period of life.

Under the current Finnish law the grounds for abortion have clearly changed. Abortions are now rarely performed on medical grounds as previously, and mostly on social grounds. One reason for this is that the new law allows for greater honesty. In 1969, a year before the new law, 60 percent of abortions were performed on medical grounds. The diagnosis in 70 percent of the cases was neurosis, overexertion, or weakness. After the enforcement of the new law these were changed to a great extent in a couple of years to social grounds. In 1991, 84 percent of those having an abortion did so on social grounds. One in every 10 abortions was on the grounds of the age of the woman—under 17 years or over 40. Only 1 percent of abortions were being recorded as being on medical grounds.

It has been an aim of the current abortion law that the abortion be performed as early as possible. This aim has been realized to a great extent; the proportion of early abortions has grown substantially. In 1969, 53 percent of all abortions were performed before the 12th week; the corresponding figure in 1991 was 94 percent.

Under the current law, access to abortion services is fairly equal throughout Finland. Previously abortions were induced less in those parts of the country where the general standard of living and state of health were the poorest. This was partly due to the attitudes of physicians living in those areas. In 1970 the rate of abortion in the southern parts of the country was two or three times that in other regions. In 1991 the rate of abortions performed in the southernmost province of Uusimaa did not differ significantly from the rate in most other provinces. The diagonal zone seen in Figure 2, with a low number of abortions in the central part of Finland, is probably connected above all with the revivalist movements that have influence in these areas. Abortion is not accepted by the Laestadian religious movement, which also has a negative attitude towards contraception.

Under the old abortion law many abortions were performed on older women. Under the current law, as Figure 3 indicates, all age groups up to 49 showed an increase in abortions followed by a decrease. The decrease was most significant in relation to older age groups, least significant in relation to the youngest women (those ages 15–19).

In 1973, when the abortion rate was highest, 15 percent of abortions were for women under 20 years of age. In 1980, when the total number of abortions had already decreased by more than 8,000, the proportion of adolescent

Figure 2
Abortions per 1,000 Births by Provinces, 1970 and 1991

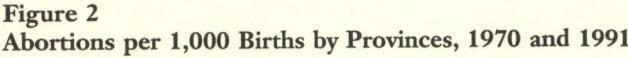

1970   1991

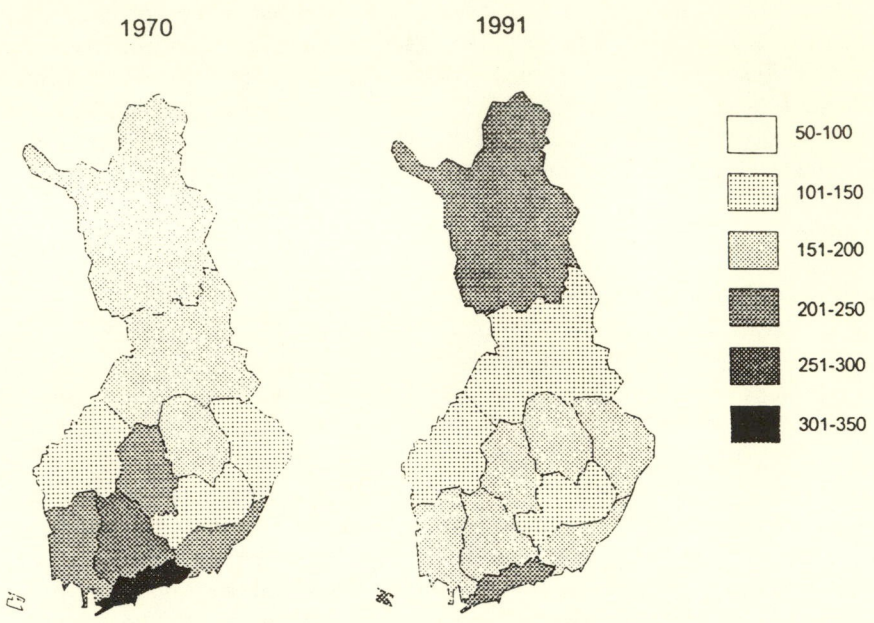

☐	50-100
▦	101-150
▨	151-200
▦	201-250
■	251-300
■	301-350

abortion was at its highest. At that time 24 percent of abortions were induced in women under 20 years of age. After this the proportion of the young started to decrease and was at its lowest in 1991—15 percent.

Between 1973 and 1987, the number of abortions decreased by 44 percent, but the decrease in adolescent abortions has only been 30 percent. As a result, abortions among young women have increased in proportion to all other abortions. At the end of the 1960s less than 10 percent of the pregnancies among those women 15 to 19 years of age ended in abortion; in 1991 the figure was 49 percent.

The relative increase in teenage abortions is obviously due to lack of motivation. Young people are well aware of birth control methods, but they do not use contraceptives regularly, and often not at all. The sexual relationships of the young are often short and therefore it is not considered necessary to use a birth control method that gives continuous protection as does the pill. The condom which is a suitable method for the young, is not used regularly in every intercourse. Often a young person trusts to luck or does not even think of contraception. The use of alcohol is often related to this.

The fact that the age structure of those who have had an abortion has become younger naturally relates to the fact that the proportion of unmarried women among them has increased. Before 1970 most legal abortions were performed on married women. However, since the 1970s their pro-

Figure 3
Age-Specific Abortion Rate, Finland, 1970–1990

per 1,000

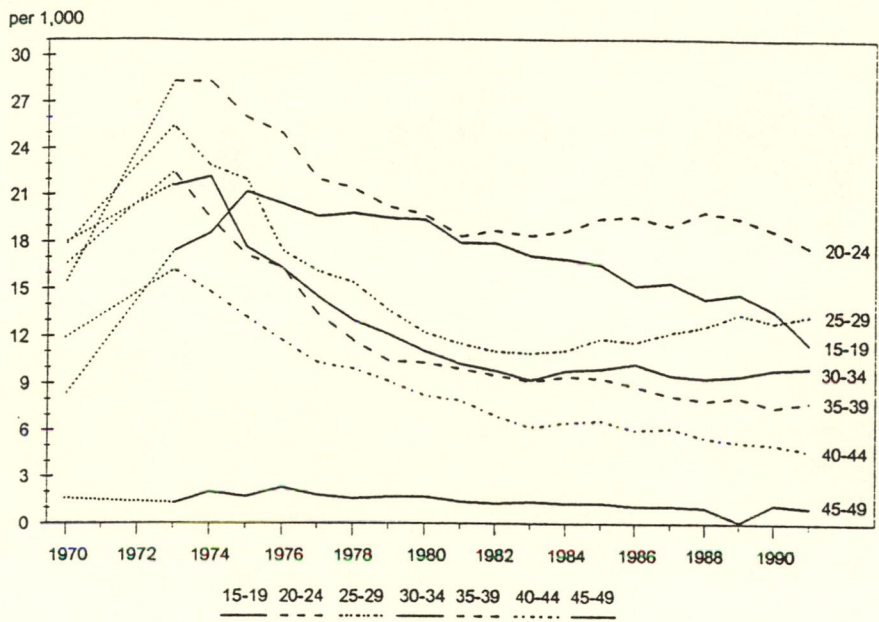

Note: Age-specific abortion rates 1971 and 1972 are missing

portion has continuously diminished and the proportion of the unmarried has grown. In 1991 about 60 percent of abortions were performed on unmarried women and under 30 percent on married women. The proportion of divorced women also increased slightly during this period, but the proportion of widows has diminished somewhat (see Figure 4).

Half of the women who had an abortion in 1991 had not yet given birth. Less than one-fifth had had one child and one-fifth had two children. Under the previous law almost 70 percent of the women having an abortion had had children before, almost one-third at least four.

In the 1950s and 1960s those women belonging to the lowest social class had more difficulty obtaining an abortion than those in the highest and middle class. Under the present law, owing to more common and equal grounds for abortion, the differences among the social classes have leveled out.

Factors Influencing Abortion

Abortion policy has been similar since the mid-1970s in all the Nordic countries. Given that, it is difficult to explain why in recent years the number

Figure 4
Legal Abortions According to Marital Status, Finland, 1969, 1980, and 1991

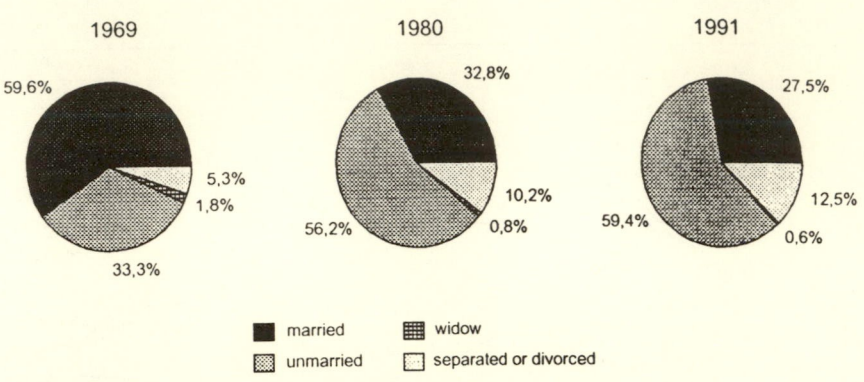

of abortions in Sweden and Denmark has increased while the number in Finland has decreased. With the exception of Iceland, Finland now has the lowest abortion rate (see Figure 5).

The explanation may lie partly in the well-organized school health-care system, which is part of the public health system. Contraceptive education is thus given to young people by qualified health professionals rather than by a teacher, usually a domestic science teacher, assigned to the task. In Finland sex education in schools starts later than in the other Nordic countries. The education depends in addition on the teacher's interest and varies considerably in different parts of the country.

The family planning services available in health-care centres are also well organised in Finland, and different kinds of birth control methods are at the disposal of those who want to use them. The media and other organisations have efficiently informed the public about the prevention of pregnancies. Also the law requires that the woman having an abortion must receive contraceptive education in the hospital; and care must be taken that she will use a reliable birth control method after the abortion.

The use of reliable birth control methods must also relate to the decrease in the number of abortions. In the 1980s in Finland the IUD and condom were the main contraceptive methods used. However, use of the pill has increased in the last few years. In this respect Finland is different from the other Nordic countries, where the health risks of the pill have caused its use to decrease.

The most common contraceptive device used by women having abortions in 1991 was the condom (43 percent). In such cases it is more likely that failure to use a condom led to the unwanted pregnancy rather than failure of the device itself. This is especially true among young people, two out of three of whom are under the influence of alcohol in their first intercourse. Of women having an abortion, 13 percent have been using the pill or IUD.

Figure 5
Abortions per 1,000 Women Ages 15–44 Years in the Nordic Countries, 1968–1990

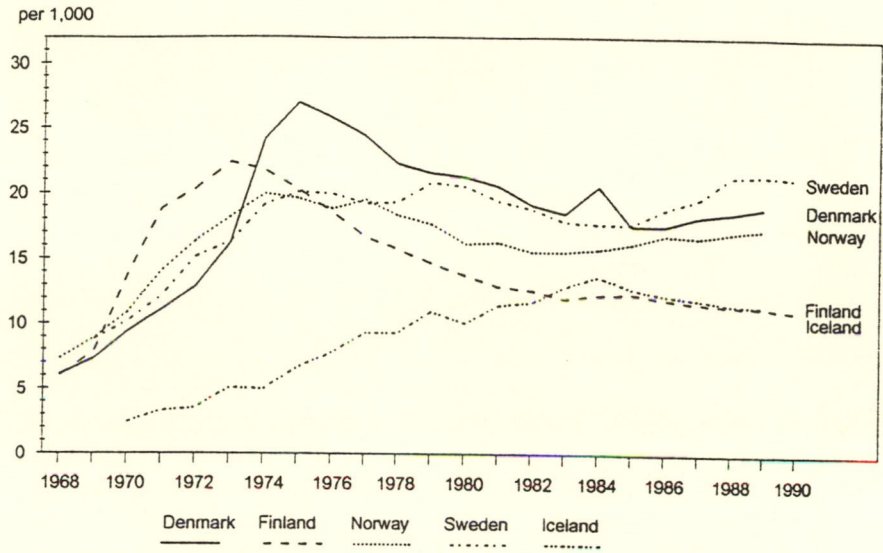

The Politics of Abortion

The present abortion law has been in force for two decades and its effects can now be seen clearly. The law has in many ways proved to be serviceable. Illegal abortions have practically disappeared and the rate of abortions has reached such a low level that it is difficult to find a similar situation elsewhere in Europe. Abortion has not become a birth control method. Women living in different parts of the country and in different population groups have experienced equality of opportunity with regard to abortion services. Abortions are also performed in the early phase of pregnancy, before the end of the 12th week of pregnancy.

The positive development of the Finnish abortion situation is probably connected to the fact that lately no strong opinions have been expressed in the media on abortion, although attitudes towards abortion have become stricter in many western countries. Most western countries are turning politically to the right, and at the same time the moral atmosphere has also become more restrictive. This development can clearly be seen, especially in the United States.

In Finland in 1978, the normal time limit for an abortion was shortened from the 16th week of pregnancy to the 12th week. This did not, however, mean any restriction in the liberal abortion law but rather was an attempt to increase the proportion of early abortions, with the objective of lessening

Figure 6
Total Fertility and Abortion Rates, Finland, 1970–1990

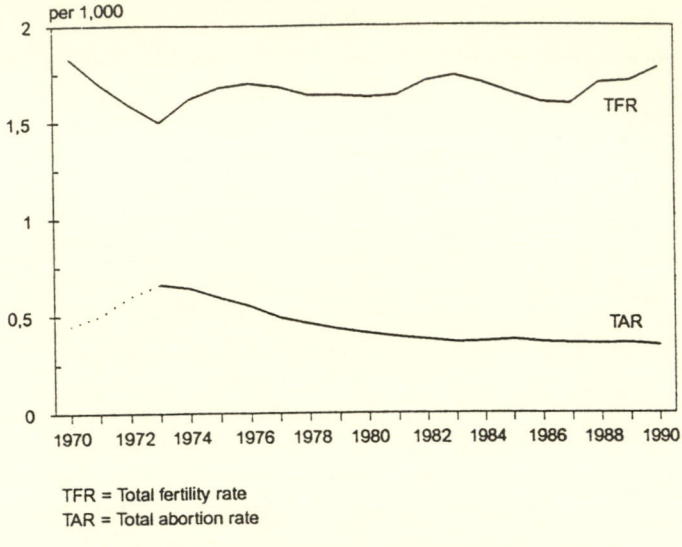

TFR = Total fertility rate
TAR = Total abortion rate

Note: Total abortion rates in 1971 and 1972 are missing

the health and other risks involved. When the current law was being drawn up, the 12-week limit was already being considered. But the level of knowledge and the physician and hospital situation were not considered to be so good in the remote areas of the country to allow for the 12-week limit.

Eight years later the situation in relation to sex education was thought to have improved enough to allow for a shorter time limit. In addition, shortening the time limit was seen in the context of the government's taking steps to improve the efficiency of contraceptive education and making contraceptives more available. Abortion has been discussed in the media in the 1980s from time to time, but it has not awakened any strong opinions for or against. The low fertility of Finland has, however, concerned some people who feel that a decrease in the number of abortions would have the effect of raising fertility. When the number of abortions was at its highest in Finland in 1973 fertility was at its lowest. Evidently the modification of the abortion law led to more careless contraception for some time. When it was possible to prevent an unwanted pregnancy legally, contraception was neglected. When the contraceptive methods became gradually more reliable, they came to be preferred as a means of birth control. Abortion rates have decreased continually, although fertility has been wavelike and clearly below the replacement level (Figure 6). In Finland no connection can be seen between abortions and fertility.

Decreasing the number of abortions is considered a goal in relation to the well-being of an individual, not for the sake of population policy. Through efficient education and reliable contraceptive methods available to everyone, it can be guaranteed that as many children as possible will be born as "wanted" children. By developing family policy, the position of those supporting children can be made easier and those who have been forced to interrupt their pregnancy mainly for economic reasons can be helped.

Satisfaction with the present abortion law is widespread and the rationale behind the law, as well as the goals set by it, are still considered to be acceptable. Although prior to enforcement of the law some women's organisations emphasised the woman's right to decide freely about her body, free abortion has not been strongly demanded in the 1980s. At the same time, the programme of the Finnish Alliance of Women says that the woman should have the right to decide about sterilisation and abortion.

The most negative attitude towards abortion in Finland is perhaps among those belonging to religious groups and revivalist movements. The majority of the population belongs to the state church, although there are not many who are active in the congregations. In the late 1970s the Lutheran Church took a negative stand on abortions granted solely on social grounds, but when the law was changed in 1979 the church's opinion was not taken into consideration.

Recently the church has been rather quiet on issues concerning abortion. It is true that the archbishop raised the issue of grounds for abortion at the end of 1992, but discussion about the matter has not continued in the media. The Christian party, which has only a few members in the parliament, has continuously kept the abortion issue in the forefront in its programme. The party opposes abortion and advocates its use solely on medical grounds. On the contrary, the other parties do not have any stand concerning the abortion law in their programmes.

Among physicians and nurses there are those who oppose abortions and do not want to perform them. They would like to include in the law a clause that states they have the right to decide whether or not they want to perform an abortion. In practice, those physicians who refuse to perform an abortion on principle probably have to make an agreement with their colleagues on how to take care of the abortions which they do not perform.

THE FUTURE

No major changes in the abortion law are likely in the near future because the existing law has fulfilled most of its aims. However, there is still a lot to do to prevent abortions performed owing to lack of information and poor availability of birth control methods. There is also reason to pay more attention to those social and psychological factors that make having a child or taking care of it a considerable strain on a woman and therefore are seen as justifying an abortion.

More psychological and social support needs to be offered to those applying for abortion. The abortion decision may be facilitated by having someone to discuss it with. Decision making also requires sufficient knowledge of abortion legislation and social support. The person planning to have an abortion should also be assisted by persons who may arrange necessary subsistence or take care of other practical problems when needed.

During the coming years attempts should be made to ensure that all those having an abortion be in an equal and uniform position. The actual practice in relation to defining social indications and the special reasons for acquiring a late abortion should be rationalised.

Abortion will most probably stay a topic of debate because it is connected with values widely prevailing in society, such as family, the status of women, and having and raising children. Those who oppose and those who accept the possibility of having an abortion are, however, of like opinion that abortion is not a good solution to the problem of an unwanted pregnancy. Birth control is the goal of both groups. Taking the opinions of both parties into consideration is the best way to ensure positive development of the abortion situation in Finland.

REFERENCES

Härö, A. S., and R. Koskela. "Laillisten raskaudenkeskeytysten viimeaikaiset kehityssuunnat Suomessa," *Sosiaalinen Aikakauskirja* 65, no. 5 (1971): 1–14.

Härö, A. S., R. Koskela, and A. Rasimus. "Aborttilainsäädännön muutos oli tarkoituksenmukainen," *Sosiaalinen Aikakauskirja* 270, no. 5 (1976): 27–36.

Jacobson, Jodi L. "Aborttikysymyksen perusteet ja ratkaisut." In *Maailman tila*, Helsinki: Gaudeamus, 1991, pp. 126–147.

Juva, Kati, Marja Jylhä, and Seppo Aro. "Aborttikeskustelu suomalaisissa lääkärilehdissä," *Suomen Lääkärilehti* 39, no. 1–2 (1984): 35–40.

Komiteanmietintö 1968: A, 11. Aborttilakikomiteanmietintö, Helsinki, 1969.

Kosunen, Elise. "Teini-ikäisten raskaudet ja ehkäisy," *Stakes*, Raportteja 99, Helsinki, 1993.

Lahti, Raimo. "Vuoden 1970 abortti-, steriloimis- ja kastroimislait, niiden soveltaminen sekä abortti- ja steriloimislakien muutokset vuosina 1978 ja 1985," *Suomen Lääkärilehti* 40, no. 18 (1985): 1809–1814.

Niemelä, Pirkko. "Finland." In Paul Sachdev (ed.), *International Handbook on Abortion*. Westport, Conn.: Greenwood Press, 1988.

Ritamies, Marketta. "Abortit meillä ja muualla," *Väestöntutkimuslaitoksen julkaisusarja D*, no 16. Helsinki, 1986.

SVT (Official Statistics of Finland), 1971–1987, Health Services, Helsinki, 1973–1989.

SVT, 1968–1988, VI A: 130–155, Population, Vol. I, Helsinki, 1970–1991.

SVT, 1968–1970, XI: 71–73, Public Health and Medical Care, Helsinki, 1970–1974.

SVT, 1993, Induced Abortions in Finland until 1991, National Research and Development Centre for Welfare and Health, Health: 3, Helsinki, 1993.

Tietze, Christopher. *Induced Abortion: A World Review.* New York: Alan Guttmacher Institute, 1986.

Vertio, Harri, Tuulikki Nurmi, and Anja Rasimus. "Muutos raskauden keskeyttämisestä annettuun lakiin," *Suomen Lääkärilehti* 34, no. 34 (1979): 1673–1677.

World Health Organization. *Abortion Laws: Report of a WHO Scientific Group.* Geneva: WHO, 1971.

Yearbook of Nordic Statistics, 1973–1987. Copenhagen: Nordic Council of Ministers and the Nordic Statistical Secreteriat, 1974–1988.

FRANCE

Colette Gallard
Translation by Elinor Neubert

THE HISTORY OF ABORTION LAW

The Era of Illegality

At the end of the nineteenth century, Malthusian organisations had started up in France explicitly demanding the right to voluntary childbearing. Marie Huot, the first woman to speak out in public, said later that she had preached "wombs on strike" to demonstrate the global, collective nature of the struggle that a strong neo-Malthusian movement was about to wage in France and abroad.

In the absence of any real popular support for the campaign for voluntary childbearing, the neo-Malthusians became progressively isolated in their battle against the increasing attacks of moralist and natalist forces. And thus the enemies of voluntary childbearing, using the political and economic contexts of the period preceding and following World War I, managed to set up a sturdy framework of legal constraints.

This took place in two stages: first, the law of 1920, which considered birth control propaganda as incitement to abortion, and thus outlawed both information on contraception and all practice of it; and then the law of 1923, by categorising abortion as an offence (to be tried in a magistrate's court) rather than as a crime, ended the relative indulgence shown by some Assize Court judges. Abortion was no longer tried before the Assize Court, and it was hoped that more severe sentences would be handed out by magistrates than by the ordinary people who made up the juries of the Assize Courts.

The laws of 1920 and 1923 marked a severe decline in social equality. Although women from the higher income groups were still able to procure contraceptives from neighbouring countries (U.K., Holland, Switzerland), and even sometimes to obtain an abortion there, working-class women faced the problems of their continual pregnancies and the difficulty of "making ends meet" for their large families in inadequate and unhealthful housing conditions, alone and with no one to turn to.

In 1927, the trial of Henriette Alquier (a schoolteacher who published a programme of sex education in *The Bulletin of the Feminist Group of Teachers*) aroused public opinion and obliged the left-wing political parties to take a clear stand. But they did it in the name of freedom of opinion and not to defend a woman's right to voluntary motherhood. As for the feminist movement, they were completely absorbed in the fight for women's civil rights. Thus it was once again left to the neo-Malthusians to organise the defence of a woman's right to voluntary maternity.

In 1933, proposals for legislative reform were put forward by Socialist and Communist members of the parliament; their aim was to "seek social protection for mothers and for children by setting up a National Maternity Fund, by instituting sex education, by the return to unrestricted propaganda on anti-conceptional prophylaxis, and by new legislation on abortion."[1]

It was an important initiative, but the support of the Communists was short-lived, for in 1936, then again in 1938, Maurice Thorez, general secretary of the Communist party, opposed free contraception and sex education by deliberately insinuating that the campaign in favour of birth control was an attempt to impose a limit on the number of pregnancies per couple, rather than making the individual's right to free choice the basic demand of the campaign.

At the same time, a young doctor, Jean Dalsace, was challenging the law of 1920 by providing women with contraceptives; and in 1935, with the complicity of the mayor of Suresnes, he went as far as to open a dispensary in the town where women could obtain information on and prescriptions for diaphragms, caps, and spermicides, which he procured for them illicitly in England. This action, however, remained an exception that did little to alleviate the general situation of oppression suffered by women around 1939.

Between 1939 and 1945, the triumph of the family as a prime ideological value and the strengthening of repressive measures against the "social plagues of drink, prostitution, birth control propaganda, and abortion"[2] contributed to the general restriction of women's rights. The law of January 15, 1942, treated abortion as treason; a launderess, Marie-Louise Giraud, was guillotined on July 30, 1943, because she had carried out abortions.

The Struggle for Decriminalisation

For most French people, the postwar period (1945–1952) was notable for the day-to-day material problems of existence. During this period, the reformist feminism of the Liberation brought in measures that did away with the most flagrant discrimination against women, thus causing a momentary lull in the activities of the feminist movement. But the feminists never abandoned their global analysis of the condition of women; the disparity between the rhetoric on equality of the sexes and the reality, as well as the systematic recuperation of the ground the feminists had gained by social organisations seeking to maintain male supremacy, became increasingly clear, and later became the ideological bases of the fight for free abortion.

In 1949, the publication of Simone de Beauvoir's book *The Second Sex* caused a scandal because of her implacable denunciation of the oppression of women. In her statement on sexual oppression she spoke extensively of the tragedies brought about by clandestine abortions and continued unavoidable childbearing. Her well-known proposition that "women are not born women, they are made into women" was the starting point, and later the reference point, of the different currents of the women's movement at the time of Liberation.

During the same period, the natalist aims of the government ("we need 12,000 beautiful babies in the next 12 years"[3]) were clearly restated, backed by practical measures to encourage a rise in the birthrate, and the Catholic Church (whose influence was particularly strong in the rural provinces), helped to discourage any change in attitudes about sexuality. A pact of silence hid the few voices trying to express the deep uneasiness felt by many young Catholic couples.

In 1953, after visiting a birth control clinic during a trip to the United States, Doctor Labroua Weill-Halle published an article intended to raise awareness of this issue in *The Hospital Weekly*. None of her colleagues appeared to notice it. In 1955, at the Congress of Medical Ethics, she made another attempt, and this time encountered fierce opposition from Catholic doctors, but also a certain current of sympathy and interest. It took the resounding shock of a trial for infanticide in 1954–55 to shake public opinion into awareness of the catastrophes that could be caused by too many, too frequent pregnancies. A journalist, J. Derogy, began a study of birth control for the newspaper *Libération* in October 1955. A series of articles that appeared under the title "Are Women Guilty?" raised the level of debate in the press and in public opinion, both deeply divided between the defenders of the status quo and the partisans of progress. The various reactions proved that women were still considered by many men as irresponsible minors, but did allow those who were interested in the idea of "planned parenthood" to get together. This was how 20 women met to lay the foundations of La Maternité Heureuse, which became Le Mouvement Français pour le Planning Familial (MFPF, the French Family Planning Movement) in 1960.

The association had no neo-Malthusian desire to influence the birthrate, but advocated effective birth control for individual couples to avoid the dramatic consequences of abortion. In spite of the interest shown by public opinion, all the institutions (the government, the legal system, the church, the medical profession) were unanimous in their opposition to any attempt to challenge what they called "natural law." The initiatives taken by the pioneers acted as a catalyst to the various opposition forces, from the Communist party to the Catholic Church, who united in a manner totally foreign to their traditional cleavages, demonstrating clearly how specific the issue was.

Gradually MFPF centres opened all over France. Volunteer workers and doctors saw increasing numbers of women and couples coming for advice and prescription, and simultaneously pursued their obstinate aim: to obtain the legalisation of contraception by keeping the issue in the public eye through meetings and debates and by political lobbying. In 1965, six weeks before the presidential election, François Mitterand took a stand as a supporter of repeal of the 1920 law and thus forced the other candidates into the argument. Slowly but surely, support for contraception gained ground and it was finally legalised (although with many restrictions) in 1967.

The 1968 revolution provided the opportunity for slogans on sexual liberation to be publicly aired; the women's liberation movement expanded and strengthened.

The idea of a woman's right to choose replaced the notion of individual birth control; the MFPF underwent a radical change of position, investing all its forces in the fight to get the 1920 law changed. In 1971 the press published a manifesto in which 343 women, including such well-known figures as Simone Signoret (their enemies called them "the 343 tarts") publicly declared that they had had an abortion. In 1972 a girl of 17, charged with abortion, was released without a sentence being passed. The press seized on the affair and gave it considerable coverage, particularly since the girl's mother and the abortionist were tried a month later. Celebrities were called as witnesses for the defence (Simone de Beauvoir, Delphine Seyrig, Nobel Prize-winner Jacques Monod, to name a few) bringing a wider perspective and a deeper level of analysis to the debate. In 1973 the *Manifesto of 313 Doctors* was published: they declared that they had performed abortions and asked to be charged. The pressure of public opinion was such that no charge was brought. But the parliament did not yield.

It took the creation of a fait accompli situation—with abortions openly performed in MFPF centres regardless of the legal consequences, the active support of trade union representatives, the diffusion of the banned film *Histoire d'A*, and the election that followed the death of Georges Pompidou— for the debate finally to take place in the parliament.

The law that was passed by the Assemblée Nationale on January 17, 1979, depenalised abortion partly, for a trial period of five years in the first instance; this law remains in force today, with only minor changes.

ABORTION: CURRENT LAW AND PRACTICE

The Law of 1979

On January 17, 1979, the French parliament passed a law that legalised abortion in certain circumstances. This law stated that a woman whose pregnancy places her in a state of distress may request an abortion. The abortion may be carried out only until the 10th week of pregnancy by a doctor in a public or private hospital. The doctor receiving her request must warn the woman of the risks she is taking and give her information on the possibilities of help offered if she keeps the child. She must consult a social worker or counsellor, who must deliver a certificate. She must wait for a week before the abortion can be carried out—the week of reflection required by the law. Unmarried minors must have the written consent of at least one parent. Foreign women must have resided in French territory for at least three months, or have a residence permit.

The penal code sets out punishment for all abortions or attempts at abortion except those carried out under the terms of this law. For the abortionist, the punishment is from one to five years in prison and a variable fine; the punishment is doubled if it involves a habitual abortionist; for the woman, the penalty is from six months to two years imprisonment and a smaller fine. These legal arrangements are suspended for abortions carried out in the limited framework of the law.[4]

The advantage of this law was that its terms indicated clearly that the woman alone was judge of her "state of distress." It also obliged doctors who were "conscientious objectors" to inform the woman at once of their refusal to carry out an abortion.

The legalisation of abortion, even though it was provisional, resulted in the demobilisation of public opinion, of the trade union supporters, and of the women's movement, who considered the battle won; only the MFPF remained to demand that the law be applied and to denounce the inadequate provision available. The association declared that any woman requesting an abortion, whether within the limits of the law or not, should find a solution to her problem; and it rallied all its forces to carry out a very detailed and rigorous national survey, aimed at bringing influence to bear when the law came up for revision in 1980.

Without using the structures of political parties, trades unions, or other groups, women alone organised a march on October 6, 1979, just before the law was revised, at which 50,000 met together for what became an enormous collective fête, where they sang, danced, and publicly declared that no one could decide their lives for them.

But the parliamentary debate was sadly reactionary. The definitive law voted was no improvement on the provisional one. The terms under which abortions could be carried out were the same, the sentences were heavier, and legal constraints were set up; doctors could make financial profit from women's problems.

It was not until the Left returned to power at the end of 1982 that abortion was covered by the Social Security reimbursement system. Since then, and because of this measure, most women have taken abortion for granted, even if they have moral or ethical objections.

The MFPF lobbied and fought for several years to raise public support for the complete removal of abortion from the penal code and for it to be simply integrated into ordinary medical practice under the health code; they met with disappointing results. Unconditional enemies of women's rights, on the other hand, have over the last 10 years reorganised, gained strength, and taken the offensive in an attempt to get abortion outlawed again. Their most spectacular initiatives have been the circulation of a video film *The Silent Cry*, raids on centres performing abortions, and the organisation of a Fête for Life in Paris in 1991.

Abortion in Practice

We consider abortion statistics to be reliable only from 1981, when there were 180,500 abortions according to the official statistics office, the INED. The most recent statistics available are for 1989 and show 162,000 legal abortions. This figure has probably remained fairly stable for 1990 and 1991. But the 4,000 or so women per year who have to go abroad (to the U.K., Holland) to obtain an abortion must be added to this figure, as well as the unknown number of illicit abortions carried out in this country, which do not appear in official statistics.

A study carried out in 1988 on 1,077 women who came to the MFPF for illegal abortions, 820 of them for late abortions, shows the reasons behind the requests beyond the legal time limit. In the six first categories, the women (739 in total) had not brought the illegal situation upon themselves.

1. 429 (52.3 percent) were for medical reasons, mainly physiological problems like "false" periods when the woman was in fact already pregnant, women who became pregnant in the postpartum period, or because of incompatibility of the pill with other medication, etc. In 78 cases, medical errors appeared to have occurred. In 39 cases where a pathology was evident, therapeutic abortion was possible. This group included mainly abortions at under 15 weeks of amenorrhea, except in the case of drug addicts.

2. 158 (19.3 percent) were due to changes of situation during a pregnancy, originally accepted if not desired: serious conflict between the partners, abandonment, death, eviction, loss of employment, accident, and other unpredictable difficulties.

3. 94 (11.5 percent) cases involved cultural problems; there would be 291 if the minors and foreign women whose pregnancies were not beyond the legal time

limit but who were in illegal situations had been included. This is the category in which the latest abortions are to be found.

4. 31 (3.8 percent) cases show poverty to have been the deciding factor. In fact, poverty is found more than a hundred times as a contributing factor and was not always noted on the survey questionnaire because it is so common. These cases are generally very late.

5. 18 (2.2 percent) result from rape and violence. This category is increasing as we learn to recognise such problems, and will increase as women learn to speak out on violence instead of keeping it secret. These are also very late abortions.

6. 9 (1.1 percent) are due to bad application of the legislation.

7. 56 (6.8 percent) carry the comment "indecision." Several were undergoing psychotherapy. We do not always know what their final decision was.

8. 25 (3 percent) speak of a woman's "negligence," with a question mark: but what does this "negligence" hide?

To sum up, of the 1,077 women excluded by French law (820 for asking too late, 197 for being minors without permission from a parent, or foreign women without the proper papers), the immense majority were not responsible for the illegality of their situation.

The figure for illegal abortions abroad covers women whose pregnancies were too far advanced (over 10 weeks) to obtain an abortion in France, minors without permission from at least one parent, and illegal immigrant women. The women in such circumstances who come to the MFPF (about 3,000 a year) are often sent to us by the public services themselves (hospitals, social workers) who are unable to help them.

The situation as regards illegal abortion in France is slightly different. The law stipulates that private nursing homes must limit the number of abortions carried out to 25 percent of their total number of operations. When they risk overstepping this percentage, some nursing homes simply include any further abortions in another category (e.g., removal of polyps). These abortions are absent from the statistics.

Foreign women without the necessary residence permits can generally find a solution in France provided they can pay (the private sector rarely checks immigration papers); if not, teams like the MFPF, who consider abortion to be one of women's rights, have to arrange some solution for them.

During the provisional period (1975–1980), a few doctors were charged with financial profiteering. There were two attempts to bring to trial social workers and the MFPF for having informed women of the possibilities available for abortion abroad. In one case, the charge was dropped, and the other came under the general amnesty for minor offences that traditionally follows a presidential election.

Abortions can be performed only in a public or private hospital structure. On the whole, the attitude of doctors and medical staff is reasonable; the personnel working in certain structures can be highly motivated (this is especially the case in the centres set up immediately after the law was passed by staff who supported the campaign).

If the public sector does not have adequate provision for the needs of women requesting abortions, the private sector fills the gap in a fairly satisfactory manner, at least as regards the number of abortions. However, this varies from region to region. Depending on local conditions, 30 to 70 percent of abortions take place in private nursing homes, where a first appointment is often given in 24 hours, instead of a week or 10 days (or even more) in the public sector.

The official public sector rates in January 1991 were 902.16 francs for an abortion without a general anesthetic and involving less than 12 hours hospitalisation, and 1,397.37 francs for an abortion with a general anesthetic and 12 to 24 hours hospitalisation. Private sector rates, which are also officially determined, are a little higher. Social Security covers 80 percent of the cost of an abortion in either the public or the private sector, but only at a public hospital can women simply pay the remaining 20 percent; at a private nursing home, they must pay the whole cost of the operation generally on entry, often with "extras" that sometimes almost double the official rates, and must then wait for three weeks or longer for reimbursement. This makes the option impossible for many women.

Extra financial coverage for abortion is provided by the private health insurance schemes generally subscribed to by employers for their staff and staff's families.

For women who have no Social Security or other coverage and who are unable to pay, application can be made for free medical aid; a special accelerated procedure is available for abortion. This is rarely accepted in the private sector.

The "social" interview that is compulsory before the abortion poses certain problems. As well as professional social workers (who have no specific training for the task and thus can project their personal ethics), marriage guidance counsellors in family planning centres are entitled to see women for these interviews. The certificate they deliver is in no way a "permit to abort," and they have no right to refuse such a certificate to any woman. But the training of marriage guidance counsellors is in the hands of various government-approved associations, some of which are close to the Catholic Church and opposed to abortion; they tend to be dissuasive, to seek to influence women, and to instill guilt feelings.

Women thus have to go through a kind of obstacle race of procedures; they must obtain a first appointment at a hospital or nursing home, get various tests done, find the necessary money to pay, or apply for free medical treatment, go through the "social" interview, return to the hospital for the operation, often needing to get organised for an overnight stay, this second appointment being possible only after a week's legally required "reflection" period between the original request and the abortion.

Most women have support from their partner or from a close relative or friend, but do not want their colleagues, wider family group, or neighbours to know. Girls under 18 who cannot or do not wish to tell either parent are often in dramatically lonely situations.

The Politics of Abortion

The strong movement of support that arose in favour of legal abortion was probably due to the number of women who had gone through or had seen other women close to them go through dramatic experiences linked to unwanted pregnancies. It was a compassionate reaction towards the many women who were led by misfortune to such extremes. The accounts of the debates that took place at the Assemblée Nationale show that it was the deliberate use of *miserabilism*—exploiting the full dramatic impact of the worst situations—that persuaded the members of parliament of the various parties to pass the law. Several years later women wanting abortions still felt they had to plead that kind of situation to explain their request and "be granted" what they wanted.

In 1982 the law on the reimbursement of abortion by Social Security was undoubtedly a milestone in the evolution of attitudes regarding abortion. Although the measure may have shocked quite a lot of people, the idea of the right to abortion was more and more widely accepted. This was all the more so as the total number of abortions did not increase (on the contrary, the decline in the rate continued—11 percent in five years, and the statistics became much more reliable), and as reimbursement normalised the financial picture by putting an end to profiteering.

On the other hand, all the groups that had struggled for legalised contraception and abortion remained persuaded that women would not be able to use these techniques as a means towards their own autonomy unless at the same time genuine sex education programmes were set up. We have continued to meet with considerable reticence in this field; information about the genital organs and reproductive physiology is now included in school science textbooks, but education on relationships and sexuality is generally barred for all sorts of reasons: parents' associations often stand in the way, arguing that it will incite the children to premature experiments in sex; contraception should be taught, but nothing said about sexuality or boy-girl relationships. In any case, the government has not made financial provision for such education to be carried out on an adequate scale. The situation on sex education was far more advanced in the 1970s than it is today.

And with the appearance of AIDS, ideas about abstinence, fidelity, and the return to moral order have blossomed, as if AIDS were an expiation for the "mad" years after 1968. Sex education is acceptable only provided it concentrates on the dangers of AIDS—in fact, on the dangers of sexuality, with no mention of pleasure.

The deterioration of the economic and social climate has pushed issues like sex education, contraception, and abortion into second position. But the marketing of the abortive pill RU 486 raised a controversy that shows how sensitive public opinion is on such questions. In April 1982, Professor Beaulieu announced to the Academy of Medicine that a new molecule was being developed that would have both an abortive and an end-of-cycle contraceptive effect. At the end of 1983, pro-life pressure groups intervened for the first time, forcing the laboratory to stop research on the new molecule as an end-of-cycle contraceptive. The use of the new pill had to be limited to abortion. In 1987, the National Committee on Ethics agreed to its use in specialised centres within the strict framework of the abortion law. (This, for the supporters of the right to choice, put an end to the hope of seeing a more flexible procedure becoming available in family planning centres, providing a solution for the cases of minors without parental consent.) An attempt was made at the beginning of 1988 to sink the RU 486 by a violent boycotting campaign in the United States and to a lesser degree in Europe against the laboratory that produced it, Roussel Uclaf.

In September of the same year, the Pharmaceutical Marketing Licence Commission of the Ministry of Health decided in favour of commercialisation of RU 486; on October 26, under the combined effects of pressure from the Catholic Church and from French and foreign pro-life movements, as well as pressure exercised on Hoechst, the main shareholder of Roussel Uclaf, the firm, fearing a boycott of their whole operation, announced they were suspending production of the pill. This announcement provoked a storm of international protest (even the World Health Organisation expressed regret). Two days later, the minister of health, asserting that RU 486 was "morally the property of women," instructed Roussel Uclaf to start distribution again. In January 1991 the Council of State, following a request from six associations opposed to abortion, rescinded this instruction. This measure did not, however, disturb the commercialisation of the pill.

Alongside these legal procedures, over the last two years the pro-life lobbies have gone in for violent action: raids on abortion centres, where they occupy the centres, cut off the telephone, chain themselves to furniture, open medical record files, tamper with sterilised material, and dissuade the women. Make no mistake about it—the commandos who are opposed to abortion are also anticontraception; in fact, they are against a woman's right to control her fertility. They base their action on the rigid doctrine of the Roman Catholic Church—"the object of all sexual acts is procreation."

Organised in several associations—Grossesse Secours, Comité pour l'Enfant à Naître, Secours Future Mères, Mère de Miséricorde, Avenir de la Culture (Pregnancy Assistance, Committee for the Unborn Child, Help for

Future Mothers, Mother of Mercy, The Future of Children)—they are linked to and are suspected of receiving financial support from various pro-life and extreme right-wing groups abroad, like Tradition, Family and Property in Brazil, which are involved in the Vatican's vast world crusade against fertility control, and, at least for the extremists, for a return to moral order.

Very determined, although in a minority, they organise their activity at different levels: assistance for women who have begun an unwanted pregnancy; awareness-raising campaigns in traditionalist circles (bell-tolling in memory of "children killed by abortion," pilgrimages to the Fountain of the Holy Innocents); campaigns directed at public opinion (showing foeti in formaldehyde); calls to have the law on abortion changed. They also have means of influencing pregnant women requesting abortion at the "social" interview through those of their members who have been trained as counsellors by approved associations; such counsellors are also entitled to take part in sex education schemes in schools.

They make only a very restricted impact on public opinion, however, although many contradictory currents of opinion are surfacing at the moment. Women generally seem to take abortion for granted and are ready to defend it if there is a real threat, but a stir was created recently over the fact that many contraceptive pills are no longer reimbursed by the Health Service, and quite a lot of negative reaction was expressed on account of abortion still being reimbursed. The present government has no wish to see the abortion issue on the table again, but with legislative and presidential elections looming there is no way of knowing what may occur if there is a change of government.

Without waiting to find out, the supporters of the right to choice are moving into an active role again; at the MFPF's initiative, associations, women's movements, trades unions, and political parties are getting together again and joining forces with progressive groups in the rest of Europe that are facing the same risks. We have chosen the slogan "Love Is Ours" to defend the rights we have fought for so long to gain.

THE FUTURE

There was a general election in France in March 1993 in which the Right gained a majority of seats. At the same time, Simone Veil, who had defended the law on abortion in 1975, was appointed Minister of Health and Social Affairs. She has asserted on many occasions that the abortion law should be fully implemented and that it should not be discussed any further in the parliament. However, the anti-abortionists are relentless in their campaign and have been trying to eliminate the government budget that permits reimbursement of abortion from Social Security. In addition, for some hospitals, implementing the law means doing so in the most restrictive way possible. And finally, the growing debate on bio-ethics will serve to raise the issue of abortion once again.

For all these reasons, it is necessary to keep a watchful eye on this basic woman's right—the right to choose.

NOTES

1. Quoted from the journal *Le Problème Sexuel,* founded in 1933 by Berthe Albrecht.

2. *Protection de la Famille et de la Maternité,* part of the measures taken by the Vichy government in 1942.

3. Charles de Gaulle, quoted in Jacques Rabaut, *Histoire des Feminismes Français,* Edit. Stock, 1978.

4. At the moment the penal code is undergoing revision, but although the women's movement had hoped that sentences for women and medical staff involved in illegal abortions would be abolished, this now seems unlikely.

REFERENCES

Khoppers, B.M., I. Brault, and E. Sloss. "Abortion in Francophone Countries," *American Journal of Comparative Law,* 38, no. 4, 1990, pp. 889–922.

Leridon, H., Y. Charbit, P. Collomb, J. P. Sardon, and L. Toulemon. *La seconde révolution contraceptive.* Travaux et Documents, cahier no. 2, September 1991.

Mossuz-Lavau, J. *Les lois de l'amour (les politiques de la sexualité en France).* Paris: Payot, 1991.

Mouvement Français pour le Planning Familial. *D'une révolte à une lutte, 25 ans d'histoîre du Planning familial.* Paris: Editions Tierce, 1982.

GERMANY

Sabine Klein-Schonnefeld

THE HISTORY OF ABORTION LAW

The All-German Historical Background

In 1871, the penal code was enacted, and within it was Section 218.[1] Since that time abortion was a felony punishable by imprisonment of up to five years; no exceptions or indications were provided. This merciless legislation caused not only an enormous amount of grief and harm but also disease, mutilation, and death through self-inflicted or backstreet abortions, suicides, infanticide, and the neglect of unwanted, unwelcomed children (see Zwerenz 1980; Amendt and Schwarz 1991).

In the context of industrialisation and urbanisation, and with a dramatic drop in the birthrate at the end of the 19th century, politicians, the medical profession, and scientists began to consider social reforms in relation to family policy, public health, and population policy. The proletarisation of great parts of the population induced, among others, Friedrich Engels (1820–1895) and August Bebel (1840–1913) to develop a Marxist theory of population and family policy. After World War I, with the defeat of the German Kaiserreich in the liberated Weimar Republic, Marxist and social democratic ideas joined, and were met by a growing and strong women's movement demanding sexual freedom and birth control. Debates on public health in particular were strongly influenced by new discoveries in the medical sciences, leading to neo–social Darwinistic theories and aiming at the controlled production of "perfect" human beings. Patriarchal thinking among the Left and a basically science-orientated conception of the world led to a tendency to see applied technologies of these discoveries as an answer to many socially caused public health problems. The sexist and racist implications widely used and elaborated on later by the Nazi regime were ignored (see von Soden 1988).

During the Weimar Republic, all these factors assisted the development of widespread public discussion of sexual freedom for both sexes, planned parenthood, and abortion. Even though the law on abortion proved to be more and more unacceptable, it was not changed. But finally in 1927 the Reichsgericht (Supreme Court) recognised emergency abortion if it proved necessary to save the life of the woman.[2]

Since the harsh, restrictive, patriarchal legislation still defined abortion as a felony, the Nazi government saw no need to change it, either. But they engaged in research on genetic engineering, on—now explicit—racist and sexist definitions of human "normality," of a "proper" course of pregnancy and birth, as well as research on hereditary diseases. Camp prisoners, especially women, were used, exploited, and often murdered as guinea pigs. The research was aimed mainly at women's bodies in order to control their reproductive and generative abilities, to use their wombs for the controlled production of standardised, "healthy" (as defined) descendants of a "pure race."[3]

Quite late in the Nazi period of power, and not accidentially at the peak of the Second World War, in 1943 the abortion law was changed to extend the sanctions against women who aborted themselves and to allow for capital punishment against assistants "if the offender had continuously damaged the vitality (or viability) of the German Nation."[4] But already in 1933 the genetic health laws had been introduced.[5] Through this regulation women were forced to have an abortion or to be sterilised if there was the possibility of hereditary disease. Hereditary diseases covered a wide range of socially unwanted behaviour and could target those who were said to be "antisocial, asocial, maladjusted, feeble minded" (see Müller 1987, 97 seq.). Psychiatric-medical definitions have seldom been derived in such an obvious way from the sociopolitical interests of power.[6]

Abortion Law in the Former Federal Republic of Germany

After World War II, the death penalty was abolished with the establishment of the Federal Republic of Germany (FRG). Several further attempts were made in the FRG to reform the Nazi abortion law, especially to lower the harsh sentences and to implement the Weimar jurisdiction in the law by recognizing the danger to the life or the physical or mental health of the pregnant women as a legal reason for an abortion. All these attempts failed during the period of restoration (see Ketting and van Praag 1985, 24f). Not until the economically prosperous period of the late 1960s—when educational and training reforms were demanded by the student movement and a new women's liberation movement demanded emancipation and equal rights, when liberalisation was on the agenda throughout Europe—did a liberalisation of the penal code become possible. Liberal and left-wing lawyers discussed in public a general reform of the penal code. Women activists started campaigns acknowledging they had had illegal abortions. Many prominent, well-known women and even more unknown women signed as well and joined the campaign. The aim was the general decriminalisation of abortion.

The chapter of the penal code concerning sexual offences and abortion was reformed in 1974. According to the new version,[7] abortions performed before the 14th week after conception would not constitute an offence on the part of the woman or the person performing the abortion. This was called the *period model*. After 14 weeks, abortion would be allowed only under particular conditions.

The original goal of the movement, the decriminalisation of abortion, had failed. Abortion continued to be regulated through penal law. However, it seemed that one of the most liberal laws on abortion in Europe had been established.

But the controversy went on. Conservative forces had by now formed their own movement, determined not to accept such a law even if it should pass the parliament (see Esser and Koch 1988). This counter-movement was led by the conservative parties, the Christian Democratic Union (CDU), the Bavarian Christian Social Union (CSU), and the Catholic hierarchy. As soon as the law reform had passed parliament, five single states of the FRG, Länder, all of them governed by Christian Democrats, appealed to the Constitutional Court. The law reform should have come into operation on January 1, 1975, but the Court published its judgment on February 25, 1975, ruling that the bill was at variance with the Constitution, and thus could not be enforced.[8]

Unfortunately, but inevitably, the Constitutional Court did not only rule out the law reform but also gave reasons that have affected abortion legislation to this day. The Constitutional Court separated the foetus from the pregnant woman, denied their physical and socio-emotional unity, and constructed the foetus as a person in legal transaction, as a holder of individual rights entitled to specific protection by Sections 1 and 2 of the Constitution, which safeguard human dignity and human life.[9] The judges held that the Constitution obliges the state to protect "developing life," the foetus, from encroachment by the mother.[10] Following the logic of the ruling, becoming pregnant means that the exercise of one's personal freedom and one's individual rights is restricted, while the foetus—the possible child-to-be—is seen as exposed to the alternative of "all or nothing," "life or death."[11] Therefore the constitutional protection of the possibly developing human being, the foetus, is violated if a woman could decide on her own whether to become a mother or not. Even though the interests and rights of pregnant women and foetuses had to be weighed against each other carefully, the legislator is certainly under obligation to provide better legal protection for the foetus (against the mother).[12]

This judgement was not decided unanimously but by a majority of the judges. Two—Justice Simon and the only female member of the Court, Justice Rupp-von Brüneck—gave a dissenting opinion,[13] arguing that the penal law as the most severe method of the state is not an appropriate way, but on the contrary a proven ineffective method to solve complex conflicts of an undesired pregnancy and therefore an inadequate method to protect the foetus; therefore no constitutional reason could be found to oblige a government to penalize abortion at any time during a pregnancy; however, the legislator is obliged to solve the problems and specifically to protect the foetus by means other than penalisation, such as granting social support for mothers as well as children.

Justice Rupp-von Brüneck argued further that to give the foetus's rights more constitutional protection than the pregnant woman's implies that to behave legally is to become overburdened with unforeseeable, long-lasting responsibilities and consequences, and to be forced into a specific kind of life one did not choose or want. Such a structure was unique and unknown in penal law. In general, a lawful life would not put further burdens on the shoulders of a citizen (see Arndt et al. 1979, 430 seq.).

However, the majority took a different direction. Even though they did not consider the criminalisation of abortion as the only means to accomplish the protection of the foetus, they held up the penal code as the most important means. As a result of this ruling, the parliament enacted a new version of the abortion law in 1976, which is the present one in the western states of the FRG.[14]

In the states of the old FRG, abortion is legally regulated in the chapter "Criminal Offences against Life," Sections 218, 218a, 218b, 219, 219a–d of the Federal Penal Law Code, as well as by the Sections "Infanticide" (217) and "Genocide" (220a). Abortion is in principle illegal. The core of Section 218 reads: "Anyone who terminates a pregnancy will be sentenced to imprisonment of up to three years or to financial penalty."

The chapter then goes on to identify different groups of offenders—for example, the pregnant woman herself or others, or those acting against the will of the pregnant woman. The sections which follow establish exceptions to the generally criminal nature of abortion and stipulate the preconditions and conditions for a legal abortion (218a); and define the penal consequences of a violation of these preconditions and conditions (218b, 219, 219a). Terminations before the fertilised ovum implants itself are legally not defined as abortions (219d), therefore use of the so-called morning-after pill is legal.

Without going into juridical details I want to point out the network of penal regulations that was assumed to be necessary to control abortion and abortionists—women as well as the medical profession. This tangled mass of regulations as a whole represents the basis of the current abortion law in the western *Länder* of the FRG and is called the *indication model.* So-called indications mark the exceptions to the general punishability of abortion. According to those exceptions, abortion is exempt from punishment if:

- the pregnant woman agrees to an abortion; and
- the abortion is necessary to preserve the life of the pregnant woman or to keep her physical or mental health from serious harm (medical indication); or
- it is expected that the child will be born with grave physical or mental defect (eugenic indication); or
- the pregnancy resulted from rape (criminological indication); or
- the woman is exposed to seriously distressed circumstances under which she cannot be demanded to carry out the pregnancy and which cannot be altered by any other means but an abortion (state-of-need indication, unfortunately colloquially called social indication).[15]

The woman who wants an abortion is exempt from punishment if:

- the pregnancy has lasted no longer than 22 weeks; and
- she has had counselling by an authorised agency at least three days before the abortion; and
- she has had further counselling by a medical doctor; and
- the pregnancy is terminated by a physician.

The abortionist—even the physician—makes her- or himself liable to penalty if:[16]

- the abortion is not justified by one of the above mentioned indications;
- the counselling requirement is not fulfilled by the woman;
- and the indication itself is not acknowledged by a different medical doctor but him- or herself.

Abortion Law in the Former German Democratic Republic

In contrast to the political programmes in West Germany, the GDR aimed to abolish capitalist laws and laws inherited from the Nazis to establish as soon as possible a newly designed legal system. However, it took some time to implement liberal legislation on abortion. This law was enacted in 1973.[17] In general the termination of a pregnancy is legal within the first 12 weeks after conception. The decision on abortion is left to the woman. The abortion has to be carried out by a medical professional in a gynaecological-obstetrical ward of a hospital. The physician is obliged only to inform the

woman of possible medical effects of the intended termination and of pre-
cautions or suitable methods of contraception. Abortion costs are generally
covered by the state.

After the period of 12 weeks, abortion can still be legal if the operation
is considered necessary to preserve the woman's life or if other serious circumstances indicate a necessity. But in these cases a medical committee has
to decide. Abortion is criminalized only if it is in violation of the above-
mentioned regulations.[18]

In the preamble to this law it is pointed out that the subsequent norms
are part of a legal system that seeks to initiate and respect the equal rights
and status of women.[19] This was proved through other laws, regulations, and
institutions. There was an entirely different approach—one which sought to
enable women to undertake and face the tasks of motherhood. Women were
provided with education and training and earned their own living. In the
former GDR, 91 percent of the women had a paid job, most of them full
time, even though 30 percent of all newborn children belonged to single
mothers and 50,000 marriages per year ended in divorce. All children were
entitled to kindergarten at the age of three. Of such children, 94 percent
went to kindergarten. The majority of younger children were able to be
cared for in crèches (see Süssmuth and Schubert 1992, 147 seq.). Pregnant
women enjoyed 6 weeks paid leave from work before and 20 weeks after
delivery (22 weeks when twins or more babies were born, or after a complicated delivery), compared to 6 weeks before and 8 after delivery in the
FRG. During pregnancy, women were not allowed to work overtime or
nighttime.[20] Mothers of children of preschool age could refuse overtime as
well as nighttime work. Women could stay home voluntarily until the child
was one year old, and received income based on sick pay.[21] This was effective
also for the father or other person—such as a grandmother—if they stayed
at home for child care.[22]

The much wealthier FRG could never (or, rather never wanted to)
compete with such provisions. West Germany ranks only in the middle of
the European Community in providing day-care places and still does not
offer all-day schooling, with the result that employment of mothers of up
to 10-year-old children ranks behind even Portugal and Greece (see Plett
1992).

However, it should be mentioned that women and men did not have equal
chances nor resources as regards qualifications and promotion. The traditional patriarchal division of labour in the so-called private sector was not
touched. But in comparison with West Germany, East Germany had installed a kind of "patriarchal equality" (Süssmuth and Schubert 1992, 148).

After unification the institutions in the East were stripped down. The
unemployment rate is still increasing, more so for women than for men, and
it is women again who have little chance of finding new employment. Therefore the traditional roles of womanhood and motherhood are reinstalled—

in the East and the West. The strategy of destroying a social system without having the means at hand to construct a new one is already affecting social welfare, education, and the health sector in the West as well—sectors which are necessary for women on their way to gaining equal status in society.

ABORTION: LAW AND PRACTICE UNTIL JUNE 1993

Abortion in Practice

Because abortion was legal in the former GDR and access to an operation was easy and widespread, illegal termination of pregnancy was unknown.

As a result of the devastating unification process, according to recent media reports there has been a significant drop in the birthrate; in addition, the abortion rate has dropped drastically. It would seem that women went not only on a birth strike but even on a conception strike.

In the West, abortion practice, including access to counselling and to physicians who were willing to cooperate, varied and still varies from one region to another. One of the main practical obstacles facing women in relation to abortion—and also facing counsellors and physicians—is the federal structure of the FRG (see Frommel 1990, 12 seq.). By law it is within the domain of the *Länder*, of each single state, to install and authorise the required counselling agencies and to enact implementing regulations. In the *Länder* ruled by more liberal governments, a network of counselling agencies, some church based, some secular, has been put in place. Some of these *Länder* also accept a combination of social and medical counselling in one place, so that a woman can have counselling by a social worker or psychologist in the same office where she consults the doctor who is entitled to attest to an indication. For example, in the state of Bremen there is one agency where all the necessary counselling is offered and where women can also obtain the abortion. Finally, these more liberal states do not interfere in the counselling process, recognising that professional counselling must be nondirective.

Conservative states create a more clerical attitude towards abortion that affects women (see Holzhauer 1988, 357 seq.), as well as physicians (see Häussler-Sczepan 1989, 132 seq.). In the southern and southwestern states in particular, especially in Bavaria and Baden-Württemberg, confessional and clerical counsellors predominate. In Bavaria only 3 secular counselling offices exist out of a total of 40. Even if the personnel do not feel morally obliged to urge women to continue their pregnancies, they are obliged to do so by state regulation.[23] From the perspective of the woman concerned, the legal obligation to be counselled thus also includes the legal constraint of having to cope somehow with a huge amount of moral pressure and to struggle with implanted guilt.

In addition, most of these states have prevented the development of multifaceted counselling agencies. Instead, they prescribe that the procedures of counselling and medical decision concerning an indication have to be strictly separate, done by different individuals in different places. A woman seeking abortion in one of these states has to pass through at least two different offices to get an abortion in a third place—if everyone cooperates. And it has to be done in less than two months.

Moreover, the third place often does not exist in these areas. Health laws are also under the legislation of the separate states. The federal abortion law states that abortion may be carried out only in licensed institutions. And some of the states have not passed licensing rules. Therefore only hospitals can be considered.[24] But in these states, especially in rural areas, many if not most of the hospitals are run by the church or ecclesiastical organisations, even though they are state funded. These organisations prohibit their medical staff from participating in abortions through their employment contracts. In these states legal abortion is, in fact, impossible.

In consequence, "abortion tourism" has emerged in the west of the FRG. Official data show that during the early 1980s, 60 percent of the women from Baden-Württemberg who officially registered for an abortion went to Hessen to have the abortion.[25] Women living near the borders of the FRG even preferred travelling to neighbouring countries such as the Netherlands or Austria, where termination of pregnancy is allowed during the first three months and where no bureaucratic obstacles and no degradation have to be endured. However, this is an illegal act and can be prosecuted in the FRG as illegal abortion if the woman cannot prove that she had received social and medical counselling beforehand, as required by German law.[26]

In general, health insurance is obliged to pay the cost of legal abortions. The health insurance system is ruled by federal law. Insurance contributions are partly paid by the employer. Since the *Länder* operate as public service employers as well, they can regulate their part of the contribution. Some of the southern states, such as Rhineland-Palatinate, decided that certain insurance policies for public servants do not cover payment for an abortion if the abortion is legalised by a state-of-need indication.[27] The state of Baden-Württemberg even attempted to challenge the federal health insurance system by appealing to the federal Constitutional Court. However, several procedural mistakes were made, so the Court was able to refuse to decide on the matter.

In summary, it has to be emphasised that women who live in the western states of the FRG have to face a restricted legal situation as regards abortion, and in addition they are confronted with very different legal and practical obstacles. One aim of the law reform of the late 1970s was to create more equality, justice, and fairness—to provide better social and medical counselling for women in need so that they would not be forced to backstreet abortionists and a corresponding health risk. The law reform failed in this respect because of structural reasons determined by the law itself. By having restrictions, the penal law served to set the interests of doctors against those of women. Such a division is unhealthy. The more liberal the public-social attitude, the more liberal the position of the administration of justice, especially in relation to prosecution; the more adequate the facilities available for women, the safer women feel in expressing their needs and the safer physicians feel in listening to these needs with sympathy; the better educated women are and the more they think for themselves, the less their convictions depend on (church-controlled) ideologies; the more money women have at their own disposal, the easier they find ways to use their rights. The present abortion law in the west discriminates regionally as well as in terms of social class (see Liebl 1990, 36 seq.).

Empirical research reveals that about 120,000 women who live in western states of the FRG terminate early pregnancies every year. Only 40 percent of these terminations are carried out legally; 60 percent are illegal. The vast majority of illegal abortions are not pursued by prosecution authorities, even if postabortion health complications lead to the notification of other state authorities, such as the Social Security office or public health department (see Liebl 1990, 177–78).

But prosecutions do occur. Between 1976 and 1986, proceedings were officially instituted in 1,164 cases (Liebl 1990, 4–5). Police or prosecutors usually became aware of the cases in the context of other, different investigations (more than 50 percent). In about 25 percent of all cases, reports indicated police activities. The other cases became known to the police accidentally—for example, through self-accusation during domestic conflicts or in the context of border control. Hardly a single case was uncovered as a result of direct police investigation. The fact that the majority of cases were brought to light in the context of different criminal investigations implies that the suspects usually were already objects of police interest. This again is an indicator for their belonging to the lower class. In fact, women investigated either (1) were very young and still attending school or (2) had the lowest possible degree of schooling. They belonged to the working class. These women are overrepresented in the context of criminal investigation on abortion.

Most investigations end with the suspension of proceedings (about 70 percent), but some suspensions carry a character of sanction. Nearly every fourth suspect must face summary punishment or even a charge, and the majority of these suspects have to expect a conviction (Liebl 1990, 154 seq.). The first main question in an investigation is if all the stipulated regulations have been followed by the women and by the abortionists. Second, the legal profession increasingly tends to re-scrutinize the indication for the abortion. Here a power struggle is occurring over the woman's body: who is going to have the last word, the final decision on the woman's reasons for having an abortion—the medical profession in their white gowns or the legal profession in their black gowns? This struggle is part of a campaign aiming to abolish the state-of-need indication.

The Politics of Abortion

After the penal law reform in the 1970s and after the liberalisation of abortion law, including the decriminalisation of abortion during the first weeks of pregnancy, was ruled out by the federal Constitutional Court, the anti-abortion campaigners sat back to consider their success for a while. They finally came to the conclusion that the result was not far-reaching enough to control women's reproductive abilities, and left far too much space for women's own decisions, especially if they were assisted by sympathetic doctors. The conservative patriarchy reorganised and attacked the state-of-need indication, the only indication which left some room to interpret the legal norm on the grounds of personal values and individual judgements.

The leading figures and organisers of this anti-abortion coalition were middle-aged or old conservative men, all of whom had high-ranking positions in public life: conservative politicians in leading party and governmental positions, highly influential lawyers, and bishops and other clerics. So neither money nor media coverage was ever or will ever be a problem for this group.

The reorganized campaign started up again in the late 1970s and was highly aggressive and offensive from the beginning. As nearly everywhere else in Western countries, they chose their terminology very carefully and in an intelligent, effective way. The termed themselves "pro-life"; who, in opposition, would want to be called "anti-life"? In this setup even the moderate feminist pro-choice position could be read as the demand to have the freedom to choose against life, "to choose to kill," as the crusaders put it. The vocabulary was deliberately propagandistic. It is cruel; it strips the problem in question of all its complexity, and—most important in achieving the effects of accusation and guilt—an individualisation is constructed: the pregnant woman is portrayed as the life-threatening enemy of the foetus. The cause of an unwanted pregnancy, the attitude of a possible father, the social make-up, the social environment of a sexist, class-structured, anti-children society—none of these are important factors of the problem anymore.[28]

This agitation involved public appearances, speeches, articles, official announcements and statements by *Länder* ministers of justice, and the like. In addition, the hierarchy preached from the pulpit that "a holocaust against children" took place every day in Germany, as Bishop Dyba put it. Cardinal Höffner called it mass murder. The Catholic Church in Fulda and elsewhere ordered the bells to be rung in honour of the "murdered children." Corresponding Protestant groups chimed in. And all this was backed by affirmative statements from high-ranking politicians (see Friedrichsen 1989, 102 seq.).

This campaign was carried to extremes by adding manipulated pictures of foetuses. They appeared to capture reality, to be just like any photograph that people would normally see. The fact that the images were illusory was far from immediately apparent. The pioneer in creating such illusions is Lennart Nilsson, a Swedish photographer and well-known reactionary ecologist and social Darwinist, whose photos in *Life* magazine (1965) were "an unprecedented photographic feat in color"—showing an 18-week-old foetus alive in his amniotic sac with placenta. These photographs, which now are very common, were taken of surgically removed ectopic pregnancies. Foetoscopy in situ—the technique of penetrating the uterus with a camera—did exist in 1965, but was not highly developed. Even today, in addition to multiple enlargement, the pictures require a series of different area shots in order to compose a glossy print of a foetus that appears as a single individual being, to all intents and purposes detached from the body of which the foetus actually is a dependent part. "Seeing on command" (Duden 1991, 22 seq.) sets in; everyone believes he or she is watching real life, not multiple enlargements and photomontage. And nobody could escape these images, this metaphorical language. Unsolicited, it arrived in your mail; posters advertising it in public were widespread.

Aside from this public brainwashing process, the legal profession was busy as well. Experts wrote articles for law journals, and these were quoted in textbooks and specialist literature, the literature which is used every day by professional lawyers, including prosecutors and judges. In this way the legal interpretation of a state-of-need indication was reduced almost to zero (see Dreher and Tröndle 1988): no personal, social, or economic circumstances could justify a personal state of emergency anymore. A single mother of four children living on Social Security could easily live on Social Security with an additional child. A mother of two could be forced to give up her part-time job. A young woman of 16 was forced to carry on with a pregnancy by court decision, even though she contemplated suicide as proved by a psychological expert; the judge related these intentions to a normal ambivalence during an early state of pregnancy and was convinced that she would overcome such depression. A circular argument was created: a personal state of need to justify an abortion could not exist since every woman still had the opportunity to have the newborn child adopted. The minister of justice in Bavaria worked on a bill by which the pregnant woman was given a "guarantee to purchase" by the state itself in case the newborn child was disabled and not fit for adoption (Friedrichsen 1989, 111). This cynical approach, which never came to a reading in the parliament, showed clearly that women should be bound to the duty of giving birth.

This well-tuned and well-orchestrated creation of opinion was established during the late 1970s and 1980s. The process was more intense in the southern states of the FRG. As with access to abortion services, a strong North-South gradient was established. This gap was even widened in 1988, when "the Witch Trial of Memmingen" took place.

In 1988 public prosecutors officially accused more than a hundred women of having had an illegal abortion. The case took place in the small, rural, mainly Catholic Bavarian town of Memmingen and is well known in Germany as "the Witch Trial of Memmingen" or "the Crusade of Memmingen" (see Friedrichsen 1989; Pro Familia 1989; Frommel 1992: 106; Frommel 1990, 12). The case started off with an investigation of (suspected) tax evasion against a gynaecologist, Dr. Horst Theissen. His files were confiscated by tax officers and handed over to the prosecution. All the women were interrogated through a long questionnaire. The questions were not simply restricted to the suspected act of an illegal abortion, but encompassed their whole personal and social biography. Most women received an order of summary punishment and paid the fine. Even though the waiver of objection implied an acknowledgement of faulty or even culpable behaviour, most women accepted it to avoid further legal proceedings, to escape publicity and a personal public appearance in court.

Some partners or husbands were also charged with aiding and abetting an illegal abortion. These were not those partners or husbands who left the pregnant women to face everything alone, but those who accompanied the women to counselling and to the doctor.

On September 8, 1988, the court case against Dr. Theissen began. His practice was not licenced to carry out abortions since no outpatient treatment was permitted in Bavaria. Therefore the abortions he performed were illegal. In addition, some of his patients had not been counselled by a separate agency and a different doctor to establish the indication for abortion. But these factors in themselves did not constitute the main problem, especially since the accused cooperated during investigation and in court. The substantial questioning of state-of-need indications became the main topic. Now, years after the situation when patients had been in a personal predicament and had revealed themselves to a doctor in good faith and in confidentiality, prosecutors and judges got down to work to review the whole situation again in a public court. The patients were called in and crossexamined in public. Those who had already accepted the summary punishment order could legally not refuse to answer, since there was no danger of self-incrimination. They were just witnesses. Partners, family members, even employers of the women were called as witnesses. That is how, for example, a Turkish husband was informed that his Turkish wife had had an abortion in Germany some years before the two had met.

On May 5, 1989, the court pronounced judgement. Dr. Theissen had been accused of performing 156 illegal abortions. Of these, 77 cases had been dropped. Dr. Theissen was found guilty of performing 36 abortions without a (state-of-need) indication. In these 36 cases, the court overruled the indication given by a medical professional—namely, Dr. Thiessen himself. The sentence was two years and six months imprisonment and a ban on his practicing as a gynaecologist or obstetrician for three years (see Friedrichsen 1989, 272 seq.).

An appeal was made and Dr. Theissen is still waiting for a new trial.[29] But in its ruling the court of appeal, the Bundesgerichtshof, has already made clear that (1) the seizure of confidential medical files and their use in a criminal court proceeding is legal and (2) a court can in principle legitimately review stated indications for abortion. The problem still in question is how and to what extent a court can do this in accordance with the law.

The Abortion Question and the Process of Legal Unification

The federal parliament was obliged by the unification treaty to enact a new law on abortion for the whole FRG by December 31, 1992. Until that date, the former GDR and former FRG laws existed side by side. The agreement stipulated that the new law must protect the pre-natal possibility of a new life on the one hand and on the other has to consider the ambivalence experienced by the pregnant women more effectively than at present under the two different existing laws. This discussion turned out to be complicated since the conflicting interests were the same as they always were—reaching from a pro-choice position of decriminalisation to a strict anti-abortion stance. In addition, further interpretations of the judgement of the federal Constitutional Court have been established, as mentioned above, further adjudication has taken place or is pending, and different interpretations of the unification treaty were up for discussion.

Some politicians, led by those in the Bavarian Christian Social Union, even interpreted the provisional clause in the unification treaty in combination with the judgement of the Constitutional Court, as a mandate to abolish any justification for abortion on the basis of a state-of-need indication.

The counterpoint was represented by the Grüne/Bündnis 90 (Greens and former civil rights activists of the former GDR). They pleaded for complete cancellation of penal provisions for abortion and took the pro-choice position of decriminalisation. They argued that the judgement of the Constitutional Court dealt only with a specific historical situation that is different today. Moreover, they considered the stand of the Court to be untenable and to encroach on the human rights of women.

Between these two positions lay a range of political propositions and legal opinions. But a kind of institutionalised women's movement did emerge in the federal parliament, despite individual party membership. An all-women coalition was founded by Uta Würfel (FDP/Liberals) to formulate a compromise in the interests of women and to ensure a majority vote on such a compromise. Women of all parties joined this group. Members of the conservative parties in particular, but also the Liberal Uta Würfel herself had to endure strong public insults. However, this group drew up a so-called Group Bill on abortion. They started out with the premise that the ruling of the federal Constitutional Court had to be accepted, that the state was obliged to protect the unborn "life," otherwise a new law would be ruled out again by the Constitutional Court. They were in favour of protection through helping. In doing so, they kept close to a point of view expressed by the dissenting opinion of the Constitutional Court's judgement. Therefore they held that women seeking a legal abortion should receive professional counselling; but after counselling and within the first 12 weeks of pregnancy, the women themselves should be the only ones to decide on the termination of pregnancy. The termination must be carried out by a professional doctor or in a hospital.

To meet the requirement of improving efforts for the protection of unborn "life," an additional bill was drafted, the Pregnancy and Family Support Act (Schwangeren- und Familienhilfegesetz), through which men and women become entitled to state-financed counselling on all questions and problems of sexuality, birth control, pregnancy, adoption, sterilisation, and the like. The act also proposed that all children be entitled to care with registered childminders or in crèches and, from the age of three years on, in kindergarten.[30]

This cluster of bills as a whole passed the federal parliament by 355 votes to 299, and also the second chamber, the Bundesrat, on July 10, 1992.[31] In the Bundesrat only Bavaria voted against the bills; Baden-Württemberg, Mecklenburg-Vorpommern, and Thuringia abstained. On July 28, 1992, the president of the FRG signed the bills. The Bavarian Landesregierung (state government) and 248 members of the federal parliament, all members of the Christian Democratic Union and Christian Social Union (CDU/CSU), did not accept that they had lost a democratic vote. Immediately after the president had signed, they filed a petition for an injunction (*Antrag auf Eilentscheidung*) at the federal Constitutional Court to prevent the specific law on abortion from being enacted. The motion was concerned only with reform of the specific abortion law by which women were obliged to counselling but had the freedom to decide themselves on the termination of a pregnancy after counselling.

The other regulations have been enacted. On the basis of this new legislation, physicians and municipal authorities are allowed to establish practices or centres to carry out abortions—even in the southern states.

On August 4, 1992, the federal Constitutional Court decided by provisional rule that the abortion law should not come into operation until a decision on the substantial legal and constitutional question has been reached. Explicitly the judges made clear that the adjournment should not be read as a prediction of the future substantial ruling. According to the judges, the Court followed pragmatic considerations. Since the legal examination of the substantial questions could possibly make further rewriting of the law necessary, it would not be appropriate to enact the new law; instead, the old laws still stood. The substantial ruling was to have been announced by the Court at the end of November 1992.[32] According to this schedule—

postponed several times—the Court would probably also have had to agree to an extension of the unification treaty since it was very unlikely that the government could draw up another all-German bill and meet the parliamentarian procedures to enact a new law for January 1, 1993.

THE FUTURE

The final Constitutional Court decision on abortion cannot, however, be predicted.[33] As far as I am concerned, a blanket confirmation of the law is improbable. That is why I want to take a closer look at the advantages of the new law.

Assessment of the Proposed Legislative Changes

The current political debate was initiated by unification and by the corresponding necessity for harmonization of two different legal systems. East German women will certainly be the losers in this alignment process. They were permitted to terminate an early pregnancy without the threat of criminalisation. Motherhood was understood as a social challenge, and corresponding social support for mothers and children was implemented in the former GDR.

The effect of recent court decisions in the west has been to severely restrict abortion, to establish a pro-life system in practice. But the new abortion law that the Constitutional Court had to consider was closer to the former East German model and could therefore have meant liberalisation of current practice in the west. Such possible liberalisation would not result from efforts of feminists in the west; rather, it would be a gift for them resulting from unification.

The newly created state obligation to provide public child-care facilities for everyone everywhere will be a great positive benefit, but will very likely fail for financial reasons. The new federal regulations will finally permit establishment of outpatient abortion centres in the south, whether or not the Bavarian government likes it.

Abortion counselling will become compulsory for women without exception. Until now a case could be dismissed even if a woman avoided counselling before an abortion if a court acknowledged afterwards that the abortion was justified on grounds of an indication. Under the new regulations the woman will commit a criminal act if she circumvents compulsory counselling. In addition, only state-approved authorities will be recognised for counselling, while hitherto any physician, including the one she had known and trusted for years, could counsel the woman.

The greatest hope is attached to the abolition of experts' acknowledgement of indications. Women themselves will have to make the decision on an abortion after fulfilling the tightened counselling obligation. This new requirement is clearly a direct political response to the jurisdiction as established, for example, in Memmingen. Yet, in Memmingen most of the women were prosecuted because they did not fulfill counselling obligations. The abortionist was sentenced for giving false indications or operating without valid indications. Therefore, the cancellation of indication regulations might work in favour only of the abortionist. Anyhow, we will have to find out how the abolition of indications will be handled in practice. In particular, Bavarian courts restricted legal indication definitions in an unbearable way. I wonder how they might misinterpret the woman's right to decide (see Frommel 1992b, 8f).

I see the main problem of the present political debate, however, as the almost complete absence of a pro-choice position. Even one of the strongest and most prominent former pro-choice campaigners, Alice Schwarzer, recently accused individuals who still put forward pro-choice arguments of jeopardizing, if not destroying, possibly the best abortion law reform ever. Everybody seems caught up in the sexist, patriarchal ideology that the interests and rights of a woman and a foetus conflict with each other. This is the anti-abortionists' point of view, which elevates the "protection of the life-to-be" and grants women under restricted, exceptional and—if possible—controlled circumstances the necessity of a decision but never the right to decide. The often unconscious acceptance of this principle became more widespread with the conviction that apparently the Constitutional Court supported this general, compulsory duty to deliver—even though that was more than 10 years ago and included a strongly dissenting vote. That is how the pro-choice voice was silenced.

In a secularised society even a Constitutional Court should not replace God the Father. In a democracy the powers of a Constitutional Court are bound to law, to the Constitution itself, and not to preceding judgements.[34] The Court should be able to acknowledge social developments and its own misconceptions. Anyway, the Court—so far—had never questioned the woman's legal status as a holder of rights (Rechtssubjekt) and never stated that the foetus is also a holder of rights, but that the foetus is an object of legal protection.[35] The baby will become a holder of rights after being born alive. That is the very moment when he or she can claim rights and titles against third parties.[36] Therefore the pregnant woman is a holder of (constitutional) rights while the foetus is not; legally a difference has to be acknowledged.

The status of the foetus as an object of legal protection does not automatically substantiate a punishment claim by the state against those who might endanger the foetus, as thalidomide (Contergan) trials have shown. In addition, the pregnant woman is not just any third party. The specific relationship of a pregnant woman and a foetus as a physical and emotional symbiosis is unique, and has to be legally accepted through de jure distinction between rights and duties (1) on the part of pregnant women and (2) on the part of other third parties towards the foetus. From the woman's angle, which is the decisive one, the criminal ban on abortion means at the very same time a legal command under the threat of punishment in the case of noncompliance. This legal command comprises all physical and mental risks of pregnancy and giving birth and the acceptance and carrying through of all responsibilities attached to pregnancy and motherhood—a legal command to assume responsibility for another human being. Such a far-reaching, one-sided, sex-based restriction on possibilities of personal development is already an infringement of the equality principle, Section 3 of the German Constitution.

The need of, not a right to, legal protection for the foetus might conflict with the individual identity of a woman and her constitutional freedom of responsible and trustworthy motherhood, which can only be chosen and which is the main protection a foetus can get. Pregnancies legally forced upon women constitute, on the contrary, a coercion that violates the dignity of the woman—Section 1 of the Constitution—as well as her constitutional right to protection of her individual sphere of life—Section 2—and her constitutional right of autonomous decisions on the basis of moral principles and scruples—Section 4 of the German Constitution (see Frommel 1991, 367 seq.).

From this point of view, the pro-choice position agrees with the Constitution. As mentioned before, only a few feminist lawyers carry on with this discussion (see Frommel 1990; Nelles 1991–92). The results of a public opinion poll in 1991 show that the majority of the population favour this stance: 55 percent in the western states and 74 percent in the eastern states of the FRG (*Der Spiegel*, May 13, 1991).

So why is there no strong movement against the sexist control imperative of some aging, conservative, clerical patriarchs? As far as I can see, the women's movement is exhausted and feels defeated. A hundred years of fighting apparently did not move a stone. All arguments on the abortion question have been exchanged and repeated many, many times. Moreover, times have changed. The sociopolitical climate in which the Constitutional Court had to decide on the latest abortion law is characterised by a growing economic crisis in both the west and the east. Women are being excluded once more from the labour market, giving paid work and corresponding income to men. Violence is exploding everywhere in sexism, racism, and wars. It is definitely not the best time to put forward feminist demands, even though they are important. The federal government is preparing a new bill to allow easier access to embryos for researchers in genetic engineering in order to place German genetic research in a competitive position.[37] At the same time, an 18-year-old woman died of brain damage[38] and the carcass was bound to machines to keep the womb "alive." The woman was in the fourth month of pregnancy; after her death, the womb was used to fulfill delivery duties. The parents of the dead woman were coerced to agree with the experiment; the threat implied was that the medical profession would go ahead anyway and that the grandparents would be possibly disqualified from looking after their grandchild if the foetus developed fully. A miscarriage ended the experiment.

Present and Future: After the Constitutional Court Ruling

On May 27, 1993, the Constitutional Court pronounced the—so far—most recent decision on the abortion question and gave its reasons on 43 closely printed pages. Once again, the decision taken was not unanimous, so an additional six pages were devoted to the dissenting opinions of two members of the Court, its vice-president, Judge Mahrenholz, and Judge Sommer. Both these judges favoured a pro-choice position, as represented, at least partially, in the proposed legislation.

The majority legal position—including the opinion of the Court's only female member—explicitly criticised the proposed legislation, as was within the Court's authority. But the six judges went further and indeed usurped the role of the legislators. They drew up a new law, and in so doing bypassed not only the government but also parliament; they decreed that their new law take effect as of mid-June 1993. In surpassing both their legal task and their professional competence, the judges left little scope for the democratic, parliamentary decision-making process. This raises major issues about the state and the rule of law far beyond the specifics of the abortion question. The parliament could (and should) overrule the Court, but the politicians seem unconcerned that the judges have overstepped their authority. The substantial contents of the new law brought about as a result of the decision of the Constitutional Court are laid out below.[39]

Abortion is in principle anticonstitutional. The proposed law passed by parliament is thus discarded.

The constitutional right to life for "the unborn" is finally created, and in addition it is put above the constitutional rights of the pregnant woman, regardless of the temporal-physical development of the foetus. They refer to "the unborn" absolutely independently of the state of a pregnancy as "the child." The judges deduced the absolute right to life of "the unborn" from the Constitution itself, not from penal law.[40]

As the absolute right to life of "the unborn" is guaranteed, even against the rights of its mother (-to-be), abortion is illegal. The guarantee of legal protection can be ensured only by prohibition of abortion in principle, backed up by the state's duty to enforce that principle.[41]

In exceptional cases the constitutional rights of "the unborn" may conflict with those of the pregnant woman—for example, with her guaranteed right of dignity (Section 1 of the Constitution), or her right to life and integrity (Section 2 of the Constitution). But the constitutional rights of "the unborn" definitely do not clash, in the Court's opinion, with a woman's constitutional right to make autonomous decisions on the basis of individual moral principles and scruples (Section 4 of the Constitution).[42] Even those constitutional rights of the woman guaranteed by Sections 1 and 2 of the Constitution may not be taken to mean under any circumstances that the state does not have the duty to deliver on its guarantee of absolute protection of "the unborn." Therefore, an abortion can be permissible only in cases of legal exception—that is, when the continuation of the pregnancy would lead to the sacrifice of a pregnant woman's life or life values.[43] As a result, the only legally acknowledged indications for abortion are the medical indication (the abortion is necessary to preserve the life and health of the pregnant woman) and the eugenic indication (the expectation is that the child will be born with grave physical or mental defect).

Even then, referring to these indications is justified only with the reservation that the pregnant woman undergo newly established advice procedures.[44] The Court required these procedures not only for those abortions that are legally justified by, for example, a eugenic indication, but also for those abortions that were formally accepted on the criminological indication (resulting from rape) and the state-of-need indication. Although both these latter indications are now outlawed, making any abortion on the basis of such indications illegal, the Court stipulated that the abortion could be allowed if the woman went through the required advice procedures. The paradox is this: abortion in the first 12 weeks of pregnancy is for the most part prohibited, but there will be no legal sanctions if the woman meets the advice requirements. Only violation of the advice requirements will lead to criminalisation. This legal construct is almost beyond comprehension and can be understood only as a result of the high-wire act by the Court's majority between the "supreme rights of the unborn" and the—more or less—reluctantly acknowledged fact that criminalisation of abortion historically has never prevented abortions.

By maintaining the general principle of the illegality of abortion, the judges simultaneously decided that health insurances—statutory health insurance as well as private medical insurance—can no longer pay for abortions since it is illegal to pay for illegal acts.[45] Women are now personally liable for their abortions.[46]

The Court ruled that protecting "the unborn" required not only the use of penal law but also the mandatory requirement of advice designed to win over any woman to the decision to deliver;[47] the advice must aim to convince the woman to carry the pregnancy through to completion. In addition, such advice has to be given in specific advice centres recognised and authorised by the state.[48] The woman will need a certificate given by the advice centre confirming that she fulfilled all her advice duties, and the advice centres will have to ensure through proper records that they can prove that all the advice requirements have been fulfilled. If the advice centre staff are not convinced that the woman involved herself properly in the advice interaction, they can withhold the certificate, which is a compulsory prerequisite to contacting a medical doctor for an abortion.

The medical doctor has to convince him- or herself that the advice requirements have been fulfilled.[49] In thus subjecting the doctor to state control and scrutiny, the ruling embodies to a large extent the dreadful standards established by the Memmingen trial. A threat thus hangs over the heads of doctors: any doctor carrying out abortions still runs the risk of criminalisation. Thus in several East German towns the medical profession has already refused to take part in such illegal acts.

In summary, I can agree with Monika Frommel: as a relatively well-paid western academic, I have access to established advice centres in the northwest of the country. I believe I could cope with the unreasonable demands of the advice requirements. I am trained and am used to dealing with political and legal paradoxes. And I can pay for an abortion.[50] All of these essentials cannot be presupposed for the majority of women in the west. It is worse in the east, where, for example, hardly any advice centres exist. As a citizen, therefore, I can only be embittered over the misogyny encapsulated in the ruling, in the characterisation of woman as unreasonable, needing control because they are portayed as potential enemies of the foetus. As a lawyer I am outraged at a ruling in which the Constitutional Court went far beyond its competence and which is full of legal contradictions. So far the counselling centres are busy trying to deal with the ruling and to meet its requirements, despite the contradiction. The medical profession is deeply uncertain if it is reasonable to expect doctors to participate in illegal—albeit nonprosecutable—acts. In the eastern states, population increase has stagnated as the number of "voluntary" sterilisations has increased dramatically. And in the western states the renewal of the phenomenon of "abortion tourism" to countries such as the Netherlands and Austria is likely.

Since the pro-choice argument has been presented repeatedly—including by the dissenting vote of the two Constitutional Court judges Mahrenholz and Sommer—but has not been heeded, the future will be characterised by more or less detailed legal discourse on how to organise and control advice centres and the medical profession. And another legal question has already been raised—whether or not the prohibition on insurance payment for abortions in which the woman has fulfilled the advice requirements conflicts with the European Community law on freedom of trade and services within the Community. What would happen if a German woman who had fulfilled the legal requirements in relation to advice had an abortion in another European Community member state and the health insurance of that country had to pay, as laid down in European Community law?[51] In such case, the German insurance scheme would undoubtedly have to reimburse the foreign insurance scheme. Privately insured German women could even leave their insurance company in favour of a foreign company which does cover abortion expenses. Maybe one day even German insurance companies will fight for the liberalisation of German abortion law in order to be able to compete in the European market.

NOTES

1. The penal code was one of the first laws enacted in the Bismarck Reich, founded in 1871, and it was more or less identical to the Prussian penal code of 1851.

2. Entscheidungen des Reichgerichts in Strafsachen, RGSt 61, 242.

3. These experiments on women formed the main foundation of eugenic knowledge and were of great interest for Western scientists after the war. There is less political-legal debate in Western countries about the eugenic indication for abortion than about any other indication.

4. Verordnung zur Durchführung der Verordnung zum Schutze von Ehe, Familie und Mutterschaft vom 18.3.1943, Reichsgesetzblatt I 140, 169.

5. Erbgesundheitsgesetze, Reichsgesetzblatt 1933 I 529; RGBl. 1935 I 773.

6. The Nazis tightened the abortion law only in 1943. Before that they had used other methods of control. Only a drastic drop in the birthrate and dramatic death rates towards the end of the war led them to use the penal law.

First, they started off with destroying the Sexuality Counselling Centres (*Sexualberatungsstellen*) established during the Weimar Republic, which had offered counselling on planned parenthood, contraception, and all problems in the field of sexuality.

Second, they introduced an ideology of motherhood and executed this ideology by expelling women—among many other social groups—from education, training, and the labour market, and by excluding them from policy making. This placed women definitively in a separate so-called reproductive sector, handing them over to private controllers such as fathers, brothers, husbands. Women lost economic independence and received in return only super-elevation of the traditional values of motherhood. Following critical sociopsychological theory (see Brückner 1972) we can argue that expelling human beings from the productive sphere leads to a mental condition of normative insecurity and uncertainty. The person lives in a closed private world, receiving all information and knowledge that is considered as important through other people; she lives an exterritorial and dependent life. That was the basis of the power of sexist ideology.

Third, racism was established as a legalised state ideology and had an important influence on the control of women as well. The discrimination, selection, and murder of the Jewish population—and other groups that were defined as inferior races and/or unfit, perverted, etc.—meant also stabilisation of the German "race." It placed German women in the position of seeing themselves as upholders of the highly valued genotype; women were valued as expensive breeding dogs. Consequently, every method of birth control was forbidden. The criminalisation of homosexuality was enforced. Homes were established—in fact, brothels (they were called *der Lebensborn*—"Spring of Life")—where young single German women were put at the disposal of (married) SS officers to breed further Germans; see Koonz 1988; Klein-Schonnefeld 1990; Panke-Kochinke 1991; Duden 1991; Beer 1991.

7. Strafrechtsreformgesetz vom 18.6.1974, Bundesgesetzblatt I, p. 1297.

8. Bundesverfassungsgerichtsentscheidung (BVerfGE) 39, 1 seq.

9. BVerfGE 39, 1, 36.

10. BVerfGE 39, 1, 42.

11. BVerfGE 39, 43, 48, 51. See also Nelles 1991/2.

12. BVerfGE 39, 53 seq.

13. BVerfGE 39, 53 seq.

14. Strafrechtsreformgesetz vom 18.6.1974, Bundesgesetzblatt I 1297 i.V.m. Strafrechtsänderungsgesetz vom 18.5.1976, Bundesgesetzblatt I 1213.

15. Unfortunately the term *social indication* has been adopted into everyday language. While the legal term *state-of-need indication* carries the literal and figurative sense of a serious state of emergency, which can be and usually is caused by a cluster of economical, social, mental, and emotional factors, the now-common expression social indication is almost reduced solely to the meaning of economic factors. This fits well in the propaganda of anti-abortion campaigners, who refer to social indications by drawing the picture of a selfish, egotistic, irresponsible woman who is just too lazy and too mean to give up some advantages by becoming a mother, and prefers to kill the possibility of a human being instead. In addition, most abortions in the western *Länder* of the FRG are legalised nowadays through the state-of-need indication, while more and more gynaecologists are restricting the grounds for a medical indication, even though they feel insecure and unsure in judging the criteria of a personal state-of-need indication; see Häussler-Sczepan 1989, 171 seq., 192 seq.

16. This law attributed some more freedom to women who needed an abortion by shifting both the responsibility of identifying the indication and the threat of punishment towards the medical profession. This "legal setting" damages the trust between a woman and a doctor and has a restrictive effect on the decision-making freedom of physicians; see Monika Häussler-Sczepan 1989, 181 seq.; Holzhauer 1988, 287 seq.

17. Gesetz vom 9.3.1973 über die Unterbrechung der Schwangerschaft, GB 1.I Nr.5, p. 89.

18. § 153 DDR-StGB (Penal Code of the GDR).

19. Gesetz vom 9.3.1973 über die Unterbrechung der Schwangerschaft, GBl. I Nr. 5, 89.

20. Arbeitsgesetzbuch der Deutschen Demokratischen Republik vom 16.6.1977, GBl. I Nr. 18, 185, § 243 Abs. 1 AGB.

21. This was between 70 and 90 percent of the net income, depending on the number of children and other conditions; see § 26 Abs. 1, 2 SVO.

22. § 246 Abs. 3 AGB.

23. In practice the vast majority of counsellors follow a professional, nondirective method and do sympathize with their clients. But the regulations put pressure on the counsellors, especially since on a number of occasions pro-lifers made appointments pretending to be in need of abortion counselling and accused the agencies afterwards of law breaking. This is also the reason why no agency in the south informs clients anymore about opportunities for easier access to abortion services in the north or even in foreign countries.

24. Because of new legislation in 1992, this situation is currently changing. For example, in Munich the first outpatient abortion centre will be opened in 1993. See the section in this chapter titled "The Abortion Question and the Process of Legal Unification."

25. The law requires that statistics on legal abortions be kept. But the official data cannot include abortions for which women crossed borders—for example, to the Netherlands or to Austria—nor the occasions when physicians in the south perform

abortions in their practice by giving the indication themselves, without being licenced, both of which are illegal. Official data are not structured by reality, but by (1) established procedures of collecting data, (2) obstacles such as restricted access to legal abortions, (3) the moral acceptance of abortion in society, (4) access and quality of contraception, (5) motivation of birth control, and (6) the specific kind of socially accepted sexual relations; see Ketting and van Praag 1985; 115.

26. In 1992 the media revealed that a woman was stopped by the border police in Northrhine-Westphalia, searched for drugs, and finally confessed—to end the searching—to having just had an abortion in the Netherlands. She was dragged to a hospital nearby (which was unnecessary since she had confessed already), was forced to undergo an unwanted gynaecological examination (which was illegal), and prosecuted. Northrhine-Westphalia belongs to the northern states that have implemented a quite liberal practice and liberal regulations. Even though this is certainly an exception, it can happen and women are aware of that fact.

27. Even referring to strictly legal discussions, there are many conflicting opinions on this point. I cannot set them out here in detail since it would take a completely new article to explain the German public health insurance system. In this context it may suffice to point out that even concerning payment for legal abortions, one cannot refer to a uniform practice, not even in the western states of the FRG.

28. In line with the control-imperative of women's reproductive capabilities and in the specific context of the abortion question, the main problem for the feminist movement during this century has been that the feminists argued from a powerless position, while their counterparts had the power. Therefore feminists always found themselves structurally in a defence position, under pressure to justify their point of view. Being put in such a place, fighting a lost battle, sophistication and differentiation sometimes get lost and stances are taken that can be as cruel as the ones used by the powerful. This is the reason why the women's movement often ignored the complexity of the abortion question, including the very difficult, but important aspect of the individual decision of having an abortion, the fact that it is unfortunately a decision *against* a possible different social life perspective that certainly would be welcomed if actual social, economic, and private circumstances were different; if the woman had the assistance of a partner; and if she lived in a society that would reserve places and living possibilities for her and her children. Therefore the individualised abortion decision is structurally a societal decision. The individualisation of all the factors involved easily creates individual guilt—and that is how the monstrous and devastating accusation of killing works so successfully; see Amendt 1988.

29. Another case is still pending: see Bay OblG, Urteil vom 26.4.1990. On the Theissen case, see BGH Urteil vom 3. 12.1991, both published in *Strafverteidiger* 3, 1992: 106 seq., with commentary by Monika Frommel.

30. Entwurf eines Gesetzes zum Schutz des vorgeburtlichen/werdenden Lebens, zur Förderung einer kinderfreundlichen Gesellschaft, für Hilfen im Schwangerschaftskonflikt und zur Regelung des Schwangerschaftsabbruchs (Schwangeren- und Familienhilfegesetz), Deutscher Bundestag, 12. Wahlperiode, Drucksache 12/2605; cf. documentation in: zweiwochen dienst Nr. 67/1992, 7.7.1992.

31. The Bundesrat is a senate of the federal parliament, with representatives from the separate German states.

32. Cf. z.B. die tageszeitung vom 6.8.1992, p.5—but later adjourned several times.

33. The Constitutional Court arrived at a decision in May 1993; for the details, see pp. 130–132.

34. BVerfGE 77, 84.

35. BVerfGE 39, 1 seq., 41.

36. This fact is indisputable and is recognised in, for example, judgements dealing with claims for damages by thalidomide (Contergan). Cf. AG Aachen, Beschluss vom 18.12.1970, in: *Juristenzeitung* 1970, p. 507.

37. This law passed parliament in September 1933.

38. When the body was brought to hospital the brain had stopped functioning. Some time ago the stopping of the heartbeat was the main criterion of medical death. Nowadays it is the cessation of any brain function. The experiment was a failure; the foetus did not survive, despite the efforts of the doctors and technicians.

39. Publication of the ruling, reasons, and dissenting votes—decision of May 28, 1993, by the second senate of the Constitutional Court—2BvF 2/90; 2BvF 4/92, 2BvF 5/92—in *Juristenzeitung* (JZ), Sonderausgabe (special edition).

40. See Leitsätze 1 and 2, page 1, op. cit.

41. See Leitsätze 3, page 1, op. cit.

42. See Leitsätze 5, page 1, op. cit.

43. See Leitsätze 7, pages 1 and 2, op. cit.

44. I do not want to use the term *counselling* for the Court-established forced advice procedures, since all substantial counselling principles are denied by the Court—for example, respect for the convictions and decisions of the counselled woman.

45. See Leitsätze 15 and 16, page 2, op. cit.

46. Women without a personal income may be able to claim supplementary social welfare benefits (see Leitsätze 16, page 2, op. cit.), which again is a strange legal construct in view of the constitutional principle of the illegality of abortion. But this does not meet the urgent need of low-paid women. Thus now the wife of a professor or manager with no income of her own might be entitled to benefits, but not a working woman on a low income. So far, only two (Social Democratic) *Länder* have organised state funds, and in Berlin a private fund has been established to assist this latter group of women. Women's ability to obtain financial assistance will thus differ from state to state in the Federal Republic.

47. See Leitsätze 11, page 2, op. cit.

48. See Leitsätze 12, page 2, op. cit. As said before, these regulations have been in operation since mid-June 1993. At that point there were almost no advice centers in the new *Länder* of former East Germany since no advice was required in the former German Democratic Republic. The liberal-oriented counselling centres in the West were quite sure that they could not meet the new requirements.

49. See Leitsätze 13, page 2, op. cit.

50. Frommel 1993; "Das Urteil zu §218 StGB," in *Wortlaut und Kommentar*, pages 142–43.

51. The retired Judge Vultejus is preparing a publication dealing with this specific problem, which should be published in *Schriftenreihe der Humanistischen Union*, number 17.

REFERENCES

Amendt, Gerhard. *Die bestrafte Abtreibung: Argumente zum Tötungsvorwurf.* Fulda, IKARU, Fuldaer Verlagsanstalt, 1988.

Amendt, Gerhard, and Michael Schwarz. *Das Leben unerwünschter Kinder.* Universität Bremen, 1991.

Arndt, Claus, Benno Erhard, Liselotte Funcke, and Kurt Brockelmann. *Der § 218 vor dem Bundesverfassungsgericht.* Heidelberg, Karlsruhe, C. F. Müller Juristischer Verlag, 1979.

Beer, Ursula. *Geschlecht, Struktur, Geschichte.* Frankfurt am Main, New York, Campus Verlag, 1991.

Brückner, Peter. *Zur Sozialpsychologie des Kapitalismus.* Frankfurt am Main, Europaische Verlagsanstalt, 1972, and Reinbek, Rowohlt Verlag, 1981.

Dreher, E., and H. Tröndle. *Strafgesetzbuch und Nebengesetze, Beck'sche Kurz-Kommentare Bd.10. Vorbemerkungen zu § 218 und Kommentierung zu § 218.* München, 1988.

Duden, Barbara. *Der Frauenleib als öffentlicher Ort.* Hamburg, Zürich, Luchterhand Literaturverlag, 1991.

Eser, Albin, and Hans-Georg Koch. *Schwangerschaftsabbruch im internationalen Vergleich*, Teil 1. Baden-Baden, Nomos Verlagsgesellschaft, 1988.

Frommel, Monika. " 'Lebensschützer' auf dem Rechtsweg," *Aus Politik und Zeitgeschichte, Beilage zur Wochenzeitung Das Parlament*, March 30, 1990.

———. "Frauen müssen nicht gebären," *Demokratie und Recht* 4 (1991).

———. "§ 218-Diskussion. Besser als das geltende Recht?" *Neue Kriminalpolitik* 3 (1992).

———. "Kommentar zur Entscheidung des Bundesverfassungsgerichts vom 28. Mai 1993," *Kritische Vierteljahresschrift für Gesetzgebung und Rechtswissenschaft* 1 (1993).

Friedrichsen, Gisela. *Abtreibung. Der Kreuzzug von Memmingen.* Zürich und Wiesbaden, Orell Füssli Verlag, 1989.

Häussler-Sczepan, Monika. *Arzt und Schwangerschaftsabbruch.* Max-Planck Institut für Ausländ. und Intern. Strafrecht, Freiburg im Br., 1989.

Holzhauer, Brigitte. *Schwangerschaft und Schwangerschaftsabbruch.* Max-Planck Institut für Ausländ. und Internat. Strafrecht, Freiburg im Br., 1989.

Ketting, Evert, and Philip van Praag. *Schwangerschaftsabbruch. Gesetz und Praxis im internationalen Vergleich.* Tübinger Reihe 5, Tübingen, DGVT, 1985.

Klein-Schonnefeld, Sabine. "On the Conceptualization of the Female Body in the FRG; Standards and Contradictions." Paper presented at the 112th Annual Spring Meeting of the American Ethnological Society, Southern Anthropological Society, on The Body in Society and Culture, Atlanta, Georgia, April 26–28, 1990.

Koonz, Claudia. *Mothers in the Fatherland.* London, Methuen, 1988.

Liebl, Karlhans. *Ermittlungsverfahren, Strafverfolgungs- und Sanktionspraxis beim Schwangerschaftsabbruch.* Max-Planck Institut für Ausländ. und Intern. Strafrecht, Freiburg im Br., 1990.

Müller, Ingo. *Furchtbare Juristen.* München, Kindler Verlag GmbH, 1987.

Nelles, Ursula. "Abortion: The Special Case: A Constitutional Perspective," *German Politics and Society* 24/25 (Winter 1991–1992).

Panke-Kochinke, Birgit. *Die anständige Frau*. Pfaffenweiler, Centaurus Verlagsgesellschaft 1991.

Plett, Konstanze. "Images of Women in the Law and the Making of 'The' Woman through Law: The German Example." Paper presented at the Feminism and Legal Theory Project Summer Conference, Women and Representation, Columbia University, New York, June 7–12, 1992.

Pro Familia/Kommittee für Grundrechte und Demokratie (ed.), *Abtreibung vor Gericht*. Dokumentation, Braunschweig, Gerd J. Holtzmeyer Verlag, 1989.

Strafverteidiger 3 (1992). BGH Urteil vom 3.12.1991, with commentary by Monika Frommel.

Süssmuth, Rita, and Helga Schubert. *Bezahlen die Frauen die Wiedervereinigung?* München, Zürich, R. Piper GmbH, 1992.

von Soden, Kristine. *Die Sexualberatungsstellen der Weimarer Republik 1919–1933*. Berlin, Edition Hentrich Berlin, 1988.

Zwerenz, Ingrid. *Frauen: Die Geschichte des § 218*. Frankfurt am Main, Fischer Tascheonbuch Verlag, 1980.

HUNGARY

Ádám Balogh and Lászlo G. Lampé

THE HISTORY OF ABORTION LAW

Pre-1950s

In 1991, over 90,000 induced abortions were performed in Hungary, in contrast to 125,000 births and 17,000 spontaneous abortions, giving a total of 233,000 pregnancies, including ectopic ones. Of all gestational events, 39 percent ended in induced abortion, giving a rate of 36 per 1,000 women and a total rate of 1,140 in a country of 10.35 million inhabitants (Henshaw 1990).

Reliable national statistics for the same period reveal that almost 75 percent of women in the fertile age group (15–44) had been using some form of contraception since the late 1970s. Of these, 60 percent used reliable methods: 40 percent pills, 20 percent IUDs (Kamarás 1990). These figures are similar to those in the rest of Europe (Riphagen and Ketting 1990). The obvious discrepancy between such a high prevalence of both contraceptive use and induced abortion needs historical explanation. Reading the unique story of pregnancy termination and analysing the present situation in Hungary might provide a lesson for other countries now facing a similar transition to that of ours.

In the modern era, the first example of a Hungarian law declaring induction of abortion as a criminal offence was the Vth paragraph of the penal code in 1878. It specified that abortion could be carried out only on medical indication. In light of this the number of illegal abortions was high. Although

Table 1
Registered Abortions and Related Morbidity and Mortality in Hungary,
Selected Years, 1931–1973

Year	Abortions		Morbidity		Mortality	
	Total No.	% induced	No.	%	No.	%
1931	16,790	6.0	732	4.36	179	1.07
1935	24,497	5.3	771	3.15	255	1.04
1940	26,492	2.4	348	1.31	171	0.65
1946	21,879	9.2	364	1.66	112	0.51
1950	35,973	4.7	381	1.06	90	0.25
1955	78,502	45.1	402	0.51	47	0.06
1960	195,959	82.8	357	0.18	26	0.01
1965	214,098	84.2	374	0.17	16	0.01
1970	222,120	86.7	293	0.13	16	0.01
1973	197,821	85.8	222	0.11	5	<0.01

Source: Ministry of Health, 1975.

since 1931 reliable statistics have been available on all registered, legal obstetric events, including abortion-related complications, the numbers of illegal abortions are raw estimates (see Table 1). The sources of this raw estimation were the hospital and criminal records of proven or suspected complications in illegal abortions.

The estimated number of clandestine abortions in the 1930s in Hungary was around 100,000 per annum (Klinger 1988). After the war, owing to both the direct and indirect loss of life, along with nutritional problems and the shocking postwar situation, the population did not reach prewar levels until the late 1950s. Immediately after the war, special committees were set up to consider abortion applications resulting from the epidemic of rape by invading soldiers and other miseries of those days.

The Era of Childbirth by Order

Social and economic reconstruction led to an increasing number of births—and of abortions. By 1950, the annual number of illegal abortions rose to an estimated 100,000 to 150,000 (KSH 1975). This trend indicated the need for more effective fertility control. Given the nonavailability of efficient contraceptive methods all over the world, the situation inevitably led to a confrontation between advocates of new, more liberal abortion legislation and those who were against abortion or who were in favour of population increase.

At that time, political leaders considered the increase in population as a desirable feature from the utilitarian point of view, declaring the need for more workers and soldiers to defend the nation and lead to the final victory of socialism. Interestingly, at the same time the voice of religious "pro-life"

Table 2
Prosecutions for Performing Illegal Abortions in Hungary Ending with
Sentences of Imprisonment, 1938–1958

Year	Total no. of Persons	Length of Imprisonment						
		Months		Years				
		<3	3-6	6-12	1-2	2-5	5-10	>10
1938	508	252	54	54	27	1	–	–
1950	433	108	23	62	40	13	–	–
1951	750	19	95	89	64	33	–	–
1952	894	17	103	86	73	60	9	3
1953	1307	1	88	119	56	156	123	3
1954	461	–	22	25	40	50	6	–
1955	557	4	23	38	41	53	3	1
1956	416	4	22	33	32	18	4	–
1957	133	1	10	17	11	4	1	–
1958	131	–	12	13	12	11	2	–

Source: Szabó 1989

movements was crudely suppressed, as were other church activities. In this way, the official interpretation in the early 1950s of why pregnancy termination was evil was a political (communist) one, and this fact undoubtedly influenced the attitude of society towards abortion later on.

Following a political campaign, the Council of Ministers issued a very strict decree on February 8, 1953 (No. 1.004/1953). They took the law into their own hands to increase the number of births by seriously punishing those who performed illegal abortions. Table 2 shows the most serious penalties during this period of abortion prohibition. The figures correlate well with those quoted by Klinger (1988), indicating a peak of 1,500 people convicted for illegal pregnancy terminations in 1953.

Abortionists received sentences of up to 15 years in the case of the pregnant woman's death. Women having abortions were also prosecuted, but in most cases were given suspended sentences. The ideal to follow was that of the Soviet Union, where a similar decree had been issued in 1935. But in the USSR this law was never taken as seriously; in Hungary, the sanctions were much cruder and enforcement reached to all regions and to social groups in the country.

The regime exerted great pressure on society to accept the seriousness of the population problem and increase the number of births. The statistics in Table 2 reveal only the tip of the iceberg. The media were full of reports of horrible backstreet abortions and they blamed the abortionists also from a political point of view. Since primarily health personnel were suspected of performing these clandestine abortions, in a number of cases they were ordered at random to attend the trials of those who broke the law in order to witness the penal consequences first hand (Szabó 1989), thus keeping them

Table 3
Number of Live Births and Spontaneous Abortions in Hungary, 1931–1990

Year	No. of Births	No. of Spontaneous Abortions
1931	219,784	15,783
1938	182,206	24,510
1948	191,907	32,280
1950	199,729	34,266
1955	213,876	43,097
1960	146,461	33,799
1965	134,525	34,023
1970	151,819	29,837
1980	148,673	19,972
1985	130,200	18,070
1990	125,679	17,596

Sources: KSH 1992 and Ministry of Health 1975.

in terror. But these criminal abortions were performed mostly by midwives, other paramedics, and, especially in slums and rural areas, by nonmedical "expert" old women. Not exceptionally, however, general practitioners and gynaecologists were also involved in such hidden practices.

Some new pro-natalist policies were also instituted at the same time, such as the extension of obligatory ante-natal care throughout the country, benefits for pregnant women and mothers (exemptions from heavy work and no night work, free time for nursing, and a 12-week paid maternity leave), financial aid in early motherhood, increased benefits for those having more than two children, increased rate of hospital deliveries, more day-care nurseries, and improved mother and child health-care nursing. Single mothers were given extra support while childless couples had to pay an extra tax. Despite the anti-abortion strategy, the programme went by the euphemistic title of Ordinance of the Council of Ministers on the Further Improvement of the Welfare of Mothers and Children.

During the period of nearly three and a half years when this law was in force, there was a slight increase in the birthrate, as shown in Table 3. It is remarkable that at the same time the number of reported spontaneous abortions rose also by 25 percent, indicating an increasing number of clandestine induced abortions. Illegal abortions are known to exert a great impact on the rate of maternal complication, in both the short and long term (Balogh 1992). This happened in the case of Hungarian women.

1956: Liberalisation

After several minor modifications, the Council of Ministers issued a completely new abortion ordinance on June 3, 1956 (No. 1.047/1956), which unexpectedly abolished the previous prohibition and its cruel penalties, and created liberal abortion legislation.

This ordinance clearly described its three major aims. First, it decriminalised abortion, provided it was performed according to legal regulations, and it defined access to abortion as a basic right. The establishment of Abortion Approving Committees was intended to express the control society would have over requests for abortion. In fact, however, abortion was made freely available, even if the committee was opposed. Second, the ordinance ordered the production and sale of contraceptives at a low price. And third, it abolished anything to the contrary in the previous decree. This law marked the beginning of a new era in population and abortion policy in Hungary.

The official explanation for the new decree was the need to protect women's health and provide choice in family planning as a human right. But since at that time no safe alternative method of birth regulation was available, those women having an unwanted pregnancy as a rule resorted to abortion. Education in sexual matters was left to teachers, who did not prove to be effective on this topic. In summary, the second aim of the abortion decree—striking a balance between abortion and other methods of family planning—was never sufficiently realised.

On the other hand, surgical abortion was readily available to everybody and was performed by doctors in hospitals at very low cost. The technical and hygienic conditions for surgical abortion were similar to those for any other surgery. In spite of this, although the rate of serious complication fell rapidly after liberalisation, there were adverse effects.

Owing to the increased number of abortions and the increase in the abortion rate, these statistically rare or minor side effects still adversely influenced the reproductive health of a large number of women. An especially bitter lesson was learned by gynaecologists when they realized their technique of cervical dilatation and curettage was inappropriate. This means of abortion resulted in a striking increase in late abortions and premature births, with pathology being a series of traumatic lesions on the cervix, resulting in cervical incompetence (Arvay et al. 1967; Madsen et al 1979).

While the official media adored the new rights, the supposed choice of other methods of birth regulation—a term widely used at that time instead of contraception or family planning—was far less clear to potential users. Beyond a limited supply of poor-quality condoms, other methods, even the traditional ones, were out of reach for most couples. Free choice was, in fact, equal to free abortion in the late 1950s. Premature liberalisation of abortion in this country in the absence of other safe methods of family planning made people depend on abortion almost like drug addicts. This very liberal abortion law was too early in Hungary. It was also premature compared to most other European countries. The situation, according to David (1970, 1981), might have played an important role in the prevalence of a high abortion rate in the country even after reliable contraceptives were widely available.

But one has to know the history of Hungary in the mid-1950s to understand an additional important factor in the evolution of the present abortion scene. After defeat of the 1956 Revolution and restoration of the pro-Soviet communist regime, it became necessary to prove the superiority of this social system. The most obvious proof would have been a higher standard of living, but there was no hope of achieving that without cheating and manipulating society.

The story began with noisy emphasis on the benefits of legalised induced abortions over illegal ones. At the same time, no moral or religious opposition to abortion was allowed. In spite of such an atmosphere, some writers (e.g., Fekete 1963) and doctors (e.g., Arvay 1967) raised concerns about the epidemic of abortions from moral, socioeconomic, and medical standpoints. However, no real debate developed on the issue.

It became clear, especially to those who caught the logic of events early enough, that this legislation was not pro-choice but anti-natalist. Abortion as the sole choice reflected the government's desire to consolidate the new and old regimes following the revolution. Free abortion was offered as a bonus—a "social benefit"—suggesting that a low number of children would result in a higher standard of living. The media did its best to insinuate that abortion was not only part of society's new basic rights but also a means to improve the living standard. Yet this argument sounded cynical in an era when most basic human and political rights were heavily suppressed.

More than 10 years passed before the first reliable contraceptive method—the pill—was generally available in Hungary. In 1967, the first contraceptive pill (Infecundin) appeared in the pharmacies. Until that date, and for many women even afterwards, termination of pregnancy remained the only method of family planning.

Surprisingly, concerns about the negative effects of the pill were given wide publicity, unlike reservations about abortion as a method of family planning. This development contributed to the survival of a pro-abortion attitude among the public. Such a long-standing mentality does not change easily or rapidly. Pro-abortion arguments continued to brainwash the people and prevent acceptance of more efficient contraceptive methods.

Major statistical data on induced abortions in Hungary are shown in Table 4. The percentage of medical indications among the total annual abortions during the this period was low—down to 2.9 percent in 1970.

1973: Restricting Abortion

In 1973, primarily because of repeated warnings concerning the high rate of pregnancy terminations and the rapidly decreasing birthrates, the government issued a new law, in the name of the Council of Ministers (No. 1.040/ 1973/X.8./M.T.) under the title Population Policy Decisions. In principle the new law restricted the previous conditions of pregnancy termination by defining them more precisely. It required a woman seeking an abortion to have three or more children or two children plus at least one more obstetric

Table 4
Numbers and Rates of Induced Abortions in Hungary, 1950–1973

Year	Induced abortions			
	No. in Thousands	Rate/1,000 Women, 15-49	Rate/100 Live Births	Rate/100 Obstetric Events
1950	2	1	1	1
1951	2	1	1	1
1952	2	1	1	1
1953	3	1	1	1
1954	16	6	7	6
1955	35	14	17	12
1956	83	33	43	26
1957	123	49	74	37
1958	146	58	92	42
1959	152	61	101	45
1960	162	65	111	47
1961	170	69	121	49
1962	164	66	126	50
1963	174	70	131	51
1964	184	74	140	52
1965	180	72	136	52
1966	187	73	135	52
1967	188	72	126	50
1968	201	76	130	51
1969	207	78	134	52
1970	192	72	127	51
1971	187	69	124	51
1972	179	67	117	49
1973	170	63	109	48

Source: KSH 1992.

event. It prescribed a more stringent condition for establishing medical indication, stressed the responsibility of the Abortion Approving Committees in assessing the required conditions, and introduced obligatory payment for the procedure. Abortion on the basis of medical indication remained free of charge and fully covered by the insurance system, while the fee for abortion on nonmedical grounds could be waived if deemed necessary. The basic fee was defined as HUF (Forints) 1,000, equal to US$20.

The maternal age limit allowed as an independent reason for abortion on request was increased from 35 to 40 in 1979, and again changed to 35 in 1982. The most recent amendment of the 1973 law was the abolition of the Abortion Approving Committees. Simultaneously, the manufacture, provision, and availability of modern family planning methods, including IUDs and newer contraceptives, improved free choice significantly.

At the same time, the media started to encourage parents to have three children. Maternity benefits, including the child benefit, were increased. But this did not exert a marked and lasting effect on the birthrate. The abortion

Table 5
Numbers and Rates of Induced Abortions in Hungary, 1974–1990

Year	Induced Abortions			
	No. in Thousands	Rate/1,000 Women 15-49	Rate/100 Live Births	Rate/100 Obstetric Events
1974	102	38	55	32
1975	96	36	50	30
1976	95	36	51	31
1977	89	34	50	31
1978	84	32	50	30
1979	81	31	50	31
1980	81	31	54	32
1985	82	32	63	35
1986	84	33	65	36
1987	85	33	67	37
1988	87	34	70	38
1989	91	35	73	39
1990	91	36	72	40

Source: KSH 1992.

rate, however, showed a dramatic initial fall in 1974, down to 102,000 from the previous year's figure of 170,000. But the decrease slowed down soon. The annual number of abortions reached a nadir of 78,599 in 1983, thereafter climbing to the present figure of 90,000 plus. At the same time birthrates continued to decline following a transitional increase between 1974 and 1980.

The child benefit and its modified versions in the long run did not prove sufficient to reverse the undesirable demographic trend. New factors such as inflation and unemployment eroded the value and attractiveness of maternity benefits. This is at least one of the underlying causes of the present miserable Hungarian demographic scene, which is experiencing a negative increase (owing to the low birth and high death rates) and a demographic shift resulting in an increase in older people. The aging of the society is obvious, and given that it is disproportionately greater in the middle class, thus threatens the labour supply and the delicate balance of the national economy. The numbers and rates of births following the recent legal regulation of abortion are shown in Table 5.

ABORTION: CURRENT LAW AND PRACTICE

The Law since 1989

One of the interesting features of the legal regulation of abortion in Hungary is the level of legislation at which the present and previous decisions were made. All these were done as government ordinances—that is, by order of the Council of Ministers instead of the parliament, in spite of the fact that Hungary was a parliamentary democratic republic since 1946. As it is known from the postwar history of this country, principles of this democratic system have often been violated by the political regime of the past four decades. This took place under the patronage of the Soviet Union, a story similar to that of the other Central and Eastern European countries.

According to the present regulation (Ordinance of the Council of Ministers, No. 76/1988/X.3./MT):

1. Termination of pregnancy may be performed on the written request of the pregnant woman—on condition that the case fulfills the requirements of the decree—if she is:

a. a Hungarian citizen and permanent resident,

b. a foreign citizen permanently living in Hungary,

c. a foreigner but wife of a Hungarian citizen,

d. the child or legal dependant of any of the above persons, or

e. a student at a Hungarian educational institution or employed in this country.

2. Conditions of pregnancy termination are fulfilled if:

a. there is a medical indication,

b. the foetus is likely to develop severe defects and/or is unlikely to survive post-natally,
  c. the pregnant woman has not lived in marital union or has been divorced for at least six months,

d. the pregnancy is the result of crime,

e. the applicant or her spouse does not own or rent a dwelling,

f. the pregnant woman is over 35,

g. the applicant has two living children,

h. the pregnant woman or her spouse is in prison,

i. her spouse is employed in military service and there are 6 months or more left, or

j. it is clearly justified on other social grounds.

3. Termination of pregnancy may be performed only until the legally defined gestational age limit.

4. The gynaecologist (who established the diagnosis of pregnancy) is entitled to confirm the existence of the requirements in cases 2.a to 2.i. In the case of other social indications, the Family and Women's Welfare Centres are entitled to make the decisions.[1] Regionally organised secondary committees (also known as Abortion Approving Committees) exist to investigate appeals against rejected abortion applications. They are authorised to approve or definitely reject these appeals.

5. A surgical abortion is paid for by the patient with certain defined exceptions.

6. This ordinance came into force on January 1, 1989.

A joint order by the Minister of Social Welfare and Health (SWH) (No. 15/1988/XII.7./SzEM) has further interpreted this law and scrutinized the details of its application. The upper limit of gestational age varies depending on the medical indication. It may be performed until the 12th week of gestation in the case of minors (below 18), up to the 18th week on any other indication. Pregnancy termination beyond the 20th week is allowed only in a small group of designated institutions—for example, at university obstetrics and gynaecology departments.

An appendix to the order of the Minister of Social Welfare and Health specifies the upper gestational age of pregnancy terminations on medical indication. No payment is required for abortions on medical indication. The procedure is authorized:

1. Until the 12th week if the risk of a genetic-teratological problem leading to severe mental or physical damage to the foetus is more than 10 percent.

2. The request is subject to approval until the 20th week—in case of delay owing to diagnostic procedures, up to the 24th week—if the risk of the above damage is 50 percent or higher.

3. There is no gestational age limit if the foetal abnormality is incompatible with its post-natal life.

In cases of suspected foetal damage, genetic consultants consider the case and advise the patients on the likely risk. They offer therapeutic abortion if justified and requested. Women who conceived while using intrauterine contraceptive devices (IUDs) are also entitled to have their pregnancy terminated on medical grounds. Those women who had participated in clinical pharamacological trials of new contraceptive methods and got pregnant during the study are also entitled to belong to this group.

Viability of the foetus is carefully taken into consideration when the upper limit of medically indicated abortion is in question. It is suggested that this upper limit be set as low as possible anyway because health risks to the woman during surgical abortion are known to increase with gestational age. The aim has been to perform abortions before the 12th week. These exceptional cases of late second-trimester pregnancy terminations have to be made under strict control in appointed top-level institutions, as indicated above.

Beyond these medical indications, there is a series of social indications also referred to earlier, some of them equivalent to "abortion on request." Payment for performing an abortion is required, the fee being HUF2,000 (equal to US$25), which may be reduced to zero if the woman's socioeconomic situation makes it reasonable.

Those who have undergone an abortion on any grounds are placed on a sick list for two days even if they show no sign of medical complications. Any further treatment of complications is covered by the national insurance system available for all employees and their dependent family members.

At the time of the first act liberalising abortion (1956), so-called Abortion Approving Committees (or secondary committees) were formed to consider the individual request and endorse or reject it. The committees consisted of the chairperson, one doctor, and/or one maternal and child health-care nurse, and one or more other person(s) "representing the society." The attitude of these committees towards the applicants changed over time, having been very strict at the beginning but then becoming more understanding, thus reflecting the changes in society from the mid-1950s to 1988. In 1988, the committees were abolished, again by a government ordinance signed by the prime minister. The Abortion Approving Committees had never been respected, especially not by women who considered them unfit to judge in such an intimate situation as a request for induced abortion.

Since 1988 it has been the duty of the gynaecologists of the Specialist Outpatient Clinics, Family Planning Centres, or Maternity Hospital Outpatient Services to judge whether the conditions for approving abortion requests are met. The gynaecologist must also keep the necessary records and file the documents, including those supporting and justifying the medical indication of induced abortion. The same doctor cannot give permission for abortion and then perform it without the approval of a second gynaecologist.

Given this increasingly permissive attitude to abortion regulation, virtually everybody could and still can have access to surgical abortion. In the light of these facts it is not surprising that no one was found guilty of violating the abortion law in recent years.

Abortion in Practice

The liberalisation of abortion law produced a high number of abortions to be performed within the official health system. Prior to liberalisation, there was no safe method of surgical abortion suitable for management of such an unprecedented high number of procedures.

After liberalisation, registered (legal) pregnancy terminations took place in hospitals and small maternity hospitals having 12 to 35 beds and called *delivery homes*. These were initially planned for childbirth in some regions of the country far from the closest district hospitals, and for basic ante- and postnatal hospital care. Later their licence was extended to minor gynaecological operations such as curettage and surgical abortion up to the 12th week of pregnancy.

In the beginning, by far the most common method used was dilatation of the cervix by a series of metal Hegar rods and emptying the uterine cavity by sharp curettage (D & C). Occasionally it was combined with use of an abortion forceps. Owing to the surgical technique itself and the fact that, because of delays, the operation was often performed close to the 12th week, initially there was a very high rate of complications. These included lacerations of the uterine cervix, especially at the internal oriface, and bleeding and retention of choriodecidual tissue in the uterine cavity.

In spite of the initial high morbidity, the mortality rate did not increase concomitantly because there were sufficient means in the hospitals to repair the injuries and treat the resulting infections. The rates of overall abortion-related mortality and severe morbidity declined steeply with the decriminalisation of abortion (Balogh 1992). However, long-term complications owing to the abortion techniques raised suspicions about an increase in large-scale health damage. At the same time, the moral concerns of the profession came to the fore.

As was suggested above, the major role of abortion in family planning is largely a consequence of several factors. Among them, the attitude of health professionals, especially of gynaecologists, is worth noting. Individual concerns were raised quite early about the uncontrolled and exclusive use of abortion for birth control. It was suspected that surgical abortion damaged the cervix and the endometrium, and caused later reproductive complications and failures (Arvay et al. 1967). Another professional warning stressed the responsibility of the surgeon when termination involved the first pregnancy of a woman, especially a teenager (Lampé 1978). Even minor damage during pregnancy termination might result in severe harm to the reproductive health of the young woman.

Undoubtedly some critics were wrapping their moral opposition in professional arguments. A debate developed on the effects abortion had on a resulting high rate of premature births. This led to the disappointing truth that cervical incompetence and related premature births were a result of inadequate technique (D & C) rather than surgical abortion per se. Less traumatic methods, such as pharmacological dilatation of the cervix and/or the use of vacuum aspiration in early pregnancy did not affect later prematurity rates (Madsen et al. 1979; Lampé et al. 1984). These preferred methods, including the use of prostaglandins, became available gradually, nevertheless the common method of induced abortion remained the D & C for a long time, gradually replaced by vacuum aspiration.

According to the Central Bureau of Statistics (KSH 1981), vacuum aspiration was introduced in Hungary in 1975, in a few selected institutions—the obstetrics and gynaecology departments of the university medical schools in Budapest, Debrecen, Szeged, and Pécs—as part of a one-year comparative study of D & C and vacuum aspiration. (In fact, vacuum aspiration had been in use in Debrecen for several years, employing durable molded-glass aspiration cannulae of various sizes. The new instruments had a safer pump system and metal cannulae.) The comparative study included 5,782 women out of a total of 6,350 pregnancy terminations, with nearly equal numbers

Table 6
**Total Number and Age Distribution of Women Undergoing Pregnancy
Termination and Percentage Rates of Teenagers Among Them in Hungary,
1957–1990**

Year	<20	%<20	20-29	30-39	>39	Total
1957	5,446	4.41	63,026	49,618	5,293	123,383
1960	8,370	5.16	90,461	64,271	7,428	162,160
1970	18,280	9.43	117,701	65,479	9,103	192,283
1980	8,182	10.12	34,453	30,572	7,675	80,882
1985	9,285	11.23	30,149	35,042	7,494	81,970
1989	11,384	12.58	33,135	37,136	8,853	90,508
1990	12,011	13.28	33,612	36,300	8,471	90,394

Source: KSH 1992.

in each of the two groups. Final results confirmed the superior safety of
vacuum aspiration.

Another point to consider is the role and significance of effective health
education, including practical guidance in sexual matters, in order to prevent
unwanted pregnancies. It is suggested that although prevention of unintended pregnancies is not a duty of gynaecologists, the profession could do
much more to counter the constant high rate of teenage abortion.

Indeed, the increasing number and proportion of teenage abortions has,
as elsewhere in the world, become a major problem, reflecting the insuffi-
ciency of sex education relative to the increasing sexual activity of this age
group. Table 6 shows the age distribution of women undergoing pregnancy
termination in selected years, including the percentage of abortions performed on teenagers. These figures are self-explanatory. It is obvious that
much has to be done to reverse the increasing occurrence of unwanted pregnancies, especially among teenagers.

The Politics of Abortion

A Constitutional Court decision in 1991 (No. 64/1991/XII.17/AB) declared that "It is the duty of the state to defend the life of its citizens;
therefore performing abortion without proper justification is against the
spirit of the Constitution." It also became clear that the earlier legal regulation on abortion contradicted the principles of the Constitution, which
divides the law-making and executive functions so that both may not be done
by the same body. The Constitutional Court demanded that legislation be
enacted at a proper level (i.e., by the parliament) by the end of 1992 at the
latest. (The Constitutional Court—unlike the Supreme Court—is a body of
judges, independent in its decision making even from the parliament. It exists

to assess whether laws conform with the intention and spirit of the Constitution of the Republic of Hungary.)

The Court intervention was the result of an action brought by the anti-abortion group Pacem in Utero (Peace in the Uterus). This movement blames the previous political regime for carrying out 4.5 million abortions, causing more severe loss of life to the nation than both World Wars (Jobbágyi 1989). The other argument of this movement, in accordance with the views of the Roman Catholic Church, characterises abortion as homicide and as a grave sin on the part of the operator and the woman who consents.

This pressure group claims that the basic duty of the medical profession is to protect human life. The foetus from the beginning of fertilisation is considered by them as a living human creature possessing all the future capabilities of a given individual human being. This philosophical-moral attitude is extended further by the definition of the foetus from the very beginning as a legally competent personality possessing all civil rights. In the view of the Pacem in Utero and the other militant anti-abortion and pro-natalist movements, abortion should be prohibited in principle by law. They consider abortion legally permissible only in a few exceptional cases, such as a serious threat to the mother's life, deadly disease or genetic malformation of the foetus, or if the pregnancy results from crime (rape, etc.). They refer to the task of saving the "precious human life" and to guiding the pregnant woman to solutions other than abortion. They also claim that a gynaecologist should not be compelled to perform an abortion if it is against his or her own moral standards or religious faith. To compensate the public in advance for the likely severe penal consequences if their proposal came into force, they promise that punishment will not be very heavy. These views are in harmony with those of the Christian Democratic party, a member of the governing coalition.

Hungarian society is rather heterogenous in relation to future legislation. The Protestant churches (Calvinists and Lutherans are the second largest religious group) look at the abortion issue from a more pragmatic point of view. Although differing in details, they usually consider abortion as permissible in certain circumstances, even by a social indication (Kocsis 1985).

The leading party of the governing coalition, the Hungarian Democratic Forum (MDF), is officially neither "pro-life" nor pro-choice, reflecting the pluralistic nature of the party. One group of MPs, led by an MDF member, has considered submitting a new abortion act, although their draft does not represent the overall view of the coalition parties. This proposal principally reflects anti-abortion or "pro-life" views. Other groups in the coalition stress the shocking effect of a serious restriction of abortion, rather advocating powerful propaganda against the epidemic of abortion with the simultaneous provision and easy availability of efficient family planning methods for everybody. There is a consensus in the majority of these pressure groups, however, that abortion not be the preferred method of family planning anymore.

The opposition liberal parties (Free Democrats' and Young Democrats' Alliances) and the Socialist party in principle do not consider abortion a good family planning method, although they underline that easy access to abortion belongs to the basic rights of women in a modern (liberal) society. This view is reflected in the proposed draft of an abortion law by a group of Free Democrat MPs (Free Democrat MPs 1992). The draft has two versions. The first allows pregnancy termination for all before the 12th week without any restriction; the second in effect proposes keeping the present legislation with slight amendments.

The major question was, when assessing any new abortion bill, how the Constitutional Court would interpret the value of foetal life versus a woman's interest?

UPDATE: THE LAW OF 1993

It was obvious in late 1992 that the majority of people in Hungary was in favour of the preservation of liberal principles in earlier legislation. If any prediction could have been made, it would have been that the new law would probably declare that the foetus possesses "limited personal rights." But knowing the recent history of events in Poland and elsewhere, one has to be cautious forecasting the future of abortion legislation in Hungary.

Finally, the new law (1992: LXXIX Act), titled "On the Protection of Foetal Life," was enacted on January 1, 1993. It turned out to be almost as liberal as the previous legislation as regards the most critical issue. It permits termination of pregnancy under the following conditions:

1. Up to the end of the 12th week (Paragraph 6, Chapter 1) if:

a. the pregnant woman's health is in serious danger;

b. the foteus suffers from a medically proven grave illness or defect;

c. the pregnancy is a consequence of rape; or

d. the pregnant woman is in a situation of grave crisis or stress.

2. Up to the end of the 18th week (Paragraph 6, Chapter 2) if the conditions laid out in 1 above are met, and if:

a. the pregnant woman lacks the ability to act independently, or has a limited ability in this regard; or

b. the pregnancy exceeded the 12-week limit for reasons beyond the woman's responsibility—e.g., unexpected disease, administrative delay, diagnostic failure.

3. Up to the end of the 20th week—or, if the diagnosis is delayed due to verification procedures, up to the 24th week (Paragraph 6, Chapter 3)—if the chance that the foetus is affected by a serious genetic or teratologic malformation reaches 50%.

4. Irrespective of the gestational age, the pregnancy may be terminated (Paragraph 6, Chapter 4) if:

a. the pregnant woman's life is in danger; or

b. the foetus suffers from a malformation that is incompatible with post-natal life.

In spite of the fact that the title of the abortion act suggests that it is a restrictive or prohibiting one, in some respects the new law is even more liberal and less bureaucratic than its predecessor. This is primarily because of Paragraph 6, Chapter 1d, which states that a situation of grave crisis or stress is a valid indication for abortion. This indication has been taken to include psychological or socioeconomic stress or crisis such as being single, suffering from other socioeconomic stress such as unemployment and poor housing conditions, feeling psychologically unable to have more children, and the like.

The indication is given by a Family Welfare Service nurse, who needs a diagnosis by a gynaecologist. The nurse's duty is to interview those seeking an abortion. He or she is independent of the doctor, a progressive step compared to the earlier situation when the gynaecologist alone judged the existence of the indication.

The fee for an abortion has been set by law at HUF 5,000 (equal to US$60), which can be reduced to half or even waived in exceptional cases.

The creation of the Family Welfare Service—on the basis of six months experience to date—has proved to be a good idea. The unit probably has contributed to the 30 percent decrease in abortions in the first 6 months of the new legislation. However, there are at least two other significant factors contributing to this trend—namely, the nationwide debate about the value of human life beginning in the womb, and the wide availability of the latest contraceptive methods. The new law declares that family planning is a right and a responsibility of parents, and urges wide-scale family health and family planning education beginning in the primary school. At the same time, it declares that the foetus and the pregnant woman both deserve support and defence.

NOTE

1. Family and Women's Centres (in fact, family planning centres) were organised by order of the Council of Ministers in 1973. These centres, including personnel and operating costs, have been run as part of the National Health Service, using its personnel and facilities on a part-time basis. In the first instance general practitioners establish the diagnosis of pregnancy and decide whether the legal conditions for abortion are present. The secondary committees (or Abortion Approving Committees) were set up to judge the claims of those women whose requests for abortion on social grounds were rejected in the first instance by committees within the Family and Women's Centres. Since 1988 the decision to agree or reject a request for abor-

tion is made by the gynaecologist rather than by a committee, and the secondary committees have been transferred to local offices of the surgeon general, which have a community health function. *Local* in this context means at town level or higher.

REFERENCES

Arvay, A., M. Görgey, and L. Kapu. "La relation entre les avortements (interruptions de la grossesse) et les accouchements prématurés," *Rev. Franc. Gynéc. Obstét.* 62 (1967): 81–86.

Balogh, A. "Early and Late Sequalae of Illegal Abortion." In S. S. Eng-Soon Teoh and Sir M. Macnaughton Ratnam (eds.), *The Proceedings of the XIII World Congress of Gynaecology and Obstetrics*, Vol. 5: Pregnancy Termination and Labour. Casterton Hall, Carnforth, Lancs.: Parthenon, 1992.

David, H. P. *Family Planning and Abortion in the Socialist Countries of Central and Eastern Europe.* New York: Population Council, 1970.

———. "Abortion policies." In J. E. Hodgson (ed.), *Abortion and Sterilization: Medical and Social Aspects.* London: Academic Press, 1981, pp. 1–40.

Fekete, Gy. "Silhouette Boxing in Twelve Games" (Élet és Irodalom), Series of pamphlets against abortion, 1963.

Free Democrat MPs. The draft Bill of pregnancy termination by Free Democrat MPs (in Hungarian), Supplement of *Magyar Hirlap*, March 14, 1992, pp. 1–2.

Henshaw, S. K. "Induced Abortion: A World Review," *International Family Planning Perspectives* 16 (1990): 59–65.

Jobbágyi, G. "Our National Fate: Abortion" (in Hungarian), *Hitel* 2, no. 15 (1989): 50–51.

Kamarás, F. "In Your Part of the World: Abortion Survey of Central and Eastern Europe, Part I: Hungary," *Entre Nous* (European Family Planning Magazine) nos. 14/15 (1990): 13–14.

Klinger, A. "[Abortion in] Hungary." In P. Sachdev (ed.), *International Handbook on Abortion.* Westport, Conn.: Greenwood Press, 1988, p. 218–27.

Kocsis, E. "Ethics" (in Hungarian), *Textbook of Calvinist Theology.* Debrecen: Calvinist Theology, 1985.

KSH 1981. *Data on Pregnancy Terminations and Spontaneous Abortions 1978–1979*, Central Bureau of Statistics, Budapest, 1975.

KSH 1992. *Demographic Year Book 1990*, Central Bureau of Statistics, Budapest, 1992.

Lampé, L. "The First Pregnancy" (in Hungarian), *Orvosi Hetilap* 119 (1978): 1331–38.

Lampé, L., I. Smid, Z. Hernádi, S. B. Hong, C. M. Par, I. S. Park, K. S. Won, M. Shin, I. O. Choo, S. D. Kim, A. Varma, S. L. Barron, and M. A. Belsey. "Secondary Infertility Following Induced Abortion," World Health Organization Task Force on Sequelae of Abortion, Special Programme of Research, Development and Research Training, *Human Reproduction Studies in Family Planning* 15 (1984): 291–95.

Madsen, M., E. Obel, E. Ostergaard, J. Philip, O. Karjalainen, M. Mandelin, L. Lampé, A. M. Davies, F. Szczotka, H. Wior, S. B. Wong, B. Geierstam, S. L. Barron, J. K. Russel, C. Tietze, A. Varma, L. Andolsek, M. Ogrinc-Oven,

M. Pompe, M. Belsey, K. Edström, P. Heiner, K. Kinnear, and Y. Russel. "Gestation, Birth-Weight and Spontaneous Abortion in Pregnancy After Abortion." Report of a Collaborative Study by WHO Task Force on Sequelae of Abortion, *The Lancet* I (1979): 142–45.

Ministry of Health. *Statistical Data on Maternity Events 1971–1973*, Ministry of Health, Budapest, 1975.

Riphagen, F. E. and E. Ketting. "Comparative Overview of Results from Eight Surveys on Contraceptive Behavior." In E. Ketting (ed.), *Contraception in Western Europe: A Current Appraisal*. Casterton Hall, Carnforth, Lancs.: Parthenon, 1990, pp. 77–110.

Szabó, A. F. "Childbirth by Order" (in Hungarian), *Hitel* 2, no. 15 (1989): 46–49.

IRELAND

Anna Eggert and Bill Rolston

THE HISTORY OF ABORTION LAW

Colonialism and Morality

A long history of colonialism has served to shape many aspects of contemporary Irish society. This is seen not only in the institutional structures that exist but also in the area of culture, ideas, and morality.

In institutional terms, the most obvious legacy of that history is that Ireland is partitioned. This occurred in 1921, producing what was then called the Irish Free State (later, after 1949, the Republic of Ireland) in the southern and western 26 countries, and the state of Northern Ireland (sometimes referred to as Ulster) in six northern counties. Both states had their parliaments. That in the south was called the Dail; it passed its own laws independently after partition. The Northern parliament was subsidiary to the British parliament in Westminster. This meant that it could not make laws in certain areas—for example, defence. Where it had an independent function, for the most part it followed legal practice in Britain itself. As a result, Northern Ireland has tended to acquire laws that are local copies of previous British ones, especially in relation to social legislation. The gap between a law being introduced in Britain and its equivalent in Northern Ireland is frequently long. For example, homosexuality was legalised in Northern Ireland in 1982, 15 years after the equivalent reform in Britain.

One reason for such conservatism is the cultural legacy of colonialism. The majority (currently around 60 percent) of Northern Ireland's 1.5 million inhabitants are Protestants, ultimately descended from the planters sent from England and Scotland in the 17th century to colonise and pacify the area. Always a minority in Ireland overall, they practically monopolised economic and political power for hundreds of years. Since the Act of Union which created the United Kingdom of Britain and Ireland in 1800, Protestants, especially in the northeast of Ireland, were Unionists—that is, in favour of union with Britain. By the end of the last century, with the rise of nationalism, Unionist power waned. But with partition in 1921, Unionists gained what the first prime minister of Northern Ireland termed "a Protestant parliament for a Protestant people." At the same time their small state of Northern Ireland appeared to them often to be at the mercy of unsympathetic British bureaucrats, nationalist politicians in the Republic of Ireland, and militant republicans in the IRA determined to end the state's existence by force. This feeling of isolation and siege was increased when Britain removed the local parliament in 1972 and established a system of direct rule. For many Protestants in the north the need for a sense of worth and security is found in religious fundamentalism. Moral issues, especially in relation to sexuality, take on profound importance in this society despite the veneer of secularism.

As nationalism grew in importance in Ireland in the 19th century, it forged close links with Catholicism, mainly because the colonial relationship had prevented the emergence of a strong middle class, especially in the earlier part of the century. By the time the Irish Free State was established, it was clear that Catholic moral teaching would have a profound influence on law and policy. This was because of the institutional links between church and state (as evidenced in church control of hospitals, schools, and the like) as well as the loyalty of the bulk of the population to Catholic religious practice. Religion had offered many nationalists comfort in the darkest days of colonial oppression, and the legacy of this is that upwards of 95 percent of the population of 3.5 million in the Irish Republic is Catholic and most of them practice their religion. There has thus been a fundamentalism in the south that mirrors that in the north. Often the issues that convulsed the society were, and are, issues relating to sexual morality. Even the partial decline of church influence, direct and indirect, in recent years has not totally severed the relationship between Catholic moral teaching and state law and policy.

Finally, nationalists in Northern Ireland were in many ways as welded to Catholic beliefs as their fellow nationalists in the south. The difference was that their church had until recently little influence on policy making in the north. In the early years of the state the Catholic Church was marginalised. Now it is at the receiving end of patronage from the state. But on many issues of morality, and particularly sexual morality, there is little difference between the official Catholic and official Protestant positions, whether or not the churches actually collaborate to influence law and policy.

Ireland, north and south, is marked by a conservatism that is often viewed as archaic from outside. Without justifying that conservatism, it is important to understand its roots in the historical relationship between Britain and Ireland.

The Law and Abortion

Irish women currently have abortions, however, for the most part, they do not have them in Ireland. In 1991, according to official British statistics, 1,777 women from Northern Ireland and 4,154 from the Republic of Ireland had abortions in Britain. However, these figures do not account for all Irish women having abortions in Britain. Many do not provide an Irish address, giving instead that of a relative or friend resident in Britain. Consequently, counsellors in organisations such as the Ulster Pregnancy Advisory Association (UPAA) estimate that the real number of Irish women having abortions in Britain is anywhere from one and a half to two times what the official figures state.

To understand why this "abortion tourism" occurs, it is necessary to spend some time unravelling the complicated legal situation in relation to abortion.

At the root of legislation in Britain and Ireland, north and south, is the 1861 (British) Offences Against the Person Act. Anyone who performs an abortion, including a pregnant woman, can be sentenced to "penal servitude for life." The 1861 act constantly refers to "unlawful" abortions. This begs the question: did the legislators in 1861 believe that there were "lawful" abortions, even though they did not specify what such abortions were? It was and is the opinion of lawyers that they did (see Davison 1983). More important, this was also the opinion of doctors. Despite the lack of definition in this law, doctors tended to believe that they had the force of common law—that is, practice from time immemorial—to back up their decision to carry out an abortion if it was judged necessary to save the life of a woman.

In 1921, Ireland was partitioned. The government of the Irish Free State now had authority to create its own laws. But for the most part, as in most postcolonial societies, it also continued to observe those laws that had been created by the previous parliament in London. As regards Northern Ireland, British legislation, and in particular social legislation, was often, but not always, replicated in legislation introduced by the local parliament. Moreover, the north did not always acquire the equivalent to British laws automatically; in the case of homosexual law reform, for example, it took a judgement of the European Court of Human Rights before the law in Northern Ireland was brought into line with that in Britain. In short, postpartition British legislation did not apply to the south of Ireland and, especially in relation to moral issues, did not apply to the north automatically.

In 1929, the British parliament passed the Infant Life (Preservation) Act, which stated that it was a crime, punishable by penal servitude for life, "to destroy the life of a child *capable of being born alive*" (italics added). The act thus specified one particular type of abortion as unlawful. However, it also went on to say that "no person shall be found guilty of an offense under this section unless it is proved that the act which caused the death of the child was not done in good faith for the purpose only of preserving the life of the mother."

In other words, the 1929 act specifically stated that an abortion carried out on a foetus capable of being born alive (defined in the act as being 28 weeks or more in gestational age), provided that the act was done to save the life of the mother, was no longer to be considered unlawful in the terms of the 1861 legislation.

The 1929 act thus raised, but did not answer, the further thorny question of whether other abortions done (in good faith to save the life of the woman) on foetuses *not* capable of being born alive were also to be considered no longer unlawful. In effect the act, instituted to end one element of legal confusion, served instead to increase confusion, for it allowed for legal abortion, albeit rarely, *at* 28 weeks gestation, but not before. Medical practitioners in Britain were now unsure of where exactly they stood in relation to the law if they performed abortions. Consequently, one doctor, Alec Bourne, in 1938 decided to test the law by challenging it directly. He carried out an abortion on a 14-year-old girl who was pregnant as a result of a multiple rape; he then presented himself to the police. He was charged under the 1861 Offences Against the Person Act. Bourne's defence was that the 1861 act, in talking of unlawful abortions, had allowed for, but not defined, lawful abortions. On this basis, Bourne argued that he had carried out a lawful abortion. The judge agreed with this defence and Bourne was acquitted.

The problem was that the judge's ruling in the Bourne case did not have the force of law. Had the state challenged the ruling in a higher court and had that higher court agreed with the ruling, then it would have widened the definition of what was no longer an unlawful abortion to include cases where the woman's physical life was not technically in danger. In the absence of the ruling of a higher court, the most that doctors could hope was that other judges would conclude similarly were they to carry out an abortion in circumstances such as those that faced Dr. Bourne.

How did this affect Irish law? In relation to the south, the answer is simple: it did not. In the north, the 1929 Infant Life (Preservation) Act was eventually enacted as the Criminal Justice (Northern Ireland) Act in 1945. The Bourne judgement, despite being a source of possible guidance, did not have the force of law; consequently, there was no guarantee that it could be used as a defence by a doctor carrying out what she or he judged to be a lawful abortion. The result was that in the north doctors found themselves in more or less the same situation as Bourne himself had been in—of knowing that abortions carried out on a viable foetus in order to save the life of the woman were lawful, but that other abortions took place in a legally undefined area.

It was precisely because of such lack of legal clarity that the 1967 Abortion Act was enacted in Britain. In point of fact, it did not overrule either the

1861 act or the 1929 act, but merely set out to say that there were certain types of abortion that could henceforth no longer be considered unlawful; that is, abortions carried out after two doctors concluded:

(a) that the continuance of the pregnancy would involve risk to the life of the pregnant woman, or of injury to the physical or mental health of the pregnant woman or any existing children of her family, greater than if the pregnancy were terminated; or
(b) that there is a substantial risk that if the child were born it would suffer from such physical or mental abnormalities as to be seriously handicapped.

ABORTION: CURRENT LAW AND PRACTICE

Abortion in Ireland, North and South

The last sentence of the 1967 Abortion Act stated "this Act does not extend to Northern Ireland." The law in Northern Ireland remains what it was in Britain before 1967. As a consequence the legal confusion and medical caution are similar in the north now to what they were in Britain 25 years ago, and without the refining influence of a local equivalent of a Bourne judgement to clarify matters somewhat.

There was no chance of Irish Republic legislators enacting their equivalent of the British Abortion Act.[1] Various factors between the wars—economic, political, and otherwise—ensured that the south became a progressively insular society, its conservatism captured in the 1937 Constitution, which ensures a special place in society for the Catholic Church and presumes that a woman's only role is that of mother. The Catholic Church was not shy about using its influence directly to shape legislation. Moreover, the loyalty of most Catholics to church teaching is one factor explaining their conservative stance on a number of moral issues. Thus, a referendum to legalise divorce in the Republic of Ireland in 1985 was rejected by two-thirds of those who voted.

Despite the differing legal histories since partition, medical practice in relation to abortion in Ireland, north and south, at least up until the mid-1980s, was similar. There were few abortions performed within the state medical system, and there was a certain arbitrariness in relation to a woman's chances of obtaining an abortion, no matter how clear her need, because of differing levels of caution among doctors. Statistical information in relation to abortion in the north is difficult to obtain; counsellors and doctors estimate that there are possibly somewhere in the region of 200 therapeutic abortions each year. The statistical imprecision is deliberate. A spokesperson for the government in Northern Ireland argues:

In Northern Ireland the term "abortion" is used to cover a number of medical conditions including incomplete abortion, inevitable abortion and miscarriage as well as therapeutic abortions. The existing hospital operation procedure codes do not distinguish between the ending of a pregnancy due to natural causes or from justified medical intervention.[2]

To allow for more precise categorisation and more accurate data would be to call attention to the fact that therapeutic abortions do occur, with potential conflict for, and perhaps even legal action against, doctors. The state's response is therefore to match the legal uncertainty with a statistical imprecision. For women this is experienced simply as medical uncertainty. There is no guarantee that an abortion will be carried out even in cases of rape or incest.

Moreover, because of the ambiguous legal situation, there is a certain reluctance to administer alphafetoprotein tests on pregnant women. The test detects spina bifida, the occurrence of which is higher in Northern Ireland than anywhere else in the world. The normal procedure in cases of detection of the ailment is termination, but given the uncertainty of obtaining an abortion in local hospitals, medical staff sometimes seem to prefer to remain in ignorance, and to leave the pregnant woman in the same condition.

There are many other ways in which the experience is a profoundly unsatisfactory one for women. Between 1968 and 1981 there were five deaths from backstreet abortions officially recorded in the north. The fact that there are not more is because of the geographical proximity of Britain. But travelling for an abortion is not a satisfactory option, adding as it does further physical, financial, emotional, and potentially medical difficulties to those already experienced by women who make the difficult decision to abort.

In the Republic of Ireland, at least up until the mid-1980s, some therapeutic abortions also occurred. The information about them is even less precise than about the north. For doctors in the south the minefield in which abortions might be carried out was made worse by the strong influence of Catholic morality on the state's laws and policies, as well as by the strong presence of Catholic priests and nuns in the running and administration of many hospitals. In this situation, backstreet abortions are not unknown, but their frequency is minimal given the safety valve of travel to Britain. And there is some disturbing evidence that infanticide not only occurred but still occurs occasionally.[3] But for the vast majority of women choosing an abortion, the only option in the south, as in the north, was and is to travel to Britain. The relationship between the ability to travel and the lack of evidence of backstreet abortions is most starkly shown by the fact that during the Second World War, when travel between the south and Britain was restricted because of the Irish Republic's neutrality, the number of backstreet abortions rose significantly (see Jackson 1983).

The Politics of Abortion: The South

The Republic of Ireland has a written Constitution. In 1983, as a result of right-wing pressure,[4] the government held a referendum to amend the

Constitution. Abortion was, as already stated, illegal. And it was unlikely, given the balance of political forces, that there would be any moves in the south to introduce liberal abortion legislation. The Right's motives in instituting this emotive and highly divisive debate were probably determined as much by factors external to Irish society as internal. As Kissling (1992, 16) points out, the anti-choice movement in the United States had failed in 1982 to introduce an anti-abortion amendment into the U.S. Constitution, despite a major effort. Consequently, "having failed in the U.S., this movement launched an international campaign designed to secure 'human life amendments' in the constitutions of a number of countries where abortion was still illegal, including Ireland, the Philippines and Brazil."

In Ireland they succeeded. In 1983, as a result of a two-to-one vote in a referendum, the Eighth Amendment to the Constitution of the Republic of Ireland was inaugurated. Instituted as Article 40.3.3 of the Constitution, the Eighth Amendment states that: "The State acknowledges the right to life of the unborn and, with due regard to the equal right to life of the mother, guarantees in its laws to respect, and as far as practicable, by its laws to defend and vindicate that right."

Flushed with success, the Right turned its attention to policing the amendment, pursuing relentlessly those who seemed in any way to support abortion, and in the process stretching to its limits the interpretation of what it meant to "respect" and "defend" "the right to life of the unborn." The list of potential targets for the Right was long: doctors considering therapeutic abortions, broadcasters who ran live talk shows on the issue of abortion, magazines that provided information about abortion services in Britain, and shopkeepers and distributors who handled those magazines. Indeed, most frightening of all was the prospect that the law could now be brought into play to prevent individual women going to England for abortions or to prosecute them when they returned. The Republic of Ireland appeared set to be a moral police state, with the well-organised and well-financed anti-choice advocates in SPUC (Society for the Protection of the Unborn Child) as the ever-vigilant moral police.

In 1985, SPUC sought an injunction against two of the main agencies in Dublin providing nondirective counselling for women. In 1986, the High Court granted the injunction against the two agencies—Open Door Counselling and the Dublin Well Woman Centre. In the view of the president of the High Court, Justice Liam Hamilton, the Constitution now outlawed the presentation of any information to women that might lead them to decide to have an abortion. As he put it, "The qualified right to privacy, the rights of association and freedom of expression and the right to disseminate information cannot be invoked to interfere with such a fundamental right as the right to life of the unborn."

The effects of that judgement were devastating and widespread. Open Door Counselling closed down. The Dublin Well Woman Centre, on legal advice, ceased providing pregnancy counselling of any kind in case what they had to say could be construed as procuring abortions. RTE, the state radio and television service, banned any live programmes in which abortion was to be discussed. Libraries removed copies of books such as *Our Bodies, Ourselves.* And social workers and similar professionals were advised that they could be open to legal action if they provided any form of abortion counselling. Abortion counselling was thus effectively forced underground. This meant that women frequently could not obtain any information in the south about seeking an abortion in Britain. Informal information networks were set up, and Northern counselling agencies experienced an increase in the number of inquiries from southern women. But the women best situated to acquire necessary information on abortion are urban and middle class. The Hamilton ruling thus accentuated the class nature of abortion. As one counsellor put it, "middle class women can get the information themselves and make their own way directly to clinics in Britain. What we're picking up is the poor ones who have no information and don't know where to get it until they stumble upon us" (cited in Herbert 1988, 19).

Often such women do not find out the phone number or person to contact until the pregnancy is too far advanced for them to obtain an abortion in Britain; counsellors in the south and the British Pregnancy Advisory Service noted an increase in the number of such women. Moreover, women who do contact others for information are worried that they themselves might be liable to prosecution.

The story of the two counselling agencies rumbled on for years. In 1988 they appealed against the injunction to the Supreme Court and failed. Subsequently they took their case to the European Commission on Human Rights under Article 10 of the European Convention on Human Rights, which advocates freedom of information. In 1991 the European Commission upheld the appeal of Open Door Counselling and the Dublin Well Woman Centre. In October 1992 the European Court of Human Rights ratified the finding of the European Commission and found the Republic of Ireland guilty of discrimination in not allowing women access to information about abortion services in other European states. While judgements of this court do not have to be obeyed by any member state of the European Community, the state concerned is under moral pressure not to ignore that finding entirely.

Despite this, in July 1993, the Supreme Court upheld the original injunction by a majority decision. Although the results of an interim referendum (see below) allowed freedom of information about abortion, three (male) judges said that until the law on abortion was changed, the original injunction stood. The one dissenting (female) judge disagreed, stating that the Supreme Court was now acting contrary to a popularly agreed amendment to the Constitution.[5]

SPUC initiated a second major legal action in October 1988. They asked the student union officers at University College, Dublin, not to print abortion information in their welfare manual. When the officers refused, SPUC sought a court injunction. The High Court refused the injunction, but SPUC then appealed to the Supreme Court, which ruled that SPUC was justified in attempting to suppress the publication of information on abortion. SPUC then turned its attention to individual students' union officers (from University College, Dublin; Trinity College, Dublin; and the Union of Students of Ireland), in the end taking 14 of them to court. The High Court rejected SPUC's action against the student officers, and again an appeal was made to the Supreme Court, which backed SPUC and gave the organisation leave to raise the matter again with the High Court. In October 1989 the Dublin High Court decided to refer the case to Europe.

The immediate effects of this legal battle were that the publication of any information about British abortion clinics was now declared illegal and unconstitutional. Despite that, pro-choice people continued to publish such information in ingenious ways; the telephone numbers of the British abortion clinics were printed on tee shirts; members of parliament used parliamentary privilege to read out the telephone numbers during debates, ensuring that they were then printed in the parliamentary record; one female rock group composed a song in which the chorus consisted solely of the most relevant phone numbers. All these actions were now potentially subject to injunctions brought by SPUC. Moreover, there was nothing to stop the state from moving independently against the people concerned and bringing them before the courts. For the most part, the state authorities seemed reluctant to enter this minefield. But this did not prevent customs officials from seizing copies of the British *Guardian* newspaper in 1992 because they contained an advertisement for the Marie Stopes clinics in Britain. Wishing to avoid the same fate, popular British women's magazines such as *Cosmopolitan* printed special Irish editions in which advertisements for abortion services were whited out.

The European Court of Justice considered the case of the 14 students in 1991. It ruled that abortion clinics in one European Community state had the right to advertise their services in any other European Community state, and that the citizens of that state had the right to receive that information. It also upheld the right of women from one European Community state to travel to another such state for an abortion. It thus concluded that Irish law was not in line with European Community standards. However, it did not find that the Irish courts had abused the rights of the students as they themselves had not been directly affected by the lack of access to information on abortion nor been stopped from travelling for an abortion. The European Court of Justice implied that the matter would have been different if a woman had appealed to them on the grounds that she had been prevented from travelling from Ireland to England for an abortion, or if she had been severely disadvantaged by lack of information about abortion services in Britain. As this was not the case in relation to the students, in effect the Supreme Court injunction stood.

Despite the success of a referendum allowing freedom of information on abortion (see below), the injunction against the student organisations has not been lifted as of this writing. As in the case of the clinics, the judges prefer to leave the difficult decisions to the legislators, despite the popular vote in the referendum of December 1992. The two cases of the counselling agencies and the student organisations had served to strain the relationship between the Republic of Ireland and Europe. It was clear that the government was under pressure to lessen the strain in the relationship somehow. That pressure reached a crescendo in 1992.

In December 1991, the 12 member states of the European Community met in Maastricht, Holland, to draw up the final blueprint for a single market. Economic unification was to be realised by the end of 1992. Each member state had then to ratify the Maastricht Treaty separately. For most of the states all that was required was a parliamentary debate. But two states, Denmark and the Republic of Ireland, would have to hold referenda. (A third state, France, decided to conduct a referendum as well.)

The Maastricht Treaty had nothing to say about issues such as abortion. Despite that, anti-abortionists both inside and outside the Republic of Ireland's government party persuaded Irish negotiators to introduce a protocol into the Maastricht Treaty to the effect that the European Community would not override domestic law on abortion in the Republic of Ireland. The addition of the protocol seemed to imply that no Irish person could in future cite the European Community's commitment to freedom of information and to freedom of movement between member states to overrule domestic Irish law on abortion. It now looked as if the South's ban on abortion was about to be underwritten by the European Community itself. Consequently, women's groups and others in the south immediately began to organise against the Maastricht Treaty.

At that point, an incident happened that no one could have predicted, but which served to unravel the whole of the Right's careful strategy to outlaw abortion. The parents of a 14-year-old girl went to the police stating that she was pregnant as a result of rape. The parents decided to take their daughter to England for an abortion, but checked first with the police if they could use the results of DNA tests on foetal tissue carried out in England in the event of a prosecution in an Irish court of the man who had raped the girl. The police reported the parents (not the rapist!) to the attorney general, on the grounds that a crime was about to be committed—namely, an abortion outside the territory. The attorney general obtained an interim court injunction restraining the girl from having an abortion in England. In fact, she and her parents were already in England preparing for the abortion and returned home, fearing severe consequences if they acted in contempt of the injunction. In February 1992 the High Court confirmed the injunction and ruled that the girl and her parents were prohibited from leaving the territory for the next nine months. The government saw a major crisis looming and persuaded the girl and her parents to appeal to the Supreme Court; the expenses for the case were paid by the government.

The five male judges of the Supreme Court heard the appeal at the end of February under intense political pressure to solve the state's dilemma of upholding the Constitution without appearing utterly callous and repressive. The Supreme Court lifted the High Court's injunction and the girl was able to travel to England for her abortion. A week later the judges delivered the text of their judgement and a huge controversy arose. Three of the five judges concluded that Article 40.3.3 of the Constitution should be interpreted in such a way as to prevent any woman from travelling to England for an abortion. However, they also decided, by majority vote, that the Constitution did not forbid abortion when there was "a real and substantial risk to the life, as distinct from the health, of the mother." In the narrow definition of that concept available under Catholic Church morality—namely, abortion only in the case of ectopic pregnancy and cancer of the uterus— the 14-year-old could not have been judged a suitable candidate for a lawful abortion. But the girl had threatened and even attempted suicide. In the judges' opinion there was a very real danger that she would take her own life if she had to continue with the pregnancy.

This was a novel interpretation of the law and Constitution that allowed the government off the hook. As Smyth (1992, 13) puts it, "The concept of the equal right to life of 'mother' and foetus enshrined in the Constitution had given way to a superior right to life for the pregnant woman in certain, admittedly highly restricted, circumstances."

Advocates of a woman's right to choice focused on the narrowness of the definition of a lawful abortion. But the opponents of choice were indignant that the seemingly total ban on abortion had been breached by none other than the Supreme Court.

SPUC immediately linked the Supreme Court ruling to the Maastricht Treaty. Their reasoning was that a protocol, which had been introduced as a result of their efforts, and which before the Supreme Court judgement seemed to muster the authority of Europe to underwrite their own position on abortion, had suddenly backfired. Now, they argued, the effect of the protocol was to have Europe recognise the republic's current law *and practice*; all that was necessary in future was for any woman to threaten suicide and she could not be stopped from travelling to England. The Supreme Court had allowed for abortion in certain circumstances and that was in effect now underwritten by Europe as a result of the protocol. It was, as far as the Right was concerned, the thin edge of the wedge. It was also, incidentally, the most spectacular example in recent Irish history of a government shooting itself in the foot.

SPUC threw all its efforts into canvassing for a rejection of the Maastricht Treaty. Feminists, liberals, the Left, and others were already canvassing against the treaty for different reasons. It looked as if the referendum would be rejected and perhaps the whole process of European economic unification derailed as a result of this protocol.

Consequently, the republic's government went back to the European Community asking to amend the protocol to guarantee freedom of travel and of information. In May 1992 the member states issued a Solemn Declaration, stating that they agreed:

That it was and is their intention that the Protocol shall not limit freedom either to travel between Member States, or, in accordance with conditions which may be laid down in conformity with Community law, by Irish legislation, to obtain or make available in Ireland, information relating to services legally available in other Member States.

It was hoped that this would not only placate the feminist opponents but also ensure that women could continue to travel as before, that there would thus never be another injunction against any pregnant woman, and that no court rulings would be produced to anger and galvanise SPUC. In effect freedom to travel meant freedom to export the problem. The Eighth Amendment could remain in the Constitution, but while Irish women were travelling for their abortions outside the jurisdiction, there would be no pressure on the government to have to figure out ways of realising the Constitution's ideals. It would be the best of both worlds: a statement of intent but no need for action.

In fact, it is unlikely that this Solemn Declaration has any legal force whatsoever. But it was a strategic move on the Irish government's part to separate the two issues of abortion and Maastricht. In pursuit of the same strategy, the government promised a referendum on abortion *after* the Maastricht referendum. Women's groups asked for the referendum on abortion to precede that on Maastricht, but the government said that the European Community would not allow this. The parliamentary opposition asked that at least the wording of the abortion referendum be made available before the vote on Maastricht, but the government declined.

A further tactic in separating the two issues of abortion and economic union was that the government cleverly played up the financial importance of the link with the European Community. The Republic of Ireland was then in receipt of £3 billion in subsidies, mostly for agriculture. The prime minister announced that a positive vote for the Maastricht Treaty *could* lead to a doubling of that subsidy. The tactic worked. Among those most likely to vote against Maastricht were the powerful farming lobby, but these were also the people most likely to benefit from increased agricultural subsidies. In the end the farmers put money above morality and voted yes. The referendum in favour of the Republic of Ireland's acceptance of the Maastricht Treaty was passed by two to one.

With Maastricht out of the way, the next task was to settle the wording of the abortion referendum to be held in December 1992. The majority party in the coalition government, Fianna Fail, decided on a three-part referendum. Part one stated that Article 40.3.3 of the Constitution should not be taken to mean that the freedom of Irish women to travel between member states of the European Community is in any way impaired. Part two ensured that the Constitution does not restrict freedom of information about services in other member states. Together these two points, if agreed on by a majority of those voting, would undo the effects of the earlier protocol to the Maastricht Treaty. They would also ensure that the Republic of Ireland could no longer be found lacking by either the European Court of Human Rights or the European Court of Justice on these matters.

It was the third part of the proposed referendum that was the most controversial: "It shall be unlawful to terminate the life of an unborn unless such termination is necessary to save the life, as distinct from the health, of the mother where there is an illness or disorder of the mother giving rise to a real and substantive risk to her life, not being a risk of self-destruction."

A vote in favour of this point would allow for therapeutic abortions, even within the confines of the Irish state. At the same time it would severely restrict the import of the Supreme Court judgement in the case of the 14-year-old rape victim by stating that the threat or even the likelihood of suicide is not sufficient grounds for making an abortion lawful.

In December 1992, the three referenda were held. Of those who voted, 62.3 percent supported the right of Irish women to travel abroad. Sixty percent agreed that information about services, including abortion, in other member states of the European Community, should be freely available to people in Ireland. But on the substantive issue, that of legalising abortion in certain circumstances, the proportions were reversed; 65.4 percent rejected the government's narrowly worded statement. In doing so, the population in effect told the legislators to work out the problem themselves through a law debated and passed in the Dail.

Despite that brief, the government has not shown much haste about introducing a bill on abortion. In July 1993, Albert Reynolds announced that the government would introduce new laws legalising the distribution of information on abortion in the autumn of 1993.

The Politics of Abortion: The North

To first appearances, the chances of abortion law reform in the north seem much greater than in the south. Technically, all that would be required would be a change in the 1967 act deleting the final line of that act, which states that it does not apply to Northern Ireland. In fact there are a number of obstacles working against those groups—such as the Northern Ireland

Abortion Campaign and the Northern Ireland Abortion Law Reform Association (see NIALRA 1989)—which propose that legal amendment.

For a start, Northern Ireland is remarkably like the south in terms of popular support for conservative moral positions. The source of such popular beliefs in the South is the Catholic Church. This church also has an important influence in the north in relation to approximately 40 percent of the population who are not just nominally Catholic but also highly likely to be regular worshippers. The majority of the population belongs to one or other Protestant denomination, many of which are heavily fundamentalist in their moral stance. Such church groups have organised against legal reforms in relation to divorce, homosexuality, and of course abortion. Where both Catholic and Protestant groups work together on an issue—an amazing phenomenon in a society riven by sectarian division—the obstacle is daunting. Throughout 1992, for example, both groups worked together to oppose the establishment of a Brook Centre in Belfast to give nondirective counselling on sexuality and fertility to young people. Abortion is another issue that has persuaded the groups to join forces periodically.[6]

Since 1972 the British government has ruled Northern Ireland directly, having removed the local parliament. Although in one sense this should have made it easier for a change in the British legislation on abortion to have it apply in Northern Ireland, the extent of local conservatism on moral matters has provided an easy excuse for the British government to refuse to extend the 1967 Abortion Act.

The reply of groups such as the Northern Ireland Abortion Law Reform Association has been that the individual decisions of at least 25,000 women since 1967 to travel from the north to Britain represents a respectable demand for abortion services, no matter what the public position of church groups or politicians. In addition, there is more direct evidence of support for abortion law reform. A British group, the Abortion Law Reform Association, sponsored two surveys in Northern Ireland, in May 1992 and May 1993, that revealed that 79 percent of those polled in 1992 and 82 percent of those polled in 1993 believed that abortion should be legal when a doctor believes it is necessary to maintain the physical or mental health of the woman. These are roughly the same grounds for abortion as apply under the 1967 Abortion Act in Britain. Moreover, one-fourth of those polled supported an "abortion on demand" position. Three months later, Francome (1992) reported on a survey of almost all the consultant gynaecologists in Northern Ireland. Of the 43 contacted, 33 replied. Nineteen of these said they would carry out abortions for foetal handicap, HIV-positive women, and those who were pregnant as a result of rape or incest.

THE FUTURE

In the Republic of Ireland, the combination of actions carried out by feminists and liberals, including the appeal to the higher moral authority of

Europe, together with tactical mistakes by the anti-choice proponents both inside and outside the government, have ensured that something that was unthinkable a few years ago is almost inevitable. The seemingly unchangeable prohibition on abortion brought about as a result of the 1983 constitutional amendment is on the way to being changed. The government is wary of entering the minefield of a new law on abortion, but the voters and the Supreme Court judges have passed on that task and it cannot be avoided forever. The law, when it is introduced, will be very narrow, allowing abortion for therapeutic reasons only.

As regards the north, the chances of liberalisation of the current highly restricted availability of abortion services are slim. While legal change is technically simple, given the fact that policy matters are decided in Britain, the British government's deference to the most anti-choice elements in Northern Ireland make it unlikely that the 1967 Abortion Act will be extended to Northern Ireland in the near future.

And as the legal wrangles continue in the south and legal inaction prevails in the north, thousands of Irish women continue to travel to Britain for abortions.

NOTES

1. The only legal change that occurred in the south in relation to abortion between 1921 and the mid-1980s was that the Health (Family Planning) Act of 1979 reiterated the ban on abortion in the specific case of abortifacient contraceptives.

2. Letter of J. Scott, Northern Ireland Office, to Northern Ireland Abortion Law Reform Association, August 14, 1992.

3. Rose (1978, 253) concludes that between 1860 and 1975, "while Ireland has had the lowest enumeration of illegal abortions, so far as was known or reported to the police, it has also had during this same period higher rates of infanticide, concealment of childbirth and abandonment of children under two years of age than any of the other areas investigated in the British Isles." Northern Ireland, he goes on to say, comes a close second.

4. The campaign to amend the Constitution began with right-wing pressure groups such as SPUC, the Society for the Protection of the Unborn Child. At the time, the government was a coalition one whose major partner was Fine Gael. The taoiseach, or prime minister, was Garrett Fitzgerald, a man who was, in Irish terms, a liberal as regards moral issues. The main opposition party was Fianna Fail. This party has been the ruling one for most of the years of the southern state to date. Some of its members were and are openly in collaboration with SPUC. Most members of the party were and are not fundamentally opposed to SPUC's moral positions.

5. The Irish Family Planning Association was never subject to an injunction preventing them from providing information on abortion. Thus when the referendum on access to information was passed in December 1992, the IFPA judged that they were now justified in providing such information. They do so openly at the same time as the Well Woman Clinic and Open Door Counselling are still prevented by the original injunction from providing information.

6. Thus, when British Liberal MP David Alton visited Belfast to explain his Private Member's Bill, which sought to curtail the 1967 Abortion Act, he was joined in a public meeting by elected politicians from the two Unionist parties and the main Nationalist party.

REFERENCES

Davison, M. "The 1967 Abortion Act and Northern Ireland." Undergraduate thesis, Faculty of Law, Queen's University, 1983.

Francome, C. "Abortion in Ireland," *British Medical Journal* 6851 (August 1992): 436–37.

Herbert, C. "Hamilton Ruling Defied," *Magill*, January 1988.

Jackson, P. *The Deadly Solution to an Irish Problem: Backstreet Abortion*. Dublin: Women's Right to Choose Campaign, 1983.

Kissling, F. "The Road from Roe to Casey: America's Abortion Wars," *Irish Reporter* 8 (1992): 16–18.

NIALRA (Northern Ireland Abortion Law Reform Association). *Abortion in Northern Ireland: The Report of an International Tribunal*. Belfast: Beyond the Pale Publications, 1989.

Reid, M. "Abortion Law in Ireland after the Maastricht Referendum." In A. Smyth (ed.), *The Abortion Papers, Ireland*. Dublin: Attic Press, 1992, pp. 25–39.

Rose, R. "Induced Abortion in the Republic of Ireland," *British Journal of Criminology* 18, no. 3 (1978).

Smyth, A. "A Sadistic Farce: Women and Abortion in the Republic of Ireland, 1992." In A. Smyth (ed.), *The Abortion Papers, Ireland*. Dublin: Attic Press, 1992, pp. 7–24.

NETHERLANDS

Evert Ketting

THE HISTORY OF ABORTION LAW

The Struggle for a Liberal Abortion Law

In the Netherlands, induced abortion was a major issue of public and political debate from the late 1960s until 1984, when a new abortion law was finally put into practice (Wet Afbreking Zwangerschap 1981). Since then the issue has almost completely disappeared from the public and political agendas. Abortion has become normal practice, and seems only of interest to the 18,000 women per year in the Netherlands who need an abortion, and to the service providers in the 18 independent abortion clinics, where most of the abortions are carried out. Abortion is almost a dead and forgotten issue in the early 1990s.

In international comparative perspective, however, the case of the Netherlands is rather interesting, and it does attract a lot of attention from abroad. This is mainly because the historical development has been quite different from other countries and because the practice of abortion looks rather paradoxical to outsiders.

Until 1981, when a new abortion bill was finally passed in the Dutch parliament (and enforced only three years later), the legal position of abortion, at least taken literally, was very restrictive.

The old abortion law dated to 1886, when abortion was included in the penal code as a capital offence. In practice, however, the law was difficult to enforce because the crime could hardly be proven. It was necessary to establish that the foetus was alive at the time of the crime, which was almost impossible. For that reason abortion was also legally declared a crime against morality in 1911. Of course, as elsewhere, the law did not really prevent abortion from being performed. Annually during the period from 1920 to 1940 about 80 people were convicted for committing this crime. This number rose to over 200 during the postwar years, but then gradually decreased to just three in 1973. After that, no convictions occurred anymore (de Bruijn 1979).

Abortion became a major public and political issue in the second half of the 1960s (Outshoorn 1986a) as part of a larger process of profound social, cultural, and political change. But there were two immediate reasons to start the discussion on abortion. First, the contraceptive pill had been introduced and became widely accepted during this period, which meant that for the first time doctors became massively involved in family planning. As a result, at least some of them felt more or less responsible for contraceptive failure among their patients and abortion requests presented to them after that. Second, England liberalised its abortion law in 1968, and Dutch women started to travel there to have their unwanted pregnancies terminated. When these travels were made public it caused some scandal, but it also initiated political pressure to change the existing legislation. Furthermore, the hospitals were heavily challenged by emerging social and feminist groups to liberalise their abortion policy, and initiatives were taken by a newly created organisation, Stimezo (Foundation for Medically Safe Abortion), to start an independent abortion clinic (Ketting 1978; Outshoorn 1986a).

On the legal front in the meantime, an initiative of extreme importance had been taken by one of the most outstanding legal experts in the Netherlands, Professor Enschedé. In 1966 he gave a completely new and, to all who were involved, highly surprising interpretation of the existing law. His argument was that the law in fact allowed for induced abortion in the case of medical necessity, although the law did not say so literally. At the time the law was passed, 80 years before, there had been a discussion in the parliament on the question of possible cases of medical necessity. The minister defending the bill at the time had argued that indeed such cases could occur, and it would not be illegal for a doctor to perform an abortion in such a case. But according to this minister, it was not up to the legislator to define these cases of "medical necessity" because medical knowledge and medical opinions would develop over time. Therefore it should be left to the medical profession to decide when an abortion would be necessary. Of course, at the time the old bill was passed, the minister had very severe (life-threatening) cases in mind, but Enschedé argued that in the 80 years since then, professional medical opinions on health and illness had changed dramatically (Enschedé 1966). Therefore the medical profession should make up its mind as to which conditions would make an abortion imperative. The relevant legal authorities basically agreed with this new interpretation of the law, and so paved the way for finding out in practice conditions that would medically indicate an induced abortion. And that was exactly what the medical profession did in the next few years. Starting in 1967, several university hospitals created so-called abortion teams that took abortion requests into consideration and tried to reach consensus on the "medical necessity" of an abortion.

The experimentation within these narrow legal boundaries developed much faster than anybody would have expected. In only a few years a practice evolved of abortion on the request of the woman (Ketting 1978). By 1973 all the abortion teams had been dissolved again because they had made themselves redundant by accepting every abortion request. The narrow legal space had been stretched out in practice to its absolute maximum, leaving politicians with the dilemma of either directly interfering in this practice and turning it back, accepting all the social and political trouble it would cause, or changing the law in accordance with the new, very liberal practice of abortion. However, the politicians proved unable to deal with the situation. It took them 14 years and seven abortion bills to come up with a solution.

The basic political problem was inherent in the Dutch party structure (Roethof 1982). During the 1970s and 1980s there were three major political parties: the Christian Democrats, the Social Democrats, and the Liberals. The Christian Democrats were and still are the centre of the political spectrum. They always participate in coalition cabinets with either the Social Democrats or the Liberals. The Social Democrats and Liberals were never together in power, although they almost always constituted a majority in the parliament because they opposed each other on the important social and economic issues. However, they shared a liberal view on the issue of abortion, in contrast to the rather restrictive stance of the Christian Democrats. As a result, the parties that constituted cabinets always had extreme difficulty forging some compromise on the issue of abortion.

It might be said that during this 14-year period of political struggle, the Liberals and Social Democrats effectively prevented the Christian Democrats from interfering in the evolving practice of abortion services (although they tried every now and then), whereas the Christian Democrats effectively prevented the other parties, through heavy political pressure, from coming up with a liberal private member's initiative and pushing it through. In principle these parties would have been able to do so, because there was definitely a large majority in parliament in favour of a liberal solution.

Only once, in 1976, a Liberal–Social Democratic private member's initiative was taken, which succeeded in the second chamber of the parliament, but then failed a few months later in the first chamber (Senate), allegedly for fear among some Liberal members of not being acceptable anymore as a coalition partner to the Christian Democrats after the forthcoming elections (Outshoorn 1986b).

Finally, after severe difficulties, the Christian Democrats and Liberals forged a basically liberal compromise on the issue in 1981, which was passed in both chambers of the parliament with the smallest majority of votes possible. Most of the members voting against it did so because they felt the bill was still too restrictive.

Since some of the most controversial elements were not resolved in the bill itself—public funding of abortion and the exact wording of the right of the woman to decide—but postponed to be settled definitely in accompanying administrative regulations, it took another three years for these regulations to be finalised and accepted. Therefore the new law came into effect only at the end of 1984.

No serious political attempts have been made since then to alter this law. The major political parties were tired of the subject and happy to close the political book on abortion. Only some very small right-wing Protestant parties, representing a small percentage of the electorate, are still campaigning for a tighter law. But these initiatives are felt by most of the Dutch people to be part of the national folklore. It is very unlikely that any legal change will occur in the foreseeable future.

Creation of Liberal Abortion Services

Before politicians were fully aware of what was actually happening, a system of liberal abortion services had been created that was strong enough to resist attempts to turn back the tide. This all happened during the socially and politically turbulent period between 1967 and 1973, a period of intense cultural renewal that provided a unique climate for change.

The creation in some university hospitals of abortion teams that collectively decided on requests for abortion was an important but only transitional stage in the development of liberal abortion services. For several reasons these teams did not work satisfactorily. First, there were not enough teams to deal with the growing numbers of abortion requests presented once the teams were known to exist. So, many women were still forced to have an illegal abortion or to travel to England. Second, work on the teams—which consisted of a gynaecologist, a psychiatrist, a social worker, the general practitioner for the woman, and sometimes some others as well—was extremely time-consuming and inefficient. And third, many women who had their request denied after lengthy deliberation turned out afterwards to have got their abortion somewhere else. This, of course, made the team feel it had done a useless job.

The work of the teams had been important, however, because as they confronted the actual misery and determination of women with unwanted pregnancies, they tended to become ever more liberal. Several of them finally reached the conclusion that only the pregnant woman herself can decide whether an abortion is medically necessary. The psychiatrists played a prominent role in reaching this conclusion (Ketting 1978).

The teams learned a lesson that was put into practice by another organisation, Stimezo, because the gynaecologists in the few hospitals where abortion teams had been active were not ready to perform all the abortions that were needed. Stimezo was founded in 1969 as a private nonprofit foundation, intending to provide safe medical abortion services. At first it tried to do this through pressure on hospitals, but later it decided to offer abortion services itself. The founders were mainly family doctors who were confronted with abortion requests in their practices, which they could hardly refer to hospitals.

Stimezo started with a large public-information campaign on the need for abortion services, culminating in 1970 in a national television programme that had a fund-raising purpose. With the private donations received through this campaign it started its first abortion clinic in 1971. As this clinic operated on a nonprofit basis and women had to pay for the services, the fees were used to start a second clinic in another part of the country, where the story was repeated. By the end of 1971 there were six abortion clinics; two years later, there were 11 of them; and in 1974, 14 were operating (Schnabel 1976). About two-thirds of these clinics were members of Stimezo; the others were independent. In only three years a strong and highly professional organisation of abortion clinics had been created.

There were four important factors that made it possible for this organisation to survive in the semilegal abortion situation. First, as has been indicated, political interference in this process was weakened by opposing opinions in the parties constituting the successive cabinets during this period.

Second, several leading gynaecologists were pleased at the creation of independent abortion clinics because it relieved them of the pressure to perform the abortions themselves. For that reason they were willing to support and defend these clinics if necessary. General practitioners, not gynaecologists, worked in these clinics. (The number of abortions performed in hospitals, compared to abortion clinics, has decreased since these early years. In 1973, 28 percent of Dutch patients were treated in hospitals; in 1988 this was only 15 percent; Rademakers 1990.)

Third, the defence of these clinics suddenly became a major goal of the rapidly growing feminist movement. In 1976 the minister of justice tried to close one of the Stimezo clinics, but did not succeed because feminist groups immediately occupied the clinic. The occupation (the clinic continued its work in the meantime) led members of the parliament to ask questions about the intentions of the minister, which finally forced the minister to abandon his initiative (Outshoorn 1986a).

Finally, Stimezo itself had grown into quite a strong political pressure group. It was well organized, had highly qualified scientists and political lobbyists among its staff, and had purposefully and effectively created an image of respectability. The organisation had decided to invest heavily in research on abortion. During the period from 1974 to 1991, Stimezo published 47 research reports, most of them on abortion and contraception, and it developed its own abortion reporting system. Furthermore, it produced several films on abortion as well as published a variety of public information material. The outcome of this investment has been an image of Stimezo as a highly professional organisation that knows all the ins and outs of abortion. The media and politicians got to know Stimezo as where a woman turns and learns about abortion. In this way Stimezo became very influential in defining the issue of abortion.

Abortion Services for Women from Abroad

In the early 1970s, abortion was still illegal in almost all of Western Europe. England was the first country to liberalise its abortion law in 1968, soon followed by Denmark (1970 and again in 1973). Austria, France, and Sweden adopted new abortion laws in 1975, West Germany in 1976, and Italy in 1978 (Tietze 1979; Ketting and Van Praag 1985). During these years tens of thousands of women from countries where abortion was still illegal travelled to more liberal countries. In fact, this was happening even before 1968. Swedish and Danish women, for instance, travelled to Poland to have their unwanted pregnancies terminated; Austrian women went to Czechoslovakia for the same reason; and several Dutch women even had abortions in Yugoslavia.

From 1969 to 1973, England became the international country of rescue for women in need of abortion. In 1969, 5,000 women from other countries travelled to England for that reason. Four years later their number had grown to 56,600, most coming from France and West Germany (Tietze 1979). But soon after the first Stimezo clinic was opened the Netherlands started to assume this role. In 1975 the number of abortions on nonresidents in England had dropped to 33,500 (Tietze 1979), whereas during the same year 84,000 foreign women had abortions in Dutch clinics (Ketting and Schnabel 1978). This means that about 300 foreign women per day sought help in the Netherlands. The enormous surge completely changed the character of the Dutch clinics. They became truly international clinics with, on average, only one out of every nine patients a Dutch citizen. Table 1 presents a historic overview of the number of foreign abortion patients who have received treatment in the Netherlands (data preceding 1975 are not systematically available).

Since 1975, the number of foreign patients has dropped year by year as a consequence of legal changes in the other Western European countries. The French legal change as of January 17, 1975, brought a sharp decrease in French women travelling to the Netherlands (or England) in the next year. The new German abortion law, which came into effect on June 21, 1976, had a much more gradual effect. This is because the law did not allow for abortion on request, and practice developed only slowly in a liberal direction. Belgium changed its legislation in April 1990; the effect of this change is therefore not yet visible in the Dutch abortion statistics. It is to be expected that Belgian women will not have to rely on Dutch clinics anymore in the

Table 1
Number of Foreign Women Having Abortions in Dutch Clinics, by Country of Residence, 1975–1988

Year	W.Germ.	Belgium	France	Spain	Other	Total
1975	61,000	12,000	9,000	**	2,000	84,000
1976	60,000*	10,000*	2,000*	**	2,000*	74,000
1977	56,500	8,500	1,200	**	2,300	68,500
1978	42,000	7,900	900	**	1,200	52,000
1979	32,000	7,500	800	**	1,100	41,400
1980	26,200	7,100	500*	2,000*	500*	36,300
1981	20,900	6,600	700*	4,000*	600*	32,200
1982	17,800	6,300	600	4,300	600	29,600
1983	14,600	5,600	600	5,800	400	27,000
1984	11,300	4,900	600	7,300	400	24,500
1985	8,300	5,000	**	6,300	1,000	20,600
1986	7,800	4,700	**	4,600	1,100	19,200
1987	7,000	4,800	**	2,500	1,200	15,500
1988	6,500	4,400	**	1,400	1,400	13,700

*   estimate
** included in "other countries"

Sources: Ketting and Leliveld 1983.
         Ketting and Leseman 1986.
         Rademakers 1990.

near future; however, a whole generation of Belgian women (particularly from the northern half of the country) has been dependent on Dutch clinics since 1971.

The legal changes in other countries have not only caused a quantitative change in abortion requests in the Netherlands but also a qualitative one. In several countries, including West Germany, France, and Spain, abortion at an early stage of pregnancy is now widely available, but it is often difficult to have a pregnancy terminated after 10 to 13 weeks gestational age. Therefore, the women still coming to Dutch clinics are increasingly those in later stages of pregnancy. In 1988, 33 percent of all foreign women treated were 11 or more weeks pregnant; among the Dutch abortion patients, the proportion is only 7.4 percent (Rademakers 1990).

ABORTION: CURRENT LAW AND PRACTICE

The Law of 1984

Unlike in other countries, abortion practice in the Netherlands was liberalised more than a decade before the old abortion law was finally changed.

The 1984 change was basically a legal approval of a practice that evolved from 1970 to 1973—a practice which is among the most liberal in the world. The new law hardly meant any change to abortion practice as it existed since 1973. Every woman can have a medically safe abortion up to about the 20th week of pregnancy, without facing significant barriers.

The structure of the current abortion law is such that abortion remains a criminal offence as long as it is not performed in a licenced clinic or hospital. In this case the person who performs the abortion is punishable with several years imprisonment. The woman herself never faces punishment. In a licensed institution the abortion is not punishable as long as a medical doctor performs the treatment.

Any hospital or clinic can apply for a licence, but it should fulfill certain requirements in order to receive and keep it. Some legal regulations are part of these requirements:

1. An abortion is permissible only if the pregnant woman is in "a situation of emergency" that cannot be resolved in another way. This means that the law does not stipulate any specific indications for abortion (as in England or West Germany), but just a general one. Furthermore, the law does not give more precise definition of this "situation of emergency." In fact, with this rule the legislator has formulated only the morality beyond abortion. It is not a rule that can be or has ever been enforced in practice.

2. The woman decides whether such a situation of emergency exists; the doctor has to counsel the woman on possible alternative solutions, and she or he has to make sure the woman has made her decision on her own free will and in a responsible manner. In the social and political debate preceding this new law, the question of who finally decides on abortion—the woman or the doctor—was the most intensely disputed one. The wording of the answer gives the woman priority over the doctor. The latter has only to check the woman's free decision.

3. The woman has to wait five days after her abortion request to think things over before having the abortion. In fact, this rule made the only real change in the practice of abortion that existed previously. Abortion service providers and feminist groups protested this heavily, but they did not succeed. The five-day waiting period more or less became the symbol of legislative power to change the practice of abortion. But even this rule has been made partly ineffective. A few years later the government accepted that so-called menstrual regulations—treatments performed within 16 days following the woman's missed period—would not need this waiting period. In practice, this was an important decision because about one in every five abortions is a "menstrual regulation" (Rademakers 1990). To prevent misinterpretation, it should be stressed here that these menstrual regulations have always been included in the abortion statistics.

4. Abortions are permitted until the foetus is viable (in practice, an upper limit of 22 weeks gestation). Hospitals and clinics that want to perform abor-

tions after the 12th week of pregnancy must meet some extra technical and organisational requirements. These are quite easy to meet, so that until now no request for this special permit has been denied.

5. There is no legal barrier to women from abroad having an abortion in the Netherlands. This is quite important, as most abortions in Dutch clinics are being performed on foreign women, although their number has gradually been decreasing as a result of legal changes in surrounding countries.

6. All abortions have to be reported to the General Health Inspector every three months. These data are strictly anonymous; only accumulated statistical data are presented.

7. After adoption and enforcement of the new law, the parliament decided that the Ministry of Health should fund all abortions on Dutch citizens. Since 1985 abortion is free for Dutch women; women from abroad still have to pay for it.

By and large, the 1981–84 abortion law changed the existing abortion practice marginally. The five-day waiting period was a defeat for those campaigning for a liberal abortion law, but the decision on government funding was a victory. Almost all other rules can be characterised as the legalisation of existing practice, thereby ridding the abortion services of their previous "semi-legal" character.

Abortion in Practice

There are hardly any obstacles for women getting an abortion. The usual way is for the woman to consult her family doctor first. (Many women have already decided by then that they want to have the pregnancy terminated; almost all women know abortion is legally available.) She discusses her situation with this doctor who, if she wants, gives her a referral note for an abortion clinic and the address and telephone number. She then makes an appointment by telephone with the clinic for the treatment about a week later (or earlier if her last period was less than six weeks before), and she is given some practical information. A few days later she goes to the clinic to have the abortion, which usually takes only about two hours (intake, medical examination, operation under local anaesthesia, and a short rest), after which she goes home again. After about two weeks she has a follow-up examination, either in the clinic or at her family doctor, the decision for which is left up to her. She doesn't have to pay for the treatment, and there is very little red tape. The abortion clinic is usually close by. (Holland is a small country and has 18 abortion clinics.) As a result, most abortions are performed very early in a pregnancy—almost 80 percent before the 8th week of pregnancy, and only 1.3 percent after the 15th week (Rademakers 1990).

Of course, there are some exceptions to this rule. Some women do not want to consult their family doctor, and a few family doctors are opposed to abortion. In that case she can either go to a family planning clinic to get

Table 2
Number of Abortions, Abortion Rate, and Abortion Ratio Among Dutch
Residents, 1971–1988

Year	No.	Per 1,000 Women 15-44 Years	Per 100 Known Pregnancies
1971*	16,500	6.1	6.8
1975	15,000	5.2	8.3
1980	21,300	6.7	10.5
1981	21.100	6.5	10.7
1982	20,700	6.3	10.8
1983	19,500	5.9	10.1
1984	18,700	5.6	9.7
1985	17,300	5.1	8.8
1986	18,300	5.3	9.0
1987	17,800	5.1	9.5
1988	18,000	5.1	9.7

* estimate

Sources: Ketting and Leseman 1986.
          Rademakers 1990.

a referral or make an appointment directly with a clinic, in which case she has to go there twice (first for a consultation and six days later for the operation). The family planning clinics refer about 7 percent of the abortion patients.

About 15 percent of all Dutch women are referred to a hospital instead of an abortion clinic, for a simple historical reason: a few hospitals continued performing abortions after they started it around 1970, and the family doctors in their vicinity are used to referring their patients there.

If a woman is rather late in pregnancy (more than about 13 weeks of pregnancy, 2.5 percent of all women), she will be referred to one of the three specialised clinics. Only if she is very late in pregnancy will she have to stay in this clinic overnight (only 0.3 percent of all abortions in clinics). On the other hand, the 15 percent who are treated in a hospital have a fair chance of having to stay there overnight (40 percent of all hospital abortions; Rademakers 1990).

It is almost needless to say that refusal of abortion requests (except in the extremely rare case of more than 22 weeks of pregnancy) or illegal abortions never occur. Only in a case where the woman is forced (for example, by her parents), but does not want the abortion herself, will she not get it.

The incidence of abortion among Dutch residents has always been remarkably low (Table 2). The abortion rate is less than half the English rate, almost a fourth of the Danish and Swedish rates, and less than a fifth of the rate in the United States (Henshaw and Morrow 1990). This is explained largely by the unprecedented high use of modern reliable contraceptives (Ketting and van Praag 1985).

Among the Dutch-born population, abortion is even lower, since 40 percent of all abortions among Dutch residents are performed on women who have immigrated to the Netherlands. These immigrants constitute only about 8 percent of the Dutch population. Abortion rates for the ethnic groups are three (for Moroccan) to nine (for Caribbean) times as high as among the Dutch born (Rademakers 1990).

The abortion rate among teenagers is also extremely low at just four per 1,000 15- to 19-year-old girls. In England and Sweden this rate is 5 times as high, and in the United States 11 times (Henshaw and Morrow 1990). This very low incidence has been attributed mainly to the general openness regarding questions of sexuality and to the availability and accessibility of contraceptive services in the Netherlands (Jones et al. 1986).

Attitudes Towards Abortion

The general attitude toward abortion grew more accepting during the process of liberalisation. In 1970, 43 percent of the population agreed that a woman should have the right to choose an abortion if she wants it; in 1980 this was 55 percent, and at that level the attitude of the population stabilised (van Delft 1991).

These figures tell us more about general tolerance in Dutch culture and society toward other people's behaviour than about people's feeling about abortion in their personal lives. Tolerance of what others want to do for themselves—as long as it does not immediately affect yourself—is an outstanding feature of Dutch mentality, which is deeply rooted in the history of the country and its culture. It is linked to a long history of trading with different cultures, with different values, beliefs, and modes of behaviour, that demands tolerance in order not to jeopardize commercial interests. It is also closely linked to the fact that the Netherlands has been half Roman Catholic and half Protestant since its emergence as an independent state in the 16th century. Dutch society could hardly exist and survive as a coherent entity without its strong sense of "let my neighbour do it his or her way, and let me do it my way." This strong cultural trait is also important in explaining, for instance, the extremely liberal attitude toward homosexuality compared to other countries. No fewer than 93 percent of the population subscribes to the statement that "homosexuals should have maximum freedom in deciding on how they want to live." But one should not make the mistake of concluding from this that homosexuality is generally accepted; this means that it is tolerated. "They" are allowed to do what "they" want (as long as it does not affect me).

The same is true, to a large extent, for abortion. In a national survey of 20- to 40-year-old women, Vennix (1990) asked these women first how they felt in general about the right to choose on abortion. Fifty-five percent of them replied that the woman (with her partner) should have this right. But when then asked what they themselves would do in the case of an unplanned pregnancy, only 15 percent said they would probably or definitely have that pregnancy terminated. This indicates that many women tolerate abortion (for other women) but do not accept it (for themselves).

When it comes to actually being confronted with an unplanned pregnancy, a larger share of women choose to have an abortion. In Vennix's survey, 29 percent of the women who had had an unwanted pregnancy chose to have an abortion; but in another survey, carried out in 1982, only 17 percent of the women replied that they had their unplanned pregnancy terminated by abortion (CBS 1984). From the annual numbers of actually reported abortions, compared to those mentioned in these surveys, it can be concluded that a significant percentage of women do not admit their abortion experience in these surveys. This indicates that many women are ashamed to admit this experience.

All these survey data point in the same direction: abortion for most women is an option, but one that should never be used. They are not ready to count on this possibility. Probably this is one of most important factors explaining the highly effective contraceptive use of Dutch couples compared to couples in other countries (Ketting and van Praag 1985) and the extremely low rate of unplanned pregnancies (Jones et al. 1988).

THE FUTURE

Abortion in the Netherlands has been and still is different from many other countries in at least two ways. Abortion was liberalised in practice many years before it was legalised, and the need for abortion among Dutch citizens is extremely low. These two features are to some extent connected to each other.

As the politicians were for many years unable to solve the legal question of abortion, the problem of induced abortion was not defined as one that should be solved by making it legal, but instead by preventing it! During the long period of political struggle and disagreement, there was general agreement that contraceptive use should be improved to make abortions unnecessary. As a consequence, investments in improving contraceptive services and contraceptive education, and in family planning research and information, have been extensive. These investments have definitely paid off. At the same time, this long period of semi-illegality of abortion strengthened the existing view of abortion as a method only to be used as a last resort.

At the same time, the incidence of induced abortion is extremely low in the Netherlands; only one out of every six women, on average, will ever have an abortion during her lifetime, and that is far less than in any other country in the world where abortion is legal. One might say that abortion is acceptable in the Netherlands but not accepted. Couples do everything they can to prevent abortion, and they are very effective in that respect, although they will not face any difficulty in getting an abortion if they wish so. The case of the Netherlands is the best example in the world to indicate that complete liberalisation of abortion can be combined with a modest need for it (Ketting and Schnabel 1980; Ketting 1982).

This current situation and its historic background make it rather unlikely that there will be any significant change in the foreseeable future. All the major political parties are satisfied with having solved the problem after so much difficulty, and they definitely do not want to start again. As far as possible, the problem is under control, after having been settled in the typical Dutch way: the pragmatic way.

REFERENCES

CBS. *Onderzoek gezinsvorming 1982* (Survey on family growth 1982). Den Haag: Staatsuitgeverij, 1984.

de Bruin, J. *Geschiedenis van abortus in Nederland* (History of abortion in the Netherlands). Amsterdam: Van Gennep, 1979.

Enschedé, Ch. J. "Abortus op medische indicatie en strafrecht" (Abortion on medical indication and criminal law), *Nederlands Tijdschrift voor Geneeskunde* 110 (1966):1349–53.

Henshaw, S. K., and E. Morrow. *Induced Abortion: A World Review*, 1990 Supplement. New York: Alan Guttmacher Institute, 1990.

Jones, E. F., J. D. Forrest, N. Goldman, et al. *Teenage Pregnancy in Industrialized Countries*. New Haven: Yale University Press, 1986.

Jones, E. F., J. D. Forrest, and S. K. Henshaw. "Unintended Pregnancy, Contraceptive Practice and Family Planning in Developed Countries," *Family Planning Perspectives* 20, no. 2 (1988):53–67.

Ketting, E. *Van misdrijf tot hulpverlening* (From crime to assistance). Alphen a/d Rijn: Samsom, 1978.

———. "Contraception and Fertility in the Netherlands," *International Family Planning Perspectives* 8, no. 4 (1982):141–47.

Ketting, E., and F. Leliveld. *Abortus en anticonceptie anno 1982* (Abortion and contraception in 1982). Den Haag: Stimezo Nederland, 1983.

Ketting, E., and P. Leseman. *Abortus en anticonceptie 1983/84* (Abortion and contraception 1983/84). Den Haag: Stimezo Nederland, 1986.

Ketting, E., and P. Schnabel. *De abortushulpverlening in 1977* (Abortion services in 1977). Den Haag: Stimezo Nederland, 1978.

———. "Induced Abortion in the Netherlands: A Decade of Experience, 1970–80," *Studies in Family Planning* 11, no. 12 (1980):385–94.

Ketting, E., and Ph. van Praag. *Schwangerschaftsabbruch, Gesetz und Praxis im internationalen Vergleich* (Induced abortion, law and practice in international perspective). Tübingen: DGVT-Verlag, 1985.

Outshoorn, J. "De politieke strijd rondom de abortuswetgeving in Nederland 1964–
1984" (The political struggle over abortion legislation in the Netherlands
1964–1984). Dissertation, Free University of Amsterdam 1986a.
———. "The new politics of abortion." In J. Lovenduski and J. Outshoorn (eds.),
The New Politics of Abortion. London: Sage 1986b, pp. 1–26.
Rademakers, J. *Abortus in Nederland 1987/1988* (Abortion in the Netherlands 1987/
1988). Utrecht: Stimezo Nederland, 1990.
Roethof, H. J. *De abortuskwestie en meer dan dat* (The question of abortion and more
than that). Den Haag: Stimezo Nederland, 1982.
Schnabel, P. *Abortus in Nederland* (Abortion in the Netherlands). Den Haag: Stimezo
Nederland, 1976.
Tietze, Chr. *Induced Abortion: 1979*, Third ed., New York: Population Council, 1979.
van Delft, M. L. E. *Sociale atlas van de vrouw* (Social atlas of women). Rijswijk: Sociaal
en Cultureel Planbureau, 1991.
Vennix, P. *De pil en haar alternatieven* (The pill and its alternatives). Delft: Eburon,
1990.
Wet Afbreking Zwangerschap. (Law on the Termination of Pregnancy), Staatsblad,
n. 257, 1981.

NORWAY

Brita Gulli

THE HISTORY OF ABORTION LAW

The Penal Code and Proposals for Reform

Women's fight for self-determination goes far back in history. In 1915, the well-known Norwegian feminist Katti Anker Møller proposed that women who tried to have an abortion should not to be punished. She did not argue for women's self-determination directly, but her demand for decriminalisation was based on this principle.[1] Her proposal was provocative at the time and was much discussed. One medical doctor argued that doctors should not be put in the position of "servants of women with erotic adventures." But this debate in the leading, conservative morning paper was stopped because it involved "terms and expressions that ought not to be printed." Morality, especially women's sexual morality, was the main concern. The debate led to no legal changes. Abortion was regarded as basically illegal and punished according to the penal code. In some very few cases, on strict medical indications, doctors performed abortions.

In 1935, a government commission proposed an abortion law to regulate and liberalise the practice of abortion. Doctors were granted the right to perform abortions. This proposal was the first effort to regulate abortion in the modern sense. This need for regulation came about for several reasons.

First, it seemed that illegal, backstreet abortions, with their dangerous medical consequences, were on the increase. This was calculated on the basis of women brought to hospitals with fever and ongoing abortions. The operations were regarded as having been performed by someone other than a doctor and therefore illegal. These calculations are, of course, always unsure, particularly since the number of hospitals was on the increase also at this time. It became more usual to use them. But medically dangerous abortions were definitely a problem, not least because economic hardship made life more difficult for women than before.

Second, the control of abortion instituted in the penal code decreased as illegal abortions seemed to increase. Most illegal abortions were not discovered anyway, and in practice the judges became less and less willing to punish women for trying to get an abortion through illegal channels.

Third, the number of abortions performed by doctors was on the increase. Abortion used to be performed as an alternative to caesarian section, a dangerous operation. One might have thought that the development of modern, safe surgery and modern hygiene, speeding up at this time, would reduce the number of abortions performed by doctors. But the actual development went in the opposite direction. Doctors expanded the medical indications for abortion, and they needed a law to regulate as well as to legalise this expansion in their medical practice. Actually, the law proposal originated from the leader of the Norwegian Association of Surgeons. The decision was put in the hands of the doctors. The scope of the medical grounds was increased and other, new indications were added: social, ethical, and eugenic. The proposal was indeed a liberalisation.

This proposal met strong opposition, but some of the indications were more provocative than others. Interestingly, the eugenic indications were not discussed much, perhaps because this way of thinking was very usual in the whole of Europe and North America between the wars. What was criticised was the independent use of social indications—meaning that a woman could have an abortion for economic reasons, an alcoholic husband, bad housing, and so on. Even unmarried women could possibly get an abortion on social grounds.

The proposed law was supported by many radical women, coming partly from the labour movement, partly from the middle class and more bourgeois backgrounds. The radical wing of feminists, from both socialist and bourgeois quarters, found even this proposal too moderate and demanded full self-determination. But the proposal was supported by many leading representatives from the legal profession. Their view was that abortion was not a matter to be dealt with through the penal code, part of a change in perspective as regards the proper use of the penal code and punishment compared to other methods of social control. In this period in Norwegian society, the penal system in general was restricted, actions were decriminalised, and a more modern view on deviant behaviour was introduced. Such behaviour should be controlled and regulated, and preferably hindered through a system of modern social policies; help was as important as control.

Several medical doctors supported the proposal, particularly surgeons, while other groups within the medical profession were much more critical.

Many were, in fact, critical of the surgeons' general tendency to operate instead of treating the patient. Some also felt that to perform abortion on social indications was outside their professional role. Many of the critical doctors were Christians as well, and much of the opposition came from Christian quarters. The fundamentalist groups in particular constituted very active opposition. Abortion should be restricted as much as possible, they argued. The beginning of life had to be protected. They feared that legalisation of the social indications would make Christian marriage break down.

The First Abortion Law, 1960

The proposed law never passed the parliament; the whole process was broken off by the war. In 1948, after the war, the Women's Rights Organisation asked the government to continue work on abortion reform. A new government proposal was presented in 1956. This was a carbon copy of the prewar proposal, including the social indications. And in 1960, the first Norwegian abortion law passed the parliament. It was not very different from the original proposal, except in one respect: when the act reached parliament, the social indications were taken out, and instead so-called sociomedical indications were introduced, stressing that abortion may be performed only on some kind of medical indication, even if this was stretched quite far compared to dominant views in the 1930s. This change reflected the interests of the medical profession and changes in their understanding of what medicine was about. They did not want an independent social indication, as this would imply that social workers would have a say in the decision. Indeed, a proposal along these lines had come from the public health authorities.

It has often been argued in Norway that the Christian opposition has had great influence in the abortion question compared to, for example, Sweden or Denmark, where Christians as a political force are much weaker. Looking at the content of this law, one has to conclude that it was a "doctors' law," even if the Christian opposition may have delayed the reform process. The law secured the doctors' professional autonomy within the context of a growing sociomedical perspective in the profession itself. This perspective had been much less pronounced in the 1930s; at that time the medical profession was split on what was technically possible and ideologically acceptable. The sociomedical perspective of the 1950s bridged that gap. The Christian opposition wanted the indications for abortion much more restricted. They also wanted a member of the local church councils (a body within the state church) to take part in the abortion commissions' decisions. They lost on both points. After the war, the Christian opposition was the only group still favouring an old-fashioned form of control—that is, extended use of punishment. With the new law, the process of redefining the abortion question, that started between the wars, of bringing it out of the penal code and into the arena of social policy, was completed.

Formally, abortion was a criminal offence for the woman herself as well as for everyone who did not follow regulations. But in practical terms it was a sleeping paragraph. Women having illegal abortions were not prosecuted; indeed, very few abortionists were punished. A total of two persons (both women) were punished according to these paragraphs in 1954. But statistics showed that criminal abortions were increasing, from 600 in 1920 to 7,300 in 1954. (The Norwegian population was about 3 million.) The redefinition of abortion reflected a basic change of attitude with regard to the legitimacy and usefulness of the penal system. The government commission even argued that doctors' commissions should be used to persuade the women who did not obtain a legal abortion not to go to backstreet abortionists. Thus, the new law was an attempt to contain "the abortion wave." Help and control were part of the same system—help for women with legitimate needs, control of women with illegitimate needs.

It was a Labour government that decided to drop the social indications and also generally side with the medical profession. In doing this, the party elite took sides against their own women's and youth organisations, who supported the social indications on the grounds that only these could actually help the 7,000 women each year who underwent illegal abortions. Why did the party elite do this? And what was the political situation among the different women's organisations? Had the agreement among feminists of different social classes of the 1930s disappeared?

A major difference between the 1930s and the 1950s was that after the war no one spoke about a woman's right to decide. "Social indications to help women in need" was the most liberal abortion demand in the 1950s. It was supported by many women's organisations from the labour movement, the Labour party, as well as the unions. After the war many of these women's organisations cooperated with bourgeois organisations under an umbrella called the Cooperation Committee.[2]

All types of groups were members of the Cooperative Committee: women's organisations connected to political parties, unions of women, Christian women's organisations like the Girl Guides, the Women's Rights Organisation, the National Women's Council, to name some. But the abortion question split this cooperative effort beginning in the early 1950s. Again, it was the social indications that became the point of conflict. Some of the Christian women's organisations managed to stop the question from being decided. They were afraid of a liberal result, a decision in favour of social indications. Meanwhile, the women's labour organisations declined to use their greater numerical power to bring about a decision to match their wishes; they did not attend the relevant meeting. Instead, they used the abortion question as an excuse to leave the committee. They relied on the Labour party, which in 1949 had done well in the general election, obtaining a majority of 85 of a total of 150 seats in the parliament.

Several factors may explain why the labour organisations dropped out. The committee had become ineffective. The abortion question was only one example of how difficult it was to get concerted action on a question. The Labour party's success in the election, and the fact that it moved from being a traditional class party to a more social democratic one, made it more attractive as an instrument for furthering the interests of labour women. Traditional loyalty must also have been of significance. The decision on the part of these women to leave the committee excluded the possibility of a broader alliance among women of different classes to work on the abortion question (see Løvik 1976).

From the perspective of numbers in parliament, the compromise made by the Labour party elite was unnecessary. The Labour majority established itself in the 1950s. In this period, it became "the carrier of the state"; every election was a sure winner. But in order to do this, the party made ideological compromises, and siding with the medical profession on the abortion question is only one example.

The abortion law of 1960 passed parliament with the support of Labour and some members of other parties, namely Conservatives and Liberals. The Christian People's party and the Centre party (agrarians), along with the rest of the Conservatives and Liberals, constituted the opposition. The compromise for the doctors had not produced wider support, after all.

The New Women's Movement and Demands for Further Change

The law was put into operation in 1964, but only a few years later the conflicts started again. The old demand of "a woman's right to self-determination" was put on the political agenda, this time by two different groups of women. In 1969 individual women from the Labour party demanded self-determination. (At this time the official stand of the women's organisation within the party was limited to supporting social indications.) By the early 1970s the new women's movement started public campaigns demanding self-determination as a political right, the old demand from early in the century.

Within the new movement, there was disagreement over the reasons for abortion. Women who were members of the Maoist party, the Marxist-Leninists, argued that the right to abortion was dependent on the social system and that abortion would not be necessary under socialism—that is, they argued from needs, and saw abortion as some kind of a sociopolitical reform. Women of a more radical—that is, feminist—persuasion argued that women had the right to decide, since they were the ones giving birth, and that this was independent of the social system. To the feminists, the idea that socialism would make abortion unnecessary was only another version of patriarchal control. Women's self-determination was a right women had as a group; it was a political right they were entitled to as women.

This discussion was important in clarifying ideological positions among the different groups and, in fact, related to the basic theoretical and political disagreements of the 1970s: was class or sex the most important factor in women's oppression? Despite disagreement over the reasons, agreement on the aim—women's self-determination—was the basis for much common political activity. Up to 1974, demonstrations were held in various parts of the country. The participants were not women exhausted by having and raising five children or women from the upper classes talking of behalf of other women. The participants were young women from differing social backgrounds, demanding—not asking—for abortion.

In the public debates, the central theme was women's rights, not needs. One important reason for this was that, in many areas of the country, particularly the more urban ones, the doctors' commissions accepted almost all applications for abortion. One could not argue any longer that doctor-controlled abortion represented "protection of life," as the Christians again did. Since the commissions accepted most applications, women might as well decide themselves, unless control was the important factor. And in many ways it seemed that this was exactly what the Christian opposition wanted, too. They talked, and still talk, about "social institutions" deciding the abortion question. But many women had experienced the humiliation of the doctors' commissions, most of whose members were men.

This state of affairs made the Christian arguments seem patriarchal. It was aggravated by the fact that there was no equality before the law. In some conservative regions the commissions' decisions were strict, while in the urban centres they were liberal, resulting in some immigration of women to the capital to get an abortion. The differences were not related to class but to where women lived; in the west and south, the doctors were more conservative. These are also areas where Christian groups are politically strong. And there were both kind and unkind doctors; some general practitioners agreed to apply on behalf of the pregnant woman while others did not. Women could not apply to the commissions themselves.

In 1974, a proposal based on women's self-determination reached the parliament, but it was voted down. Again, the Christian opposition managed to delay the process. Only in 1978, after a parliamentary election, did the new law pass.

ABORTION: CURRENT LAW AND PRACTICE

The Law of 1978

Norwegian women have the right to self-determination until the end of the 12th week of pregnancy. After that, the decision-making power is transferred to a commission of two medical doctors. The indications for abortion after the 12the week are medical, sociomedical, eugenic, and so-called criminal or ethical (if the pregnancy results from rape or some other form of sexual intercourse forbidden in the penal code). After the 18th week of pregnancy, abortion is allowed only for very serious reasons. If there is a chance that the foetus may live, abortion is forbidden. Abortion after the 18th week is legal on eugenic grounds and based on the outcome of amniocentesis, a test which cannot be performed early in the pregnancy. There is no obligatory counselling procedure that the woman has to go through. On the contrary, the law supposes that women are offered advice and information.

Abortion is always performed free of charge and is obtained through the national health system. Illegal abortion is not punishable in the case of the pregnant woman herself; indeed, women who have had illegal abortions have not been punished since the 1930s. Other people who perform an illegal abortion may still be punished with fines or three months in jail. But illegal abortions in the traditional sense of backstreet, medically dangerous abortions do not exist in Norway anymore. What has alarmed public authorities, and people in general recently, is the expanding use of amniocentesis and ultrasound which leads to abortions. I discuss this further in the final section of this article.

Women's self-determination was introduced into the law in 1978. It is now easy for women to obtain medically safe abortions within the first 12 weeks. The old class differences between women are gone. The law also gives the health worker the right to refuse to participate in the operation, and this may have made it difficult for some women in the more Christian areas of the country; but on the whole, a woman's right to decide within the first 12 weeks is well established.

Abortion in Practice

An argument frequently used against a woman's right to decide has been that the number of abortions would increase. The Norwegian experience shows that that is not the case. In Figure 1, the data before 1979 include all accepted applications for abortion. After 1979, the figures include all abortions performed by doctors, since the system for applying for an abortion disappeared in 1978. While the number of abortions rose in the late 1960s and early 1970s, the number stabilized before the new law was instituted. And after the new law, the number of abortions went down to about 15,000 per year.

The rate of abortion is dependent on many factors. Because doctors accepted most applications for abortion in the period before the new law, the predicted increase did not come about. In addition, there is the demographic factor. The number of abortions as a proportion of the number of women in child-bearing ages decreased beginning in 1977. Only in the late 1980s was there a slight rise, and then only in absolute numbers. This increase is probably due to an increased number of women of childbearing age; the relative number of abortions changed very little in the 1980s.

Figure 1
Number of Abortions, Abortions per 1,000 Women 15–49 Years of Age, and per 100 Pregnancies, 1968–1989

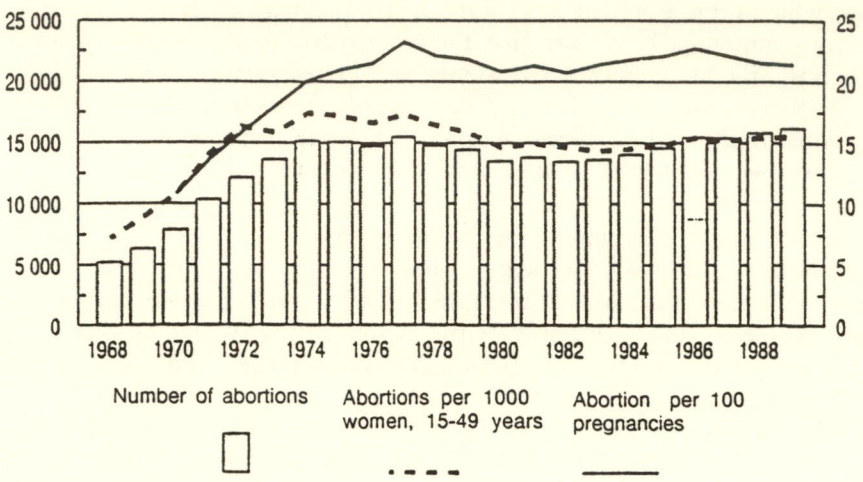

Source: Kristiansen 1991.

Seen in relation to the number of pregnancies, the number of abortions in Norway has decreased. This is due to a slight baby boom in the last few years. Whether this baby boom will continue is uncertain, since some of these births may be due to so-called postponed childbearing. Among those seeking abortion is an increasing number of young women, between 20 and 29 years and particularly between 20 and 24 years. Teenage abortions have not increased. Among women above 30, the figures are stable or decreasing. This development means a change; older married women with several children used to seek abortion in the early 1970s. At that time, however, the legal regulations meant that it was easier for these women to obtain a legal abortion on so-called sociomedical grounds.

The women having abortions are also, to a great extent, single and without children. A survey by the Norwegian Central Bureau of Statistics (Kristiansen 1991) suggests that the increased frequency of abortion among young women is because these women experience unwanted pregnancies during higher education. Relative to the population of women as a whole, the young women are more likely not to be married or cohabiting, nor capable of supporting a child financially. Sales of contraceptive pills have not decreased. Incidentally, it should also be noted that more women students than ever before have children and study on a part-time basis.

Figure 2
Number of Abortions per 1,000 Women of Childbearing Age in Nordic Countries, 1975–1989

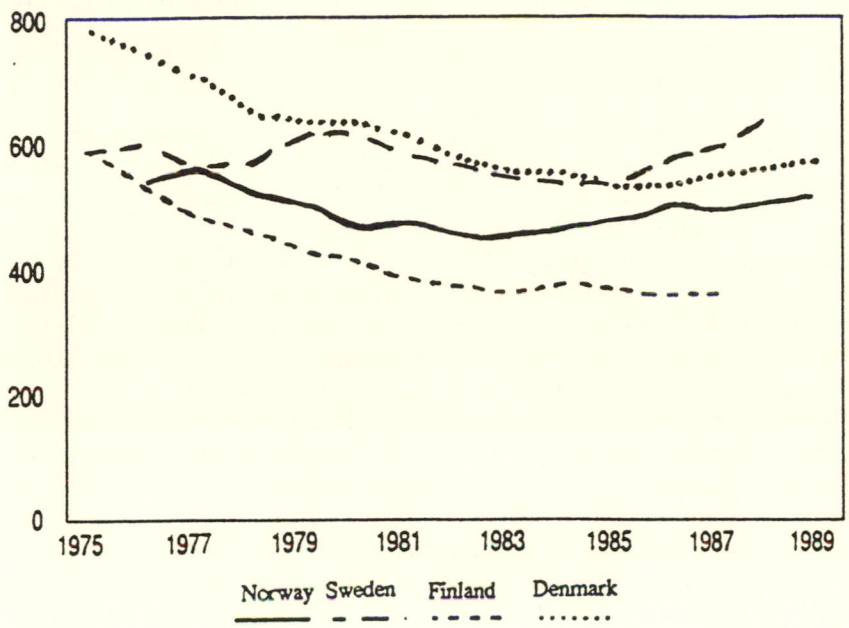

Source: Kristiansen 1991.

One way of getting the number of abortions down—an aim everybody agrees with—would be to improve government-subsidised student loans, as well as to improve the present levels of social security payment for single mothers. Single mothers—those not cohabiting with the father—have a legally defined right to support by the national social security system until the child is 10 years old. The money, however, is not enough to live on, particularly in big cities. For this reason, many single mothers apply for supplementary benefits. Proper payment plus proper development of day care for children would improve the situation.

As Figure 2 reveals, the Norwegian abortion figures are not particularly high when compared to other Nordic countries. This takes into account the changing age composition of the population, and therefore the proportion of women of childbearing age. As can be seen, all countries show a decrease in the number of abortions after 1975, and then an increase later in the

1980s. But Sweden and Denmark introduced self-determination for women earlier than Norway—at the beginning of the 1970s. (Finland still has legally regulated indications.) The number of abortions is therefore not directly connected to the legal situation. As history shows, other factors are at work.

The Politics of Abortion

A women's right to decide during the first 12 weeks has become an accepted right in Norway, even though the Centre party and the Christian People's party are still against it. But even within these parties the attitudes have become more liberal over the last 20 years. Another case illustrating the acceptance of this right is the fact that two priests employed by the Norwegian state church (Protestant) lost their jobs after having used extreme and emotion-laden actions to agitate against the new law. (They buried small dolls and used the Sunday sermon to argue against the law.) One of them also lost the right to preach.

In this way, the state church wanted to demonstrate its authority over dissident priests. The anti-abortion actions have also embarrassed more liberal priests. Recently several conservative priests within the state church have organised; they are against the present law as well as against woman priests. (We now have many women priests, and are discussing the first woman bishop.) Of course, this makes the battle lines pretty clear and confirms the suspicion of many women that conservative priests are against a woman's power to speak and decide. The actions of these priests do not reflect concern over the increased number of abortions, since these numbers did not rise after the present law was passed. Recently, a proposed new law from the Christian People's party to restrict abortion was voted down in the parliament. This action expressed the attitude and power of many women, including women politicans who favour the present law. Women members now constitute 34 percent of the Norwegian parliament.

THE FUTURE

In many Eastern European countries a woman's right to choose is now under attack. In Poland, the attack comes from the Catholic Church and from Solidarity, the union famous for its radical actions. This organisation has decided that there is a "need to protect unborn life," and it recently stopped its own women's group from speaking out against the proposed restrictions on abortion. In Slovenia, a concern over the "holiness of life" relates to nationalism. And similar tendencies are found in Turkey. In France, the abortion issue is related to ethnic and racial conflicts. As West German prohibitions on abortion are introduced in former East Germany, a woman's choice will be further restricted. It is, of course, nothing new that women's creative ability—the power to create babies—is important for a male group's quest for power, particularly when it comes to nation building. Women are indispensable for group continuity. They give birth; they are the connection between the generations. But when these groups become nationalist groups—that is, to the extent that group identity and personal identity are tied to the creation or continuation of a specific political system, state, or nation—women's self-determination comes under siege.

But there is also a new abortion debate under way related to the new gene research and reproductive technologies. This is an international development that implies new medical possibilities for intervention, earlier and more deeply into the pregnancy. Feminists have pointed to an increased tendency to sever the connection between the women and the foetus, and to fragment the meaning of motherhood.

Technological changes have their legal counterparts, too. Owing to the increased possibilities of intervention, the "rights of the foetus" are increasingly debated. In several countries laws have been passed to regulate research on foetuses and embryos resulting from IVF (In Vitro Fertilisation) procedures. What is forgotten is that the medical technology and the research are being performed on women's bodies.

Norwegian laws regulating these new technologies are comparatively strict. Research on embryos is forbidden. Egg donation is forbidden. Surrogacy contracts would be contrary to adoption laws. But public authorities as well as the general population have been alarmed by the increase in so-called late abortions performed after amniocentesis—long after the time limit for self-determination. The government has asked for more restricted practice on the part of the doctors' commissions that administer the law, but the law itself has not been changed. Some people even argue for a restriction on a woman's right to self-determination before the 12th week, on the grounds that new methods of discovering genetic diseases before this time will mean an increase in abortions on genetic grounds.

Recently the government has proposed allowing both egg donation and research on fertilized eggs. What is important, from the woman's point of view, is that the new technology (and it is the medical profession and medical researchers who are the dynamic factor here, not women) brings to life again a very old argument: women are not capable of deciding themselves, now because of complicated technology and the ethical dilemmas involved. Selective abortion, through amniocentesis and other methods, is certainly a scary consequence of the new genetic technology. But instead of people discussing the principles involved, the technology is introduced pragmatically and the decision making is vested in the medical profession and the ethical committees. This situation is the bases of much criticism of the present abortion law: the new genetic technology should be used, but should be controlled by boards and ethical committees, not by women as individuals. Future abortion debate will center on these problems.

For women, many questions arise. What type of technology should be introduced? How can we ensure that the technology introduced is not used to restrict a pregnant woman's freedom, instead of restricting technological expansion? Is technology that women cannot control acceptable at all?

NOTES

1. This historical overview is based on my thesis, "The History of the Abortion Law," Institute of Political Science, University of Oslo, 1979.

2. *Norske kvinneorganisasjoners samarbeidsnemnd.*

REFERENCES

Kristiansen, J. E. "Okende abortfrekvens?" (Increased frequency of abortion?), *Samfunnsspeilet* (The Social Mirror) 1 (1991).

Løvik, M. "The Norwegian Women's Organizations Cooperation Committee 1945–1953," thesis in history, University of Bergen, 1976.

POLAND

Jolanta Plakwicz and Eleonora Zielińska

THE HISTORY OF ABORTION LAW

The Era of Liberal Abortion

Poland traditionally has had relatively liberal abortion legislation. Already in the 19th century, the first sovereign penal code of 1818, in line with the views of the Enlightment, reflected a humanitarian approach to punishment for abortion.[1]

In 1932, after a long and heated discussion dominated by physicians, criminologists, and journalists, the penal codification of independent Poland abandoned the idea of complete protection of the foetus as a human being. Exceptions to the prohibition of abortion were introduced, and the penalty for illegal abortion was set at three years of imprisonment for a woman and five years for a practitioner, provided the abortion was performed with the woman's consent. The draft included the following indications: danger to the woman's health, pregnancy resulting from a criminal offence (e.g., rape and incest), as well as social indications described as "the difficult economic situation of a woman." The last of these was quite unusual for the time. The social indication was not included in the final text of the code, but its appearance in the draft meant that the authors were aware of the problem.[2]

After World War II, the provisions on abortion in the penal code remained untouched for the next 11 years in spite of the change in political system, as well as the fact that the abortion debate was soon resumed. In the beginning, the debate was dominated by people demanding further restrictions on abortion. The reasons cited included the need to restore the population, which had declined as a result of the war, and as was claimed in Catholic circles, to stem the number of illegal abortions (Wolińska 1962, 12–15). The debate, like all other public discussion, was silenced at the beginning of the 1950s in accordance with the hardening of Stalin's party line, and was revived only after Stalin's death.

In 1955, when a liberal law was reintroduced in the Soviet Union, voices calling for liberalisation of the abortion law started to be heard in Poland as well. The new law, which is still in force, was introduced in 1956.[3] It allowed medical and legal indications for abortion, and at the same time included a woman's difficult living conditions as justification for the termination of pregnancy if performed by a physician. It decriminalised self-induced abortion and lifted punishments for women seeking clandestine abortions.[4]

The 1956 law was strongly criticised by various groups, in particular the Catholic Church. Arguments against the law emphasised the sanctity of human life and the need to protect it from the moment of conception. The Catholic press warned on the one hand of moral damage (for instance, the increase in extramarital relations and a cynical approach to love), and on the other of Polish women becoming sterile as a result of the liberal abortion law.

The years 1956 to 1959 marked a period of severe conflict over the law's enforcement. Resistance on the part of some doctors, who had a legal monopoly on performing abortions, accompanied by the imperfect executive regulations of 1956[5] and the lack of proper facilities, resulted in an increasing number of illegal abortions. New executive regulations were issued in 1959;[6] practically speaking, they made abortion accessible on request, provided there were no medical counter-indications. At the same time, a family-planning campaign was launched, which included information and legal and medical counselling on birth control.

In the next 20 years, the abortion debate was revived several times, however the topic remained within the framework of demographic policy. So-called demographic reasons often served as justification for the manipulation of women according to the needs of the labour market (Zielińska 1987, 293–95).

The penal code of 1969 reflected the 1956 abortion law provisions: women were not to be punished in cases of illegal abortion.[7]

In the early 1970s, the Catholic Church put pressure on the communist parliament to reassess the abortion law. The move was initiated by the Polish episcopate on June 18, 1970, with an open memorandum addressed to the government on biological and moral threats to the nation. But no changes in the law were introduced at that time, except for a constitutional provision calling for special protection of motherhood.[8] The Catholic Church then launched an education campaign against abortion aimed at adolescents, young couples about to be married, physicians, and medical students. Cardinal Wojtyla (the present Pope John Paul II), the author of a foreword to the Polish translation of the encyclical *Humanae Vitae*, organised several joint conferences of theologians and doctors on the protection of the unborn.

With the emergence of Solidarity in 1980–1981, the Polish anti-abortion movement left the churches and became active in public. As a result, the minister of health and social welfare changed the abortion regulation, making gynaecologists and obstetricians its sole providers.[9] The ministerial instruction, issued in 1981, was aimed at complicating the abortion procedure.[10] Then martial law, imposed in December 1981, suppressed the abortion discussion along with all other public debate.

Legal Attempts to Restrict Abortion

In 1989 (with the country still under the communist regime), the first anti-abortion draft, signed by 78 deputies, was introduced in the parliament.[11] The draft on "legal protection of the unborn from the moment of conception" proposed a complete ban on abortion and a penalty of three years' imprisonment for both a woman and her physician. The proposed law stirred up massive debate, antagonising the whole society. In the face of protests and street demonstrations, and supposedly because of forthcoming crucial elections on June 4, 1989, the communist parliament decided to shelve the proposal (Zielińska 1990, 64–69).

Solidarity won the election, and a few months later the anti-abortion campaign started anew. The Bishops' Family Council urged parliament to continue work on an anti-abortion draft, which was reintroduced by 37 senators in December 1989. A modified version was passed by the senate in September 1990.[12] During 1990 and 1991, several drafts on "protection of the unborn" were prepared by different parliamentary bodies,[13] but their supporters did not manage to get them passed in the lower chamber of the parliament (Sejm) before new elections in October 1991.

Parallel to the work on the anti-abortion draft, the parliamentary constitutional commission agreed that the right of the unborn to life from the moment of conception be included in the new draft Constitution.

In April 1990, the minister of health and social welfare issued a new executive regulation restricting access to abortion by introducing a requirement to consult three physicians and a psychologist before getting permission for termination of pregnancy.[14] The regulation also provided for a clear time limit (12 weeks) for legal abortion on the grounds of a woman's difficult living conditions, while abortion for medical reasons was allowed at any time. It also introduced the conscience clause for physicians, with the exception of a case when the woman's life was at stake. In the same year, the Ministry of Health introduced payment for hospitalisation in regard to abortion in state hospitals, previously covered by health insurance. However, women still did not have to pay for the actual medical procedure.

On December 14, 1991, the Polish Doctors' Corporation, meeting in congress, approved a new ethics code (enforced since May 3, 1992) that forbids physicians from performing abortion for reasons other than danger to life and health or in the case of pregnancy resulting from a criminal offence (*Gazeta Wyborcza*, December 16, 1991). The ethics code was criticised as arbitrary (approved without sufficient professional consultation) by some physicians who were members of the Doctors' Corporation, and by lawyers as contradictory to legal regulations still in force. The latter argued that since the law of 1956 permits abortion for social reasons and in cases of foetal deformity, a situation should not be created whereby a physician who obeys the law is punished by the Doctors' Corporation for violating its code of ethics. It was also stressed that the ethics code is inconsistent with the penal code draft of December 1991, as well as with the anti-abortion draft being discussed in the parliament (*Gazeta Wyborcza*, December 18, 1991).

It is worth mentioning that the December 1991 penal code draft prohibits abortion but provides for wider indications such as "important social circumstances."[15] At the same time, abortion after viability is qualified as homicide (Article 125 §2) and any harm to the foetus (whether intentional or not) is punishable (Article 134).

The new anti-abortion draft was again very restrictive. It declared that each human being has a right to life from the moment of conception, and proposed a penalty of up to two years' imprisonment for a practitioner terminating a pregnancy except to save the woman's life. The anti-abortion draft reintroduced penalties for self-induced abortion, and also prohibited anyone from causing harm or damage to the foetus.

In the spring of 1992, a group of parliamentarians introduced an abortion draft that guaranteed the right to family planning and access to abortion as a last resort. At the same time, the draft of a national referendum on abortion was presented. In July 1992, both drafts were rejected and the anti-abortion draft was directed to the Extraordinary Parliamentary Commission; the draft is still pending.

The physicians' ethics code was appealed by the ombudsman to the Constitutional Court in January 1992. As of September of the same year, the case was still pending even though the code itself had become operational the previous month.

ABORTION: CURRENT LAW AND PRACTICE

Abortion in Practice

For the whole period of legalised abortion in Poland, official statistics from the Ministry of Health stated that the number of abortions never exceeded 140,000 per year.[16] However, these data are not reliable because they do not include abortions performed by private doctors, who never report all abortions in order to avoid taxes. The estimated number of abortions for this period differs depending on the source. For instance, the Catholic Church claims 600,000 to 1 million per year; according to most Polish demographers, it is 300,000 to 500,000 per year.[17]

The public accepts that the number of abortions has been decreasing gradually since 1982. The minister of health reports that both the abortion-to-birth ratio and the abortion rate are lower as well. (The rate was 27.4 percent in 1962 and 13.4 in 1987; the abortion ratio in 1962 was 33.3 and in 1987, 22.2.) However, it is difficult to predict whether the decrease will continue. Several gynaecologists have reported recently that some women have decided to terminate pregnancy in advance, fearing that soon this family-planning option will be taken away from them.

The estimated abortion rate in Poland is much higher than in the West, lower than in the former Soviet Union, and more or less the same as in Bulgaria, Yugoslavia, and Hungary (Zielińska 1987, 268 ff). The major reason cited to explain the high abortion rate in Central and Eastern Europe is the insufficient use of contraceptives. Research shows that more than 80 percent of women respondents claim they use contraception; however, the methods chosen are usually unreliable, such as withdrawal or the calendar rather than the pill or IUD.[18]

Opponents of choice are also trying to restrict access to contraception. It has been reported that contraceptive supplies in smaller towns, although never sufficient, have diminished. To avoid conflict with local Catholic priests, some pharmacists have given up stocking either all or the most effective contraceptives. Owing to intervention by the Governmental Plenipotentiary for Women's Affairs, the trend seems to have stopped.

Abortion in Poland may be performed in three types of health institutions: public hospitals, so-called physicians' cooperatives (semiprivate outpatient clinics), and private doctors' offices. The abortion procedure is free of charge (covered by health insurance) only in public hospitals. In the remaining two institutions, abortion is fully paid and performed on an outpatient basis.

The majority of abortions are justified by the woman's difficult living conditions. The number of abortions performed because of other reasons has been very low. For instance, only 1,460 abortions on medical indications were reported in 1987. (This number seems reliable, since such abortions should be done in hospitals.)

Until 1990, access to abortion was relatively easy, especially in big cities. In spite of the fact that private abortion services were quite expensive (the payment has always been around an average monthly salary), the majority of women avoided public hospitals because of a lack of choice as regards procedure, a lack of privacy, and poor sanitary conditions.

The executive regulation issued in April 1990 substantially complicated access to abortion, however. In the public health service, women now have to visit three doctors and a psychologist before getting permission for an abortion. Because doctors are overburdened, each visit may require a long wait or several attempts to get registered. This creates the danger that abortion will be performed at a late stage and thus illegally.

Doctors' cooperatives seem to be better organised, since the woman can get permission for the abortion with one visit. (Doctors' cooperatives employ not only physicians of required specialisations but also psychologists). The majority of private doctors seem to pretend that the 1990 ministry regulation does not concern them. Silent tolerance on the part of the authorities for those practices confirms that conviction. As a result, well-to-do women can avoid these restrictive abortion procedures, which discriminate against poorer women, especially those living in remote areas.

Access to abortion services is also limited in some regions of Poland by the fact that several public hospitals refuse to provide them. However, as in Cracow, some doctors who made use of the "conscience clause" while working at a hospital have invited women to have abortions in their private offices. Then, as of May 3, 1992, all state hospitals refused to perform abortions for any reason. The ombudsman reported one case to the public prosecutor, in which an abortion on medical indications was refused at a Warsaw hospital. Some private doctors still perform abortion, but the price is now five times higher than previously.

Since abortion is a highly politicised issue in Poland, it is difficult to define the attitude of medical practitioners. There is a substantial number of physicians—especially those representing the National Chamber of Physicians, the regulating body for all doctors—who feel it is their right to decide exclusively on the permissibility of abortion. This is confirmed by a successful attempt to introduce more restrictions on abortion via the physicians' ethics code. Some doctors feel superior to the existing law and consequently deny women the right to abortion in the case of foetus deformity or difficult living conditions. On the other hand, the majority of gynaecologists are reluctant to get involved in the debate. This may mean that they do not want to display any personal interest in the maintenance of legal abortion—or the opposite, that they are interested in the delegalisation because it would increase their income (because of the "crime tariff").[19]

The introduction of payment for hospitalisation in regard to abortion in public health institutions, although relatively low, raised the price of abortion in the free market. The price depends on the method applied, the stage of pregnancy, and the facilities offered. Some gynaecologists violate Polish law by openly advertising their services.

Along with the more restrictive abortion policy begun in 1990 came four deaths resulting from self-induced abortions, registered in one of the biggest Polish towns. No such cases had been reported in the previous 20 years. On the other hand, restrictions seem to have had no significant impact on the rate of infanticide, which has been quite stable since legalisation of abortion.[20]

Although abortions are not viewed as deviations in Polish society,[21] it seems that the majority of women keep it secret from strangers, children, employers, and often the fathers of their fetus. The main reason seems to be a prevailing feeling of shame. In the case of teenage girls and single women, abortion is evidence of sex "without the sanctity of marriage." As for married women (who are the main group seeking abortion in Poland), the shame relates to guilt about failing to avoid an unwanted pregnancy. It is difficult to define why Polish men feel ashamed of their partner's abortion, but it is evident that they keep silent on the subject, too. The fact that 92 percent of Poles declare themselves to be Catholic could be one reason why people are reluctant to reveal abortion.

The attitude of the Catholic Church stops people from discussing abortion in public, but not from seeking termination of pregnancy. First, statistics prove that the estimated number of abortions could not be as high as it is if Catholic women were not included. Also, research shows that one-fourth of women respondents, while believing that religious prohibitions should be observed, confess that in the case of an unwanted pregnancy they are ready to break the rule (Zielińska 1987, 284–85).

After legalisation in 1956 there seems to have been no problem with illegal abortions in Poland. The statistics show fewer than five cases per year; in some years there were none at all. And usually they involved late abortions that resulted mainly because of health complications.

The Politics of Abortion

In spite of a considerably liberal law and free access to early abortion, the woman's right to choose has never been directly recognised in Poland. The 1956 abortion law states in its preamble that the aim is to protect women's health against illegal abortion. The comments by the Ministry of Health, issued almost simultaneously with the law, stated that "the woman has the full freedom of deciding about her motherhood only by way of preventing a pregnancy. Once the conception has taken place, the will of the woman ceases to be an exclusive or decisive factor in regard to termination of pregnancy" (Krotkiewska 1956, 8).

The debate from 1989 to 1992 revealed that public awareness of a human right to choose is surprisingly low and usually is not considered to be the core of the abortion issue. Protection of a woman's health is viewed as a more convincing argument against delegalisation of abortion; so is rape, foetal deformity, housing shortage, and difficult living conditions.

The debate also revealed deeply rooted prejudices against women, especially as regards female sexuality and reproduction. Women are often perceived as sex objects and/or as purely biological creatures. There is a double standard for men and women in the area of sexual behaviour. Also, Catholic teaching is strict in this respect: women should be virgins, wives, and mothers only; sex is mainly for procreation, and every artificial way of avoiding conception is condemned.

As was emphasised earlier, the Catholic Church constitutes the main source of anti-abortion policy. Not surprisingly, all the new Christian as well as nationalist parties promote anti-abortion legislation. In 1990, the Second Congress of Solidarity trade unions approved a resolution calling for the protection of life from the moment of conception. The Polish Doctors' Corporation seems to be dominated by supporters of legal protection of the unborn.

The communists, who were in power for more than 40 years, permitted abortion as a means to achieve other goals—for instance, to increase female employment and restrict it when necessary to change the birthrate. The post-communists declare their opposition to the anti-abortion bill, however it is too early to say whether their attitude is based on recognition of a woman's right to choose. A number of small socialist parties argue for women's rights in this respect.

Respect for this right is clearly demanded by the Polish women's organisations (Plakwicz 1992, 88–91). It is worth mentioning that in the transition period, the women's movement in Poland has evoled significantly. Instead of one token communist organisation, nearly 30 associations of different background, political views, and aims were established. The erosion of women's rights during the transformation has strengthened and integrated the different women's organisations. Women have organised within male-dominated public institutions. For instance, a women's club was established in parliament and the women's section of Solidarity trade unions organised a protest of the 1990 congress resolution (as a result of which these women were expelled from the union).

At the beginning of the anti-abortion campaign, the media seemed to sympathise with the opponents of the draft. However, when chided by the Polish bishops, some of them, especially state television, took a more reserved position. Meanwhile, public opinion polls carried out in 1991 showed that 51 percent (February) and 58 percent (May) of respondents were against the draft banning abortion, and about 40 percent were in favour of the right to abortion (*Gazeta Wyborcza*, February 27, 1991 and April 11, 1991).

The winning party in the 1991 elections, the Democratic Union, has taken no official stand on abortion; the right-wing fraction within the party supports an anti-abortion bill, and the left seeks compromise. The other parties have also successfully avoided taking a decisive stand regarding abortion regulation. This may be a result of a lack of clear party line; on the other hand, such ambiguity allows the representatives to vote according to their political interests. At present the most vocal parliamentary deputies are those belonging to the Christian National party, part of the government coalition. Supported by the Catholic Church hierarchy, the Christian National party may have a decisive impact on future abortion law.

Each political force in Poland has its strategy, tactics, and means. The Catholic Church's hierarchy showed no restraint in their support for the restrictive anti-abortion draft. Church prayers were organised, priests actively participated as experts in public and parliamentary discussions on the bill, and deputies who declared themselves opponents of the bill were criticised from the pulpits in their electoral districts. The Pope's visit in 1991 was nearly suspended because the Polish parliament showed no consensus on "protection of the unborn." These are only some examples of direct church activity in order to get the law passed in Poland.

Advocates of the anti-abortion draft argue that the delegalisation will be a big step towards de-communisation and de-Stalinisation, and would bring the law into conformity with Christian values. The de-communisation or de-Stalinisation argument finds strong social resonance in the present political situation. However, the history of abortion policy in communist countries proves that a complete ban on abortion was, in fact, characteristic of the Stalinist era.

While using the rhetoric of human rights, advocates of delegalisation mean an absolute right of the unborn to life and neglect a woman's rights completely. Such an approach, as with any fundamentalist perspective, excludes the possibility of compromise. Rational evaluation of the benefits and costs of such a legal change would, in their opinion, lead to an immoral situation in which human life is relative and not of the highest value. At the same time, the opponents of delegalisation are placed in the position of being immoral people—"killers of the innocent."

The strategy of the opponents to the anti-abortion draft was defensive. It was not planned in advance, but rather dictated by the offensive moves of the other side. In the beginning, the pro-choice side was under the illusion that their opponents were seeking some reasonable solution to a socially unacceptable phenomenon—that is, abortion. However, they soon realized that supporters of the anti-abortion draft excluded any possibility of compromise and were not inclined to negotiate anything but purely stylistic modifications. Consequently, arguments against the ban—such as a woman's right to choose, to self-determination, to privacy—or evaluation of the costs (financial, social, and legal) of the proposed change in the law, or its incoherence with the theory of criminalisation (namely, that the criminal law should be used only as a last resort) were *eo ipso* rejected.

This became especially obvious during the debates in the Extraordinary Parliamentary Commission, formed in January 1991 to discuss the draft. Since the commission was dominated by supporters of the anti-abortion draft, an even more restrictive version was approved despite resistance from the commission's minority. Then, based on the rejected minority motions, an alternative draft of the abortion law was proposed (Parliamentary Print no. 798). It recognised the right to responsible decisions on parenthood and provided for relatively liberal conditions for abortion. However, as it was signed by post-communist deputies only, from the very beginning it was labelled communist and had no chance of being approved (*Zycie Warszawy*, April 18, 1991).

The parliament approved the motion of the opponents of the anti-abortion draft to hold public consultations on the issue. Surprisingly, and contrary to public opinion polls, their results showed that 89 percent of the people who signed petitions and letters to the parliament were in favour of an anti-abortion bill (*Gazeta Wyborcza*, April 11, 1991). The results of the consultations proved once again the organisational skills of the Catholic Church in Poland. It was clear that from among 1 million people who took part in the consultations, only 11,000 sent individual letters. It was also revealed that the number of collective letters received more or less corresponded with the number of Catholic parishes. It was well known as well that in some of those parishes the priests imposed direct or indirect pressure on people in order to collect signatures.

The next step the opponents took was to place a motion for a nationwide referendum on abortion. It was tabled to the parliament by 17 deputies representing different parties from a Solidarity background (*Gazeta Wyborcza*, April 25, 1991). The church expressed strong opposition to the idea of voting on a moral issue, calling it "not only anti-Christian but anti-Polish and inhuman as well" (*Polityka*, April 11, 1991). The church hierarchy seemed not to see the illogical basis of this argument, since parliamentary decisions are also a result of voting. It was noted that the church's resistance to the idea of a referendum might stem from its ability to more easily influence the vote of 500 representatives in parliament than 30 million Poles (*Gazeta Wyborcza*, May 16, 1991). Despite the clear church position on the referendum, public opinion polls showed that 76 percent of respondents were in favour of holding the nationwide vote (*Gazeta Wyborcza*, May 15, 1991).

The abortion debate reached a stalemate. With so many options, no one was able to predict the result of the vote. With the expected visit by the Pope, to whom the anti-abortion bill was supposed to be a gift, the majority of deputies greeted with relief a proposal by the Democratic Union party to postpone the vote until a new draft was prepared. The Democratic Union party also put forward a resolution calling for, among other things, the government to prepare a general programme on sex education and contraception, for the Ministry of Education to introduce the topic of "preparation to family life" into the school programme, and for the Ministry of Health to cancel the right of private doctors to perform abortions (*Zycie Warszawy*, May 17, 1991; *Gazeta Wyborcza*, May 18, 1991).

In June the new abortion draft (less restrictive than the senate's) was presented to parliament but withdrawn soon after without a reason given. Thus, the abortion discussion was postponed until new elections took place in October 1991. In December 1991, a sufficient number of signatures was collected to introduce the anti-abortion draft again into the parliament (*Gazeta Wyborcza*, December 27, 1991). In addition to this frontal attack, supporters of the anti-abortion bill have been involved in a series of steps aimed at gradually eliminating all behaviour contrary to Catholic teaching, such as abortion, artificial contraception, donor insemination, and divorce.

Adding to the restrictions on abortion in the physicians' ethics code and the 1990 ministry regulations is a draft of a law regulating physicians that proposes excluding abortion facilities from private doctors' offices. It is not yet clear, however, what kind of restrictions on contraception are being prepared. The rejected proposal for the physicians' ethics code could suggest minimal regulation. Contraceptive counselling would be offered to women in two cases only: when there are therapeutic indications and/or when a woman demands it explicitly. The code of ethics introduced certain limitations on pre-natal diagnostics and suggested a conscience clause for physicians in the case of artificial insemination. Finally, it is proposed to introduce into the family code two types of marriage—civil and church—with the possibility of legal separation instead of divorce in the case of a church marriage.

UPDATE

During a vote in the Polish parliament on January 7, 1993, the highly restrictive draft of a new abortion law was rejected.[22] The new law, however, is much more restrictive than the 1956 legislation inasfar as it abolishes the social indication for abortion and bans abortions in private clinics. The parliament accepted seven modifications liberalising the draft law on the protection of the foetus, and in doing so used some of the wording of the liberal counter-draft—an influence indicated in the title of the new law: "On Family Planning, Protection of the Human Foetus and Conditions of Permissibility of Interruption of Pregnancy." Thus the new law is an unsatisfactory merger of two drafts representing diametrically opposed ideologies. The pro-lifers find it too liberal, the pro-choice lobby too restrictive. The lawyers—irrespective of their moral judgement on abortion—find it inconsistent, if not contradictory. And the Polish Doctors' Corporation is faced with the fact that the law is now more liberal than the 1992 code of ethics.[23]

The new law declares that the life and health of the unborn should be protected from the moment of conception, and it provides for the deprivation of liberty for up to two years of anyone (except the pregnant woman) who "causes the death of the conceived child" (Article 149 of the penal code). At the same time, it states that the physician does not commit an offence if the abortion is performed in a public hospital and if:

1. two other doctors have confirmed that the pregnancy endangers life or is a serious risk to the health of the pregnant woman; or

2. prenatal diagnosis, confirmed by the opinion of two doctors, indicates the existence of serious and irreversible damage of the foetus; or

3. there is a justified presumption, confirmed by a prosecutor, that the pregnancy has resulted from a criminal act.

The penalty of deprivation of liberty from six months up to eight years is provided for causing the death of a conceived child against the will or without the consent of its mother (Article 149b of the penal code) and up to two years for causing injury that endangers the life of the conceived child (Article 156 of the penal code).

The law also provides for modification of the civil code in the sense that unborn children have gained legal capacity, with the reservation that their financial rights and obligations may be executed under the condition that they are born alive (Articles 8 and 2 of the civil code). After birth, children could also demand compensation for prenatal damages (Article 446.1 of the civil code). In addition, the law obliges the state to provide for the assistance of pregnant women and conceived children; assure sex education in school that urges "conscious and responsible parenthood and the value of family and conceived life"; guarantee free access to "methods and means for conscious procreation."

The situation as regards abortion has turned out to be what could be called an optimistic scenario. However, the question has not been resolved. There is a possibility that providing information about abortions available abroad may be illegal; there is also a question concerning the legality of some contraceptives—in particular the pill and IUD—on grounds that they may be deemed to be early abortives. On the other hand, the intense conflict over abortion has galvanised women's groups in Poland to the point where they are now better organised and more active than ever before. The Federation for Women and Planned Parenthood was formed in 1992, and was active in organising support for the referendum. The federation is now working for the re-establishment of women's choice on abortion, for widely available contraception, and for sex education.

In addition, victory by post-communist and leftist parties in the parliamentary elections of September 1993, which was partly due to their stand on church-state relations and abortion, gives hope for a return to more liberal abortion law. The assumption is based not only on the declarations of the winning parties but also on public anxiety resulting from relatively new social phenomena such as "abortion tourism" and clandestine abortions,[24] as well as from the lack of implementation of those provisions aimed at preventing unwanted pregnancies.[25]

NOTES

1. According to Article 130 of the 1818 penal code, abortion was considered a crime if performed without the woman's consent (the punishment was specified as 3

to 10 years hard labour). In other cases (self-induced abortion included) it was qualified as a misdemeanour and punished with 1 to 3 years of house detention (Article 323).

2. Articles 231–34 of the 1932 penal code. According to L. Peiper (1933, 628), the code's commentator, the exclusion from the draft of the so-called social indications as justification for abortion was done by the Ministry of Justice.

3. Law no. 61 of April 27, 1956, which determines the conditions under which interruption of pregnancy is permissible. See *Dziennik Ustaw Polskiej Rzeczypospolitej Ludowej (Dz.U.)* no. 12 (1956). English translation in *International Digest of Health Legislation (IDHL)* 9, no. 2 (1958): 321.

4. Before World War II pregnant women and other people involved in illegal abortions were rarely punished. For example, between 1920 and 1924, only 16 people were charged with this offence at Warsaw District Court. In all cases the punishment did not exceed one year in prison. Between 1947 and 1956 the average number of persons punished annually was 354.

5. Ordinance no. 68 of the Ministry of Health, May 11, 1956, on the interruption of pregnancy. *Dz.U.* no. 12 (1956): 81; *IDHL* 9, no. 2 (1958): 321.

6. Ordinance no. 15 of the Minister of Health, November 19, 1959, on the interruption of pregnancy. *Dz.U.* no. 2 (1960); *IDHL* 14, no. 3 (1963): 454.

7. Law no. 94, April 19, 1969. *Dz.U.* no. 13 (1969); *IDHL* 22, no. 4 (1971): 971.

8. The amendment (Law no. 36, February 16, 1976. *Dz.U.* no. 7 (1976) concerned Article 5, item 7, and Article 78, item 1, of the Polish Constitution Law no. 232, July 22, 1952; *Dz.U.* no. 33 (1952).

9. Law no. 110; *Dz.U.* no. 26 (1980).

10. Instruction no. 11/810 of the Ministers of Health, Transport, National Defence, and Internal Affairs, September 1981, on requirements in regard to termination of pregnancy in social health service establishments; *Dziennik Urzędowy Ministerstwa Zdrowia i Opieki Spolecznej* no. 11 (1981).

11. Published in *Tygodnik Powszechny* no. 10 (1989).

12. Senate's draft, Parliamentary Print no. 553. For more on this debate see Szawarski 1990.

13. The final draft was approved by the Extraordinary Parliamentary Commission in April 1991; *Gazeta Wyborcza*, April 25, 1991.

14. No. 178, April 30, 1990, on qualifications of physicians performing abortions and on the procedure of issuing permits for abortions by the physicians (*Dz.U.* no. 29).

15. Prepared by Codification Commission of the Ministry of Justice, December 1991, Articles 130–33.

16. Between 1957 and 1989, the highest incidence of legal abortion was in 1962 (199,429). Since 1967, the annual figure has never exceeded 150,000. Since 1980, the figure has never exceeded 138,000. In 1987, it was 122,536 and in 1989, the incidence dropped to 83,000. Approximately half of all registered abortions were performed in public hospitals.

17. According to Okólski (1988, s. 208), in 1977 about 600,000 abortions were performed in Poland. This means that every second pregnancy was terminated.

18. According to the results of a so-called Family Survey in 1987, 10.9 percent of married women did not use any birth control method, 36.9 percent used withdrawal

only, 29.4 percent used natural methods and contraceptives, and only 11 percent used contraceptives (Central Statistical Office, Warsaw 1987. See also Okólski 1983).

19. By "crime tariff" is meant that the price for a medical procedure increases relative to the risk of discovery of its illegality. For more on the side effects of the anti-abortion bill, see Błachut 1991.

20. Before World War II the infanticide rate was close to 1,000 annually, before 1956 around 80, and recently has not exceeded 30. See Wolińska 1962, 108.

21. Research on social deviation carried out in 1973 showed that abortion was not condemned very strongly. See Kojder and Kwaśniewski 1975.

22. The law, which is published in *Dziennik Ustaw*, no. 17 (1973), item 78, took effect on March 16, 1993. For further information, see Nowicka 1993.

23. The dilemma facing the physician is which norm to obey—that of the professional code or that of the general law which holds that a physician who performs an abortion in conformity with the law but in violation of the ethical code cannot be subject to professional sanctions by the medical association (judgement of the Constitutional Court, March 17, 1993).

24. Recent public opinion polls indicate that a majority of people are in favour of more widespread access to abortion. Of those polled, 81 percent favour abortion when a woman's life is in danger, 80 percent when the foetus is incurably deformed, 74 percent in the cases of incest and rape, and 53 percent when the woman is experiencing difficult financial or social circumstances. Twenty-three percent support abortion on request (see Nowicka 1993).

25. No sex education was introduced in schools in 1993–94 and an alternative youth health movement sex education programme was refused financial support by the government. Contraception is not fully accessible. Aid for pregnant women and their families exists on paper only. Moreover, public hospitals have refused to perform legal abortions, and this has caused some interventions by the Ombudsman (see *Gazeta Wyborcza*, September 9, 1993, pp. 2 and 3, and September 15, 1993, p. 4).

REFERENCES

Błachut, J., and K. Krajewski. "Projekt ustawy o prawnej ochronie dziecka poczętego. Kilka uwag kryminalnopolitycznych i kryminologicznych" (The draft law on legal protection of the conceived child. Some criminal policy and criminological remarks), *Państwo i Prawo*, no. 5 (1991): 36–47.

Kojder, A., and J. Kwaśniewski. "Wzory reakcji no zachowania dewiacyjne i ich uwarunkowania" (The reaction patterns towards deviant behaviour and conditions), *Studia Socjologiczne*, no. 3 (1975).

Krotkiewska, L. *Warunki dopuszczalności przyrywania ciazy. Teksty i kimentarz* (Requirements of Permissible Abortions. Text and Commentary). Warszawa: Ministerstwo Zdowia, 1956.

Nowicka, W. "Two Steps Back: Poland's New Abortion Law," *Planned Parenthood in Europe* 22, no. 2 (1993): 18–20.

Okólski, M. "Abortion and Contraception in Poland," *Studies in Family Planning* 14, no. 11 (1983).

———. *Reprodukcja ludności a modernizacja społeczeństwa. Polski Syndrom. Książka i Wiedza* (Population reproduction and modernisation of society: The Polish syndrome). Warsaw: Ksiazka i Wiedza, 1988.

Peiper, L. *Komentarz do kodeksu karnego* (Commentary on the penal code). Warsaw: 1933.

Plakwicz, J. "Poland: Between Church and State." In C. Corrin (ed.), *Superwoman and the Double Burden*. London: Scarlet Press, 1992.

Szawarski, Z. "Poland Moves Against Abortion," *Bulletin of Medical Ethics*, no. 62 (1990).

Wolińska, H. *Przerwanie ciąży w świetle prawa karnego* (Termination of pregnancy in penal law). Warsaw: Wydawnictwo Prawnicze, 1962.

Zielińska, E. "European Socialist Countries." In S. Frankowski and G. Cole (eds.), *Abortion and Protection of the Human Fetus: Legal Problems in a Cross-Cultural Perspective*. Dordrecht, Boston and Lancaster: Martinus Nijhoff, 1987.

———. *Przerywanie ciąży. Warunki legalności w Polsce i na świecie* (Abortion: Conditions of legality in Poland and the world). Warsaw: Wydawnictwo Prawnicze, 1990.

PORTUGAL

Duarte Vilar

THE HISTORY OF ABORTION LAW

From Dictatorship to Democracy

Portugal was governed by a conservative dictatorship between 1926 and 1974. This regime had a religious component, and identified itself with the values of the Roman Catholic Church. The Lisbon Patriarch was a personal friend of the dictator Antonio Salazar, and all the acts of the regime were publicly supported by the religious hierarchy. A concordat between the Portuguese state and the Vatican was established in 1940.

In this context, legislation on all matters related to moral issues—family relationships, the rights of women in general, and sexual and reproductive rights in particular—was made according to the ideology of the regime. Contraceptives were forbidden (except for medical use!). Divorce was legally impossible and women's submission to men was enshrined in the family code and in labour legislation.

In the late 1960s the Catholic Church was shaken by the debates produced by Vatican Council II and the encyclical *Humanae Vitae*. However, the main question was not yet that of abortion but of the use of contraceptives and birth control. Catholics were seriously divided, but the hierarchy maintained all the traditional positions on these issues. In this kind of regime, the mere discussion of the problem of abortion (like other polemical subjects) was considered subversive and almost illegal.

In 1974 a military movement overthrew the dictatorship and effective freedom of expression and organisation were installed in Portuguese society. Deep changes were made in the state and the law, which included legislation on divorce (which became possible) and equality between men and women in the family and other areas of society. With the Constitution of 1976, Portugal became definitively a representative democracy and the Portuguese state was confirmed as a secular one.

Since 1974 questions of sexual and reproductive rights have been the subject of important debates. However, in spite of these social changes and public debates, 17 years later, Portugal remains with a serious problem of illegal and unsafe abortion. The law approved in 1984 seems to be unable to solve this problem. One can say that, with the latest changes in Spain and Belgium, Portugal and Ireland are now the most problematic countries in Western Europe and have similar situations in this respect, but, while Irish women are obliged to search for an abortion in foreign countries, Portuguese women were always able to find someone easily to perform more or less expensive and unsafe abortions.

Pre-1974: Widespread Illegal Abortion

Being an illegal fact, there are no general statistics on the number of abortions in recent decades. However, the literature, common knowledge, the testimonies of health professionals, and studies available after the change in government show that abortion as a method of birth control is widespread in Portugal.

Data collected in the two main hospitals in Lisbon for the years 1967–1969 show that there were at least 200 abortions for each thousand births among the women studied. The same study revealed that in those three years, around 7,000 women were assisted in these two Lisbon hospitals because of abortion complications. In the same years, 69 women were officially recorded as having died as a result of abortion.

In 1976, when the first legislation was passed to make family planning services available, the health secretary estimated the number of illegal abortions performed each year in the country at between 100,000 and 120,000. In that period abortion was the third major cause of maternal death in Portugal, and often its consequences were partly hidden in other diseases, such as pelvic or general infections. This attitude was partly justified in terms of protecting women from legal prosecution.

In the first book about abortion in Portugal, *Aborto: Direito ao Nosso Corpo*, there were impressive testimonies from several midwives who performed abortions. They spoke about the number of abortions they performed, some around 200 per month. The testimonies of women who had had abortions were also included, revealing feelings of guilt, fear, and distress; the serious complications with infections owing to unsafe abortions; the feeling of loneliness when they had to face an abortion; the severe criticism they sometimes met in the hospitals where they had to go when they were not able to stop the bleeding or reduce the fever; and the economic and domestic complications when they had to pay often more than the minimum wage for having an abortion. Some of them had more than 30 abortions in a lifetime!

Antónia Fiadeiro (1983), a pro-choice journalist and militant, dramatically described the illegal abortion experience:

The 50 to 100 escudo notes put aside in the pocket. This time she had enough money for anaesthesia. The last one that she had done was so painful. . . . That clandestine room, full of distressed and worried women, some of them still unconscious, others already relieved. . . . The laments, the sighs, the crying . . . the silence in the midst of talking. . . . All this remained in her mind and in her eyes. How many thousands of escudos spent in half an hour . . . ? How many thousands of escudos as a profit for each body, for each belly? Had her aunt (who was with her kids) believed her lie? And her man, who had immediately said nervously that it was her problem . . . not his. . . . What a humiliation to be a woman in this way . . . and knowing so little about the facts of life. . . .

The legal prohibition on abortion did not come with the dictatorship. The Portuguese penal code of 1886 punished the abortionist and the woman who had the abortion with a penalty of two to eight years' imprisonment. However, the facts show that the practice of abortion in Portugal was also tolerated. In fact, even in such a repressive regime (where opponents were systematically persecuted and put in jail), the number of abortion cases judged in the courts remained low: one or two per year. The situation was totally different *de jure* and *de facto*. The addresses of the abortionists were publicly known, and in several cases there was evidence that they had police protection. This was the way the regime preferred to avoid social conflict, not interfering with traditional practices while supporting hundreds of illegal abortionists.

These abortions were performed mainly by nurses and midwives, and in some cases physicians. In some central hospitals abortions were performed when there was a risk to the life of the mother, or for some evident eugenic reasons. Also in these cases many hospital boards preferred to ignore the situation. Portuguese abortionists also assisted thousands of Spanish women.

The practice of abortion was closely related to the lack of information and the difficulties in obtaining safe contraception. Contraceptives were available in the main cities and in some official outlets. The pill was (and is) often sold in pharmacies without a medical prescription. However, the practice of safe contraception was not widespread. The National Fertility Survey of 1980 showed that only 33 percent of married women aged between 15 and 49 years used safe contraception; withdrawal was the most popular method of birth control used by Portuguese couples.

Post-1974: Breaking Down the Wall of Silence

After the fall of the dictatorship, freedom of organisation and expression became effective. Political parties and other civic organisations were now legal and censorship was abolished. In late 1974 and early 1975, the needs of all social groups were articulated and expressed. Everything that did not exist before and was socially needed seemed to be possible and attainable in the short term.

Issues relating to women's rights and public health were subjects of compassionate debate. The first legal feminist organisations were formed. All the left-wing parties included to different extents statements on contraception and abortion in their political programmes and activities.

Among the occupations of houses, factories, and farms, a group of women took possession of an old palace near Lisbon and opened the first clinic where abortions were performed almost without charge. Contraceptives were distributed free. (This clinic closed some time later.) At the same time, public debate about contraception and abortion was promoted by feminist groups and other women's organisations. At the time, the main protagonists of these developments were from the extra-parliamentary Left. The opportunity to fight to legalise abortion was a question that divided the extreme Left from other left-wing parties at that time. It was only some years later that left-wing parliamentarians approached the problem.

The intense ideological fight in Portuguese society continued. In 1976, elections for a new president, parliament, and local authorities were held. The question of abortion marked the political distinction between Right and Left, and in this context occurred the case of the journalist Antónia Palla. She was responsible for a women's television programme where the subject of abortion was treated. Some images of an illegal abortion were shown. The legalisation of abortion was defended by some feminists. After transmission, some conservative political parties and the College of Physicians protested the programme, and the journalist was prosecuted for moral outrage and encouragement of crimes.

Another case encouraged public discussion. A young nursing student, Conceição Massano, faced a court trial because one of her teachers discovered in her diary that she had had an abortion. Both cases finished in 1979, with the discharge of the two women and public recognition by the judges of the gap between law and reality. "Illegal abortion is a significant problem; it cannot be solved through silence." With these words the judge of Antónia Palla guaranteed the right to debate the question. But in the case of Conceição Massano, the judge discharged her, denying the facts of the accusation; as far as the judge was concerned, Conceição was mistaken in believing that she had had an abortion.

These events contributed to public awareness of the problem. The years 1977 through 1979 saw a strong campaign and public debate conducted by several feminist organisations, such as the Women's Liberation Movement (MLM), Revolutionary and Anti-Fascist Women's Union (UMAR), Democratic Women's Movement (MDM), and other groups and individuals linked to left-wing movements. The FPA (Family Planning Association) Lisbon branch promoted a series of conferences and defended the legalisation of abortion. Some trade unions took positions for the first time, supporting the existence of free and legal abortion. However, the first conference of the trade union confederation on the topic of working women refused to include support for this position in their final statement.

In 1977 a petition was presented to the parliament urging free and legal abortion. In April 1979, together with the trials of Antónia Palla and Conceicão Massano, the National Campaign for the Right to Abortion and Contraception (CNAC) made its public appearance. The CNAC promoted a declaration signed by more than 3,000 women who declared that they had had an abortion.

As a result of this three-year campaign, the issue of illegal abortion could not be ignored anymore, either by the public or among the political parties represented in the parliament. In other words, after three years an extra-parliamentary social movement, independent of the major parties, was able to force the leftist parliamentary parties to face the issue.

In the years following the overthrow, the Catholic Church continued to appear as a powerful institution, mainly in the northern part of Portugal, with significant ability to influence political decisions. This influence was both direct and indirect. Some politicians were ready to defend church interests, while others were afraid to defend certain positions that could be criticised by the church.

The Socialist party, in spite of having in its programme support for the legalisation of abortion, was unable to do anything, in fact, about legalisation because its minority governments were too vulnerable, and because in 1978 they formed a coalition with the Christian Democrats, the party most opposed to legalisation.

The Communist party, free of governmental compromises, was also afraid to approach this issue because such a polemical question could bring moral and political isolation.

These were some of the resistances that were broken down as a result of the pro-choice campaigns of 1977–79. At the end of 1979, for the first time the Socialist party, the Communist party, and the Popular Democratic Union announced in parliament that they were preparing proposals for laws on the right to legal and free abortion. However, in 1980 a general election gave a conservative coalition of Liberals, Christian Democrats, and Monarchists an absolute majority. This meant postponement of any legal reform on abortion.

At the beginning of 1982, the Communist party presented a proposal to the parliament to legalise abortion, together with proposals on the protection of parenthood and the right to family planning and sex education. This action was clearly influenced by the 1977–79 campaign, but it was also a strategic question that could divide Liberals and Christian Democrats, who were experiencing difficulties in the conservative coalition. While the Christian Democrats were totally opposed to legalisation, some Liberals were in favour and others were neutral.

The Communist party proposal was that abortion on request be legal, under medical advice, in the first 12 weeks of pregnancy, on the grounds of rape, danger to the physical or mental health of the woman, malformation of the foetus, and social and economic difficulties in the family. Abortions would be performed in state clinics or hospitals, or in private specially authorised hospitals. The penalties for illegal abortion were reduced, but they were maintained if the abortion was performed without the woman's consent. The penalty for illegal abortionists was increased (from 8 to 12 years). With this proposal a very live discussion of the abortion issue started again.

The pro-choice groups and all the parliamentary and extra-parliamentary left-wing parties defended the proposal with public statements and a new campaign. For them it was not only the matter of reducing or abolishing the penalties for abortion, because in Portugal abortion was *de facto* depenalized. The main point was to guarantee women access to easy, free, and safe abortion, performed in official institutions.

The Catholic hierarchy said that they were "obliged to fight by all legal means against the project . . . so that parliament might preserve the traditional defence of the respect for the sacred value of human life." The Bishops' Conference also advised that "the legalisation of abortion will increase and not decrease the number of abortions." The College of Physicians said that they were "one hundred percent against the proposal," that they "would maintain respect for human life from the moment of conception and even under duress would not use their professional skills against human rights."

However, even among health professionals and Catholics, these positions were not unanimously supported. A weekly journal published the results of a survey: only 19 percent of the people questioned did not support abortion in any circumstances; 34 percent were totally in favour of legalisation of abortion, and 37 percent allowed for abortions in certain circumstances, including economic difficulties. Thirteen percent of practicing Catholics and 44 percent of nonpracticing Catholics were favourable to legalisation. Older people, people who did not live in the big cities, people in lower classes, and the unemployed were least in favour of it.

During three days in November 1982, the parliament discussed the Communist party proposals, as well as the Liberal party proposal relating to family planning. The proposal to legalise abortion was defeated by 127 votes to 105. Only two parliamentarians of the Liberal party refused to vote with their colleagues against the Communist party proposal. The Communist party proposal for the protection of parenthood and the Liberal party proposal on family planning were passed.

In 1983, new elections for parliament changed the political scene. The two major parties, the Socialists and the Liberals, formed the government, with the largest majority ever to exist in parliament. At the end of 1983, the Communist party presented their proposal again. In fact, the former parliament did not have time to approve the final texts of the laws on family planning and the protection of parenthood. So once again, sexuality, sex education, family planning, abortion, and protection of the mother were hot subjects in the Portuguese parliament.

The Socialist party, however, following the Spanish experience, proposed the legalisation of abortion only in cases of rape, danger to the woman's health, and malformation of the foetus, thus excluding the so-called social causes. A proposed law on sex education and family planning was also presented by Socialists and Liberals, showing the limits of the possible consensus between the two parties in power. The Liberal position was that abortion should not be legalised but prevented through a good policy on family planning and sex education.

The pro-choice groups (National Campaign for Abortion and Contraception, Committee for Abortion Legalization, and Family Planning Association) and anti-choice groups (Movement for the Defence of Life, Family Associations Confederation) campaigned again. Professional organisations also defined themselves as pro-choice (doctors' and nurses' trade unions and judges' trade union) or against legalisation (College of Physicians).

A new book about the abortion situation, *Abortion: The Crime Stays in the Law*, by journalist Antónia Fiadeiro, was published. Meanwhile, the anti-choice movement and the more conservative parties argued, as in 1982, that those supporting legalisation were pro-communist. Stalin and Afghanistan managed to come up in the arguments used against legalisation of abortion.

The proposals of the Communist party were again rejected, and the proposal of the Socialist party regarding abortion was approved with strong opposition by Liberals, Christian Democrats, and social groups such as the church, its Pro-Vita movement, and the College of Physicians. The other proposals on sex education and family planning and the protection of the mother were also approved. The first of these—the right to sex education and family planning—was approved without support from the Christian Democrats.

This is how the first law to make abortion legal in certain cases came about. The pro-choice movement was divided in its assessment of the law. Some were positive about it on the grounds that it was possible to include all the social causes under the category of danger to the mental health of the woman. For others, the law was just a small and very restrictive step that would not solve the problem of illegal abortion in Portugal. Unfortunately, reality has agreed with the latter opinion.

ABORTION: CURRENT LAW AND PRACTICE

The Law of 1984

In the law of June 1984—Exclusion of Illegality in some Cases of Voluntary Termination of Pregnancy—illegal abortion is punished with three years' imprisonment. However, if the abortion is done to avoid "social criticism" from family, neighbours, or friends, or for some other serious motive, the penalty will not exceed one year. The performers of illegal abortions will also be punished.

Abortion may be legal in the following cases:

- It is the only way to prevent the death of the pregnant woman or serious injury to her physical or mental health.
- It may help avoid the serious danger of death of the pregnant woman or serious and durable injury to her physical or mental health.
- There are sound reasons to believe that the unborn child will suffer, without any possibility of cure, a serious disease or malformation.
- There is serious evidence that the pregnancy resulted from a rape.

In the first two cases and the fourth, the abortion cannot be performed after the first 12 weeks of pregnancy. In the case of malformation, the abortion may be performed up to the 16th week of pregnancy. The abortions must be performed in official health institutions or in other recognised private institutions. If the abortion is performed in a state hospital, it will be free of charge or at a very low cost. Health professionals may refuse to participate in abortion operations on grounds of conscience, in which case they will have to submit a written declaration.

Abortion in Practice

It is not possible to provide an exact description of the current situation as regards abortions performed in Portugal. No national data are collected or available. The data that exist come from several local studies. National statistics provide inexact figures, using ambiguous concepts such as "lost pregnancies" (National Fertility Survey 1980) or "nonsuccessful pregnancies" (National Health Survey 1987).

Nevertheless, in spite of the difficulty in collecting information on an illegal event, all the available data show that illegal abortion still affects a very significant number of Portuguese women. On the other hand, in the official data the number of legal abortions recorded as performed in state hospitals seems to be ridiculously low. In 1980, the National Fertility Survey concluded that 16 percent of women had had a lost pregnancy. But at the same time a study of the FPA Lisbon branch, done in one area of Lisbon, revealed that around 30 percent of women respondents had had at least one abortion in their lives. Eleven percent of them had had more than five abortions. The majority of abortions were carried out for economic reasons. A significant number of women had had an abortion without their husband's knowledge, and half of them had postabortion medical complications. Sixty-six percent of the abortions were because of failure to use contraception. This confirmed the suspicion that abortion is still used as a method of birth control in Portugal.

In a contemporary study of women working in a big factory in Lisbon, around 33 percent of the sexually active women had had an abortion. Again, the women over 40 years of age used abortion as a method of birth control; half of their pregnancies were terminated.

In 1982 and 1983, around 10 women each day were assisted in the emergency units of one of the main hospitals in Lisbon because of postabortion medical complications. In 1988 the main gynaecology emergency hospital in Lisbon assisted 159 girls under 19 years old because of abortion complications. In 1983, a national survey of young people between 15 and 25 in age found that 5 percent of the girls who had had sexual intercourse had experienced an abortion. In 1987, a study in the Coimbra region (north-central Portugal) found that 25 percent of the women respondents had had at least one abortion. Finally, in 1987 the National Health Survey revealed that 24 percent of married women in the fertile age group had had at least one nonsuccessful pregnancy.

All these studies reveal that, in spite of progress in the knowledge and use of contraception, in spite of the positive attitude and policy that the state developed during the last decade and especially after 1984, illegal abortion of unwanted pregnancies is still practiced by a significant proportion of Portuguese women. In fact, the most recent data on the use of contraception have shown that only 50 percent of married women between the ages of 15 and 49 use a safe contraceptive method. If the pill is now the most common contraceptive method used in Portugal, withdrawal is still used by 20 percent of couples and nonuse of contraception still exists for 24 percent of the sample.

The 1984 law did not change this situation; it did not provide legal abortion for the thousands of women who have to face unwanted pregnancies. There are a number of reasons for this failure.

First, since the law was approved in the face of strong resistance from some political groups, the church, and significant professional groups, its implementation was difficult without other steps taken in the health services. Second, the law did not clarify the kind of services necessary for its implementation, and was not subject to further regulations that could have made it more concrete. Health ministerial teams did not define clear policy or programme to implement the law.

Third, no information campaigns or counselling services were organised or supported by the government. Fourth, according to the law, no specific measures were needed to ensure implementation of services; however, the right of conscientious objection contradicts this and in fact is one of the main obstacles to realising the law.

Fifth, the text of the law made it difficult or impossible to obtain an abortion in a large number of cases of foetal malformation. Sixteen weeks is not long enough to confirm many such malformations; some examinations are only available later than this. (The Spanish law, originally similar to the Portuguese, was rapidly corrected on this point, allowing eugenic abortions until 22 weeks of pregnancy.)

As a result, it is not surprising that information collected by the FPA reveals minimal official abortion service:

1. There is a very low public awareness of the possibility to have a legal abortion under the 1984 law.

2. Legal abortion is possible only in the central hospitals of the cities of Lisbon and Coimbra, and in some provincial hospitals. Of 67 hospitals contacted, 15 could not perform abortions because they had no obstetric service; 19 did not perform them in spite of the existence of these services, claiming a lack of resources, conscientious objection, or absence of requests. Only 17 hospitals stated that they perform abortions, 3 of them in Lisbon, 1 in Coimbra, and the others in smaller cities.

3. The number of abortions is incredibly low when compared to the figures mentioned above on the practice of abortion. Since 1984, only around 400 legal abortions were performed in the country, the majority of them owing to malformation of the foetus (43 percent) or danger to the woman's health (44 percent). Abortions in cases of rape were 0.5 percent, while 12.2 percent were performed for other reasons. Eight-six percent of abortions were performed in the central hospitals of Lisbon and Coimbra.

4. All requests for abortion are evaluated by ethical or technical commissions specially constituted for this purpose. But there are no common standards to evaluate the requests. A request could be accepted in one hospital and refused in another. One-third of the requests were refused by the few hospitals that perform legal abortions.

Clearly the law is not being implemented in most hospitals and when it is, it happens under the severe and subjective control of medical committees. Because of this, illegal abortion is easy, unsafe, and expensive. The main result of this law has been to legalise several kinds of abortion that have always been performed in the hospitals, thus protecting the doctors who previously were risking their careers for eugenic or therapeutic abortions. The law also offers greater protection for the private clinics that perform abortions. In fact control of these clinics is much more difficult and inspections are infrequent.

For their part, the state and the health services did not assume their responsibilities to implement the law, even if those duties were restricted. When the law was passed, the health minister (from the Socialist party) did not support legalisation. He was one of the signatories of an anti-choice statement, contradicting his party's position on the issue. The health ministers who followed were liberals, some supportive of more extensive legalisation but who had difficulty convincing the rest of their party.

In the state hospitals, although the law legalised certain medical performances, it also placed the performers of abortion under strict control and scrutinisation by their many anti-choice colleagues and the hospital boards. Sometimes some of them experienced more difficulties than before the law. In some cases, mainly in provincial hospitals in more religious regions, there were only a few doctors prepared to perform abortions among a majority who declared or nondeclared conscientious objection. "This is not Lisbon; here you would be automatically identified as an abortionist" is an opinion often heard among these professionals.

For many health professionals, abortion remains an uncomfortable subject they prefer to ignore. This is true even for those who agree in principle with abortion. On the other side, the pro-choice movement in effect delegated the task of implementing the law to the politicians and the health professionals, and almost disappeared, believing that the fight was over. Similarly, some feminist groups declined and ceased, while others turned their attention to other priorities.

These factors may explain why, with a similar law, the situation in Spain is totally different and women have the possibility of having a legal and safe abortion in a state hospital. In 1988, 26,000 legal abortions were performed in that country.

In 1987, the Liberal party obtained an absolute majority in the parliament. Together with all the constraints mentioned above, the new health minister—a woman in favour of legal abortion—had to face severe professional conflict with health professionals and reform was again forgotten. From time to time, parliamentarians remember that the abortion law was not being implemented, but no new initiatives were undertaken.

THE FUTURE

At the end of 1990, several organisations raised again the question of illegal abortion when it was known that legal proceedings were being organised against more than 1,000 women whose names were found in the files of an illegal abortion clinic. Some of these women submitted to medical examinations to confirm the accusations. This process was condemned by all the women's organisations affiliated with the consultation council of the

Commission for Equal Rights (an official department). Some professional organisations and some groups formerly involved in the pro-choice movements began to organise a new public debate on the question. This debate will probably propose some changes in the existing law, but it will also propose practical measures than can provide information and services to make legal abortion possible.

In 1992, revision of the penal code was begun. The group working on this recommended some changes in the abortion legislation, namely expansion of the time to have an abortion in the case of foetus malformation (22 weeks), and also the inclusion of some new motives linked to sexual abuse. Since the new code must be approved by the parliament, it is probable that public debate will start in 1993, even if these are quite small changes in the law.

The pro-choice groups will have to again face their ideological opponents of abortion legalisation. They will also have against them the heavy and silent influence of lots of abortionists who have become wealthy through illegal abortions. They will have to deal with all the politicians who prefer to be quiet (even if they are not opposed to legalisation), rather than risk their political careers. They will have to counter the traditional attitudes of important professional sectors.

On the other hand, they will have with them the strength of public opinion and support by important professional sectors. They will have as evidence the results of Portugal's ambiguous attitude towards abortion. They will also have seven years' experience with the 1984 law and its limits. Will they be able to achieve significant changes in this situation?

REFERENCES

Aroso, A., et al. *Aborto e Contracepção em Debate*. Lisboa: Instituto Superior de Ciencias Social e Politicas, 1975.

CLA, *Dossier Aborto*. Lisboa: Comissão para a Legalização do Aborto, 1982.

Correia, I. "O Aborto," *A Sexologia em Portugal* (1987).

Cruz, F. A., et al. "Contracepcão em Coimbra," *Planeamento Familiar* 41 (1988).

Diário da Assembleia da República, 10, 11, 12, 59, 67, 68, 75, 1g Série, Lisboa 1982 and 1984.

Diário da República 109, I Série, Lisboa 1984.

Delegação Regional de Lisboa da APF. "Conhecimento Documentado da Zona Piloto," *Planeamento Familiar* 9/10 (1980).

Fiadeiro, Antónia. *Aborto, o Crime Está na Lei*. Lisboa: Ed. Relógio de Água, 1983.

Metrass, C., et al. *Aborto, Direito ao Nosso Corpo*. Lisboa: Ed. Mulheres em Luta, 1975.

Miguel, N., and D. Vilar. *Afectividade e Sexualidade no Novo Contexto Social e Cultural*. Lisboa: IED Cadernos "Juventude," 1987.

Ministério da Saúde. *Avaliacão do Programa de Planeamento Familiar*. Lisboa: 1987.

———. Dep. Estudos e Planeamento de Saude. *Inquérito Nacional de Saúde*, Vol. 1. Lisboa: Ministério da Saúde, 1989.

Teixeira, M. S. "Fertilidade e Contracepcão numa Unidade Fabril de Lisboa," *Planeamento Familiar* 15 (1982).

Victor, A., et al. *Contracepcão e Aborto*. Lisboa: APF, 1977.

SPAIN

Encarna Bodelón González

Translated by Nuala McKeever

THE HISTORY OF ABORTION LAW

The Republic and the Franco Era

To understand the background of abortion in Spain, we must first look briefly at two main historical periods: the Republic and the Franco dictatorship.

It was during the Republic that the major issues affecting women first emerged in public, such as women's right to vote, the first divorce legislation, and concern about family planning, contraception, and abortion. In what was then still a very Catholic society, abortion became one of the most divisive issues. Because of this, and because of the ambivalent attitude of some leftist parties towards the subject, abortion was not legalised at a national level. In Catalonia, however, there was one particular ruling that made abortion possible. A bill passed on July 25, 1936, permitted termination of a pregnancy for therapeutic, eugenic, or ethical reasons. This law was introduced in an attempt to reduce the number of backstreet abortions. The law in Catalonia differed from that in the rest of Spain for sociopolitical reasons. There was a strong women's movement in Catalonia that was heavily influenced by anarchist thinking. Within anarchist politics, the right to choose motherhood freely and the right to birth control were seen as an important weapon in the struggle for women's liberation.[1] But the importance of anarcho-syndicalism in Catalonia was not widespread throughout the Republic.

Partly because of civil unrest at that time, the call to emancipation was not seen as a priority by all women.

The end of the civil war in 1939 and the start of the Franco dictatorship marked the beginning of a dark era for women. The year 1941 saw the introduction of a law "for the protection of the unborn, against abortion and contraceptive propaganda," out of which arose the concept of abortion as a criminal offence. This concept is partly reflected in our present legislation. For 40 years women had to contend not only with the illegality of abortion and the threat of criminal prosecution but also with a complete lack of access to contraception.

With the advent of the 1960s and the influence of feminist movements in Europe, those women who had hitherto concentrated their efforts on political protest now began to intensify their fight for women's liberation. In addition, the 1970s saw an increasing number of women travelling to other European countries to have abortions.

Democracy and Women's Struggle

The transition to democracy in 1975 and the Constitution of 1978 raised expectations of a change in the abortion situation. The feminist movement set out to reclaim its demand for the right to abortion, together with decriminalisation of the use of contraceptives and access to sex education and sex information. The development of feminist thinking on the abortion issue led to a realisation of how the role of motherhood interacts with other factors in patriarchal society. At first, the pro-abortion campaign concentrated on the issue of legalising abortion and giving support to those women who had suffered. The famous Bilbao judgement, in which 11 women were accused of the crime of having an abortion, highlighted a widespread problem. This judgement marked the beginning of a period of great activity within the women's movement, and led to much debate in political circles.

Within the women's movement there was growing awareness of how the problem of abortion was completely bound up with other issues like sexuality. As a result, the feminist movement saw that abortion was not negotiable. They refused to accept that a woman's freedom to exercise this right should be limited by restrictions such as age, the interference of doctors, judges, colleagues or relations, the need to prove necessity in particular cases and circumstances, or by imposition of terms for having an abortion. This interpretation of the right to abortion was an attempt to place this issue alongside other demands, highlighting the right of women to make their own decisions.

In 1982, the Socialist party (PSOE) won the general election. In 1983, the first Socialist plan for partial legalisation of abortion met a strong reaction from the feminist movement—those to the left of the PSOE and the unions. In that initial period of optimism, those women who criticised the plan were to be of particular importance. (Since then we have seen that it was a crude neo-liberal plan.)

The partial legalisation of abortion did not come about until 1985. Women had been waiting for recognition of their right to abortion, but as we shall see, the law did not provide this recognition, but rather continued to presume that a woman is not capable of making a decision about her own body. This is the norm to which there are only a few exceptions.

ABORTION: CURRENT LAW AND PRACTICE

The Law of 1985

The 1985 reform did not bring about a complete reform of those clauses within the penal code that cover abortion. The basic principle that abortion is punishable by law still stands. However, the new law contains three immunity clauses:

1. If the abortion is necessary to avoid serious threat to the life, physical or mental health of the woman (therapeutic reason)

2. If the pregnancy is a result of rape

3. If it is suspected that the foetus will be born with severe physical or mental deformities (eugenic reason)

Besides these three conditions, further requirements have to be met. The abortion must be carried out in an approved public or private health centre and must have the woman's consent.

Each of the three categories has its own further requirements. In the case of therapeutic abortion, a doctor other than the one who performs the operation must certify that there is a risk to the life or mental or physical well-being of the pregnant woman. Most abortions fall into this category. The expression "grave danger to the mental health of the mother" has provided wide discretion in the application of the law. This has meant that medical opinion can be very important in applying the law. The interpretation of a particular case can vary widely according to the personal convictions of the doctor and the pressures to which he or she may be subjected. Women's groups have condemned the restrictive and discriminatory way in which this clause of decriminalisation has been applied. Further, they have deplored the fact that many women, whose only problem is that of wishing to have an abortion, have had to appear as suffering from mental problems or have had to claim such problems in order to have an abortion. Women are forced to express their wishes as if they were the result of madness or mental imbalance.

In the second category, that of abortion because of rape, the most striking fact is that very few women have cited this as a reason. This is not strange if one realises that abortion in this case must be carried out within 12 weeks of conception and the rape must have been reported beforehand. The problem is that women who are raped often do not report the crime right away. In Spain it is still widely believed that reporting a rape will do no more than create further problems for the victim, forcing her to relive the horror of the rape.

The third category, eugenic abortion, must be carried out within the first 22 weeks of pregnancy and must be approved by a doctor other than the one carrying out the operation. Few women have had abortions in this category.

With the above exceptions, abortion is still a criminal offence in Spain. If a woman has an abortion for reasons that do not fit one of the three categories, she can face a prison sentence of anywhere from six months to six years. The person who assists with the abortion also risks a jail sentence, the length of which depends on whether or not the operation was done with the woman's consent and the degree of medical expertise involved.

The reform pleased no one. As far as the Right was concerned, the timid reform would pave the way for abortion on demand. For women's groups, left-wing parties, and diverse socialist movements, the partial decriminalisation was inadequate, offering no solution to the abortion problem. The government line was based on the idea that Spanish society was not ready to accept broad legalisation or decriminalisation, and besides, broader decriminalisation might aggravate relations with conservative sectors of the population. As always in recent Spanish history, so-called moderation was imposed in the name of a hypothetical consensus. There never was any consensus, and the reaction of the Right and the Catholic Church was just as strong as it would have been had decriminalisation been broader. Once again the opposition tried to impose, politically through the state, standards that are a matter of ethical and moral consideration for the individual, in this case women. For the Left, partial legalisation was one of the first frustrations of their hopes for the "socialist plan." From the start, women's groups and groups on the left came out in opposition to the reform, highlighting the problems that it would create—namely that the majority of abortions taking place would not be covered by this law and would continue to be illegal.

Abortion in Practice

The 1985 reform allowed for a specific range of decriminalised abortions to be carried out in approved public and private health centres. Government figures from 1991 show that 4 percent of legal abortions are carried out on women under 25 years of age, and 13 percent on women between 15 and

19 years old—which reflects the high incidence of unwanted pregnancy in adolescents and young women.

Public health care in Spain is quite broad, however 98 percent of the abortions that have been carried out legally have taken place in private health clinics. There are several reasons for this. On the one hand, the law allowing partial decriminalisation left room for a wide range of medical objections. Many doctors have refused to carry out abortions, often owing to pressures on them because the law is so ambiguous. In some regions it is impossible to have an abortion on the health service since all the doctors have objected to carrying them out.[2]

But there are more fundamental reasons for the high number of abortions done in private clinics. The bureaucracy involved in having an abortion in the public sector is complex. In addition, 90 percent or more of the abortions in Spain are done for therapeutic reasons, mostly under the "grave danger to the mental health of the mother" clause. This means that whether or not a woman can have an abortion depends on a doctor's interpretation of that clause. Therefore, women go directly to private clinics, where the clause is generally interpreted more broadly.

Obviously this has given rise to a strange situation. Although the public health service can cover the cost of an abortion, the bulk of decriminalised abortions are in fact being excluded from the health service and paid for directly by the women involved. The cost of an abortion in a private clinic in Spain is between 35,000 and 50,000 pesetas (approximately £175–£250). There has been strong criticism of the fact that these costs are prohibitive for women of low income and that in reality abortion remains outside the public health service.

Feminist groups and representatives from private medicine estimate that the total number of abortions in Spain is over 100,000 each year. This figure includes abortions carried out illegally either within the state or abroad, meaning that approximately 70 percent of abortions in Spain are carried out illegally. The high incidence of illegal abortion is due to limitations in the current law. The partial decriminalisation does not include the majority of cases and so most women have abortions illegally.

The figures for illegal abortions could be higher were it not that some doctors interpret the law widely. Continuing protests by conservative groups against private clinics that carry out abortions has ensured that this broad interpretation of the law does not grow broader yet. Faced with the threat of legal intervention or protests, many clinics either refuse to carry out certain abortions or do them illegally.

Illegal abortions are not just taking place in Spain. Many women follow the so-called abortion trail abroad. Before the 1985 reform, most abortions took place outside Spain. Many women resorted to backstreet operations in awful conditions, but if the woman could afford it, she might go the Britain, the Netherlands, or France. It is estimated that by the end of the 1970s and the beginning of the 1980s, 33,000 Spanish women per year travelled abroad for abortions.[3] After 1985, this number went down.

It must be remembered that women seeking illegal abortions find themselves in a wide range of situations, personally, economically, and culturally. In some cases, the illegality of an abortion is a much greater problem than in others. For socially and economically deprived women, access to abortion is difficult and many terminate under very dangerous conditions. The current law is, therefore, discriminatary and unjust.

As we have seen, administration of the 1985 reform has involved legal prosecution of doctors, patients, and hospitals by certain conservative and Catholic groups. Various anti-abortion groups have attacked private health clinics, alleging that they have carried out illegal abortions. This has resulted in court orders and police records, even though in most cases the court orders have later been overturned. Members of the medical profession have condemned the lack of protection afforded by current law, under which a judge has the power to decide whether or not a doctor has acted illegally. Similarly, the law fails to protect patients, who can discover that their medical records have been examined and their right to privacy has been invaded.

The Politics of Abortion

When the 1985 reform took effect, many people declared that Spanish society was not ready to accept broader decriminalisation and that the reform went against people's beliefs. In 1992, surveys show that 80 percent of the population approve of the circumstances in which abortion is decriminalised. Also, a high percentage think the present law is not wide enough and would be in favour of either a fourth decriminalised category relating to socioeconomic conditions or a law that allows abortion more or less on demand within an as yet unspecified time limit.

There has been ongoing debate about broadening the law. This debate is characterised on the one hand by clear opposition to the present legislation, as demonstrated by the women's groups, and on the other by the ambivalent position that the Socialist party has held since it came to power. At the time of writing, press reports indicate that the PSOE government plans to change the law on abortion within the next few months (see section on the Future). But first, it is important to remember what the women's movement has tried to achieve on the abortion issue.

Since 1982, various member groups of the Coordinating Body of Feminist Organisations of Spain have defended their proposals for an abortion law based on two fundamental principles: a woman's right to decide freely on the termination of her pregnancy, and consideration of abortion as a medical operation equal to other medical operations, provided by the public health service.

This right to choose motherhood freely is linked to freedom of sexuality, and because of this, women's movements in Spain have always insisted on access to contraception and sex education. In this regard, it must be remembered that sex education is virtually absent in the state education system and that, although great changes have come about as regards information on contraception, not enough has been done. Until 1978, artificial methods of birth control (the pill, etc.) were prohibited in Spain. Although they are much more widespread in recent years, no great effort has been made to make information available to women generally. Proof of this is the fact that 56 percent of women using some type of contraceptive do so with no medical supervision. Another important statistic is that in 1985, 52 percent of women of childbearing age were not using any contraception. It is not surprising, therefore, that the women's movement links the question of abortion with issues of sex information and contraception. It is significant that when government bodies deal with the abortion issue, they isolate it from this context.

Another important point in the legal proposal drawn up by the Coordinating Body of Feminists is the absence of any insistence on a medical opinion prior to an abortion and rejection of any system of diagnosis and categorisation.

THE FUTURE

Women's groups have not been the only critics of the 1985 reform. Left-wing political parties, civil movements, unions (including the Socialist union, UGT), and even members of the PSOE have pointed to the law's inadequacies. Shortly after the measure was passed, discussion began on the possibility of extending decriminalisation to a socioeconomic category. It was even suggested that the current law be replaced by one that allows for abortion more or less on demand within an unspecified time in early pregnancy.

In the last two years, and before the ever-imminent reform of the penal code, speculation has been rife. At last it seems that the Socialist government plans to undertake abortion law reform in the autumn of 1992,[4] and reform will involve widening decriminalisation to include this socioeconomic category, together with a system of abortion on demand in early pregnancy. But none of this has yet been decided at the time of writing.

All indications are that the new regulation will deal differently with the matter of medical objections. While respecting the rights of those in the medical profession, it will attempt to resolve some situations that characterise the present scene. On the other hand, it appears that new regulations will retain the insistence on medical diagnosis prior to an abortion.

One new modification may be particularly important. According to recent statements by the minister of health, the public health service would no longer cover abortions costs. This would mean development of the private sector, as started by the 1985 reform, with all its inherent discriminations.

The Socialist minister argues that the costs of abortion should not be covered by the health service since abortion is not a basic health need, but this argument highlights the attitudes that lie behind the new plan.

The question that now arises is why these changes have come about. The answer should be found in all the problems that have resulted from the 1985 reform and the social attitudes that brought them about. Partial decriminalisation only exacerbated the problems the law was supposed to solve. Furthermore, the facts prove that Spanish society accepts or tolerates the practice of abortion, and is ready for change.

Even if decriminalisation is widened, it will not end the abortion issue, since Spanish women will find ourselves in but a new phase of the struggle that began when women reclaimed their right to abortion.

NOTES

1. The Communist and Socialist parties viewed these issues as secondary. They believed that women's liberation was bound up in the liberation of the proletariat.

2. The Spanish state is organised on a regional basis similar in many ways to a federal structure.

3. See *Commentaria Sociologico. Estructura Social de España*, 55–56 (July–December 1986): 778.

4. Because of a general election in the interim, this deadline was not met. As of the end of August 1993, there had been no change in the abortion law.

REFERENCES

Butlletí epidemològic de Catalunya. *Avortament legal a Catalunya*, Generalitat de Catalunya, Barcelona, 1990.

Colectivo. "¿Que está pasando con el aborto en nuestro país?" *Hinojo y Perejil*, marzo 1992.

Coordinadora de Organizaciones Feministas. *Proyecto de Ley de Aborto*, 1982.

Ibanez, J. L. *La despenalización del aborto voluntario en el ocaso del s. XX*, Ed. Siglo XXI. Madrid, 1991.

Jiménez Blanco, J. "El aborto. Una interpretación sociológica," *Ley del Aborto. Un informe universitario.* Bilbao: Universidad del Deusto, 1985.

Mir, S. (ed.). *La despenalización del aborto.* Barcelona: Universidad Autónoma de Barcelona, 1983.

Montero Corominas, J. *Problemática social de la ley de interucpción voluntaria del embarazo.* IV Congreso Estatal de Planificación familiar, Sevilla, noviembre 1989.

Pineda, E., "Las razones de las feministas," *El País* 10 (noviembre 1988).

Sáez de Santamaría, G. "El poder y el aborto," *El País* 1 (febrero 1990).

Scanlon, G. *La polémica feminista en la España contemporánea.* Madrid: Ed. Akal, 1986.

Uria, P., E. Pineda, and M. Oliván. *Polémicas Feministas.* Madrid: Ed. Revolución, 1985.

Varios. *El aborto. Un tema para debate.* Madrid: Seminario de la Fundación Investigaciones Marxistas, 1982.

SWEDEN

Katarina Lindahl

THE HISTORY OF ABORTION LAW

The Era of Illegal Abortions

It was a long journey to reach the current Swedish law on abortion. The situation for women was hard until the middle of this century. In the 15th century, women with knowledge of contraceptives and methods of abortion were burned as witches. Their knowledge almost disappeared. As late as the 19th century, an unmarried mother was considered a whore, degraded by society. She had to go to church to make an official apology, and the father of her child was never sought. The strain of the experience often meant that a woman who just had given birth, or even a pregnant woman, took both her own life and that of her child or foetus.

Industrialisation brought big changes to society, but single mothers were still the weakest group, very poor and marginalised. Four out of five single mothers would give away their children, and the children were placed in foster families in the country. Another solution was to leave the child to so-called angel makers—old and poor women to whom the mother gave a small amount of money to take care of the child. But the angel maker usually mistreated the child, giving it almost no food and no love; this killed the child in a short period of time. Her role was to make "angels" out of small children, and everyone knew that that was her purpose.

Meanwhile, illegal abortions were widespread and led to death or serious illness for many women. It was obvious that abortion was a question of class distinction. A pregnant woman had no right to keep her employment, so many poor women were forced to abort in order to maintain their income. Sex education did not exist. It was even forbidden (as a result of a 1910 law) to provide information about contraceptives (condoms and diaphragms). But it was not forbidden to use them. This, of course, meant that well-to-do people learned where to get them and how to use them. They also could pay to be anonymous while they delivered the child in a proper hospital, and they could pay for child care afterwards. For a poor woman, however, the only known solution was an illegal abortion, with its great physical risks and heavy mental strain. Feelings of shame and guilt were often strong, while the man involved usually did not give any support at all.

The Fight for Legal Abortion

Some individuals in the labour movement and women who fought for women's rights tried to provide information and education on matters concerning contraceptives. However, the actions were both difficult and dangerous; they could be put in prison.

During the 1920s and 1930s, there was intensive discussion about these matters. This was mainly a result of the educative work of Elise Ottesen Jensen, one of the founders of the International Planned Parenthood Federation (IPPF) and the Swedish Association for Sex Education (RFSU). She travelled all around Sweden teaching sex education to every one who wanted to listen, but the majority of her audience were poor people in desperate need of more knowledge.

The RFSU had a radical programme from the beginning. One of its main points was the right to legal abortion, on both medical and social indications. It also agitated for sexual counselling, the legal right to information about sex education and contraceptives, and free contraceptives to everyone who needed them.

In the first law to allow abortion in Sweden (1938, amended in 1946), the indications for abortion were:

• Weakness or illness that made the woman unable to go through a pregnancy (medical and sociomedical grounds)

• Pregnancy after rape

• An obvious risk that the woman could give the foetus a serious illness and the risk of mental retardation

The law did not consider abortion a basic right for women. Also, it did not stop illegal abortions; in fact, they increased. It is estimated that in the 1940s about 25 percent of the resources of a large gynaecological clinic in Stockholm were allocated to postabortion medical care—that is, to medical damages after illegal abortions. In the 1940s and 1950s, an abortion was a very unpleasant and often painful experience. The law was humiliating to women. A lot of shame and guilt were linked to an abortion, and many doctors were rude to women who asked for an abortion.

The 1960s were in many ways the beginning of a new era. Society was turning to more radical politics, and a movement for women's rights grew. Both political parties and the new movements agitated for women's rights economically and socially, for the right to work and for a salary big enough to provide a good living. It became more and more difficult to force women to give birth to children they did not want to have. When the pill came (1964), for the first time in history women could control their own fertility and pregnancy.

Changes in political attitudes were combined with a decline in the influence of religion. Conservative Christianity lost power. People started to live together without being married; attitudes towards single mothers changed in a positive direction; new laws and rules were introduced to give single mothers better economic and social conditions.

This was the decade of the so-called Polish affairs. Women who were refused an abortion in Sweden went to Poland to get it. In those days, an abortion was often late, as a result of bureaucracy. A woman needed positive approval from the National Medical Board, a gynaecologist, a psychiatrist, and a counsellor. There were occasions when the different parties did not agree with each other, and the woman had to have an illegal abortion.

ABORTION: CURRENT LAW AND PRACTICE

The Law of 1975

The present Swedish abortion act came into force in 1975, and is a wide and liberal law. Abortions are performed by medical doctors in a hospital or in other medical institutions approved by the National Board of Health and Welfare. The law entitles the woman to decide before the end of the 18th week of pregnancy whether or not she wants to complete her term. Up to the 12th week the woman is not asked any questions about her reasons. No one can stop her and no one has the legal possibility of forcing her to change her mind. But the law stipulates that she meet a counsellor if she has the abortion between the 12th and 18th week, although she still makes the decision herself. If it is obvious that there are no obstacles to the abortion, the woman and the gynaecologist can together decide that she does not need to meet a counsellor. The fact is that the talk with a counsellor takes place in less than half the cases. Some years ago a parliamentary committee suggested that this condition be replaced by an offer to meet a counsellor.

It is also possible to have an abortion after the 18th week of pregnancy, but then an approval from the National Board of Health and Welfare is necessary. The situation of the woman or the foetus has to be very serious—medically, psychologically, or socially—for permission to be given. The National Board give their approval in about half of all cases—about 100 a year are granted. Approval is not granted if the foetus is judged to be viable, and today this means that approval is never given after the 22nd week. This changes if new methods are found to keep a younger foetus alive. If there is a serious risk of the woman's death if she continues with her pregnancy, all possible efforts are made to keep the foetus alive outside the woman.

Abortion in Practice

Sweden has kept reasonably reliable statistics on abortion since 1955. However, before 1975 there were many illegal abortions, and the statistics show only the legal abortions. In the early 1970s, the figures became more reliable, with statistics showing that since 1975 late abortions have decreased dramatically. As a result of its liberal law, Sweden does not have any illegal abortions and therefore there is no punishment for illegal abortions.

Abortion is available to every woman living in Sweden who asks for it. There are no formal restrictions on availability, nor are there restrictions regarding class, age, or region. In addition, there are no known informal or secret restrictions.

During the last 30 years Sweden has received more immigrants than ever before. Some of them come from countries with a traditional—more conservative and negative—view on abortion and sex education. When women in these groups want an abortion or the pill, they can experience difficulties because of the attitudes of their husbands or fathers. Thus, it is important both to support the women and educate the men. Immigrant families often criticise the fact that professionals in youth clinics have to observe professional silence. This means that a young girl can get contraceptives and obtain an abortion without her parents knowing about it. But the midwives always try to find out if it is possible for the girl to tell her parents, in order to get support from them. It is always the girl, however, who makes the decision on these matters.

All costs for an abortion are paid through the national health service available for everyone in Sweden and the costs are low. The woman has to pay when she visits the doctor (£12 in 1991) and when she has the abortion (£12). She also has to pay a smaller amount (about £8 a day) if she has to stay in the hospital. But nowadays most women go home on the same day. The costs are the same if a woman comes to hospital for a broken leg or for an abortion. If she has to stay home from work after an abortion, she gets the usual compensation through the national health insurance. This means that in terms of cost, an abortion is comparable to any other kind of health service or illness.

When the present abortion law came about in Sweden, in 1975, many people were worried that the rate of abortion would increase rapidly. This did not happen, because the abortion act was accompanied by a big programme for the prevention of unwanted pregnancies. Youth clinics were opened, and today we have them all over Sweden as a part of the primary health care system. The youth clinics give counselling free of charge to young people in matters of sexuality and contraceptives.

A major programme for good sex education in school was also started. It was often midwives who gave the information, however it was important that teachers also were positive towards sex education, and most of them were. Schoolteachers in Sweden have traditionally taken a radical view on sex education. Sex education varies in quality, but the important goal is to talk naturally about sexuality. Sex education has been mandatory in Swedish schools since 1956.

Steps were taken to give information about contraceptives to adult women. When the midwives got the right to prescribe contraceptives, it became possible to shorten waiting lists and to combine prescription with good information. The result of this preventive work was that figures for unwanted pregnancies did not increase after enactment of the new law. The figures for teenage pregnancies even decreased. Since the middle of the 1980s, the rate of unplanned pregnancies and abortion has increased slightly, also among teenagers. However, recent figures are very positive and show that the abortion rate decreased by 2 percent during the first six months of 1991, and for teenagers by 7 percent during the same period. This trend has continued since 1991.

Moral Attitudes

Most women do not consider abortion a matter to be ashamed of, but they do not talk much about it, either. It is important that more women try to be open about their own abortions. Otherwise it is possible to label women who have abortions as a small and irresponsible group, which works in the interests of those who want a more restrictive law. In reality, abortion is an experience that at least 30,000 women in Sweden have annually; every second woman in Sweden has an abortion during her lifetime.

Kristina Holmgren, former medical supervisor of the RFSU Stockholm clinic, interviewed women who had abortions at a hospital in Stockholm. Her results reveal a lot about how women look at the question of abortion. The results confirm experiences that midwives, other health workers, and women have had. She also considers an interesting theory about male and female ways of ethical thinking.

The male world is considered as the norm, and the female as divergent. The traditional male way of dealing with a moral conflict is to divide it into smaller parts, and analyze one part at a time with a perspective of logic or justice, in order to create rules. The male way of dealing with abortion often comes out as a series of efforts to answer critical questions about the foetus: "Is the foetus a living being? When does it become a living being? Do we have the right to terminate a pregnancy after the twelfth week?" and so on. These issues are the main ones debated. But in reality the abortion dilemma is more complex.

New psychological studies show that women asking for abortions seem to have a broader spectrum when making moral judgements. They analyse the moral dilemma as a question of relationships and the responsibility of maintaining close human relationships without hurting anybody. To the woman, the foetus is a part of a network of human relationships, and she expresses a responsibility for the maintenance of this network, both taken as a whole and in a long-term perspective. "Will my child have a father? What quality of life can I offer this child?" These are examples of questions that women put on the agenda. Instead of asking when life starts, they ask how life will be. This way of looking at a moral dilemma as a question of relationships, responsibility, and care is considered to be a female phenomenon. It should be observed, however, that some men also have this outlook.

Studies have also been done on the psychological effects of an abortion. These studies show that women experience psychological problems very rarely. Fewer then 5 percent have problems like depression a long time after an abortion. The studies also show that this mainly applies to women who have had problems before the abortion; their problems are often related to the man. But even if women in general do not experience psychological problems, they do not look at abortion as a minor affair. It is considered as a big decision by every woman. However, no one is better at making this decision than the woman herself.

The view of what is right and what is wrong is formed by interaction between people over many years. It is usually not influenced by law and education. Experiences among relatives and close friends can often offer more useful advice or help than a moral code set by strangers. When the difference between personal moral conceptions and legislation is too wide, close friends come out as most important.

The official attitude towards sexuality in Sweden is very open. Nearly all Swedish children at the age of seven know where children come from. The attitude is that children must get honest answers to their questions. When the children become teenagers, most parents are much more afraid of criminality and drugs than of sexuality. As a result, it is common and accepted that teenagers let their boyfriend or girlfriend stay overnight.

Sex education in school is usually concrete, but it is often criticised by the pupils for being too technical and with too little talk about emotions. This is rather typical. Swedes talk openly, but rarely about sexual joy or how love feels. Even if there is openness, there is a lot of privacy involved. Too often sex education concentrates on diseases and unwanted pregnancies instead of sexual joy. We teach teenagers what to fear rather than what to care about—fertility, sensuality, and a joyful sex life. Since teenagers have a positive view of sexuality, the preventive work must start with that and not with the threat of fear.

Nearly all people who get married or live together have had prior sexual experience. It is common that they have had several sexual relationships, and this is accepted. Many people marry when they have lived together for a long time, often when they are expecting a child or have just had one. Divorces are common, and most of those who divorce marry someone else later. Often the parents have shared custody of the children after a divorce.

In Sweden we have high ideals about faithfulness, however this does not mean that infidelity is unusual. There is a difference between men and women in their way of handling unfaithfulness. It is not unusual for men to have long parallel relationships without intention of divorce. It is not so common that women have long relationships alongside their marriages. Women instead fall in love and want to divorce rather quickly. Women often take the initiative to divorce when they feel that they are fed up with their marriage.

Single mothers are accepted and get support from society, both economically and in other ways, such as help to get a place to live. But single mothers still have a hard time. If the father has disappeared, it is difficult to handle all the responsibility for the child. Otherwise, it is common that the father takes care of the children on certain days of the week. In Sweden there are very few teenage mothers.

Prostitution is allowed; only pimps can be punished. In the present debate, a common argument is that the man who pays to get sex should be criminalised. This argument has growing support, even if many people do not care about prostitution. Local authorities take some measures to minimize prostitution, but not enough. Most prostitutes on the street are drug addicts. Pornography is allowed if it does not show hard violence. Pornography with children is forbidden. There is an ideological discussion about pornography.

The Politics of Abortion

Before the abortion act came into force there was intensive discussion in Sweden. Afterwards, some years followed with practically no debate. But still some members of the parliament annually suggested that the act be made more restrictive, though they have no support from the majority in parliament. The professional politicians seeking to change the law have recently got company.

Before describing the resistance, it is necessary to point out that an absolute majority of Swedish people think that the country has a good abortion law. In spring of 1992, research showed that 84 percent of Swedish people questioned were positive about the abortion act. Three years earlier, the figure was 64 percent. Yet this increase in support occurred during a period when opponents of abortion became more vocal. In addition, most Swedes agree with the point that no one is better at making a decision about abortion than the woman concerned. Most people also agree that an abortion is an emergency solution, and that adequate measures to prevent unwanted pregnancies are important. Many people say that it is important to decrease the number of abortions, but they do not think that the best way of doing this is to have a more restrictive law. The acceptance of the law is the result of many years of hard work for openness in sexual matters and sex education. In general, more men than women criticise the law. In the debate, it is often a man who says that there are too many abortions and suggests that the law should be restrictive. One problem is that after an abortion the woman receives a prescription for a contraceptive but usually not a time for another appointment. A new appointment has been shown to be one way to reduce the number of repeat abortions.

Since 1975, attitudes have changed. Today it is much easier to ask for an abortion. Most doctors meet the patients in a professional way. One problem is that the doctor perhaps does not have or does not take enough time to talk to the woman. Many women, and certainly young girls, want to discuss their decision, but it is often difficult to get the time from the doctor. If she asks for it, she will possibly be put in contact with a counsellor.

No doctors like to do abortions and because of that, many abortions are performed by the youngest and least experienced doctors, who cannot chose their work in the same way as their more experienced colleagues. This does not mean that the medical care is insufficient, but maybe the psychological care could be better. Many women claim that they got their best support when talking to other women in the same situation.

We also know that nurses and assistants who clean up after an abortion can find this work difficult. Some of them condemn women who have had abortions. There is a myth about irresponsible women using abortion as a contraceptive, but this comes from a minority among the staff. Many women find that they are well taken care of and say that they got good help in the hospital.

The working conditions of the medical staff have been used in the latest attempts to attack the abortion law. It is said that it is such awful work to clean up after an abortion that the health workers want to change the routines. Lately the National Board for Health and Welfare made a recommendation about burying the remains of the foetus. This was a much criticized recommendation when published in 1990. Those who are critical claim that only human beings are buried, and the consequence of this recommendation is that a foetus is a human being so abortion must be murder. This was also seen as a way to blame the women. To answer the critics, it was said that the recommendation was asked for by medical staff, but the fact is that these same arguments have been used in many countries by the opposition.

In all political parties represented in the parliament there are members who are against abortion and who think that the law should be more restrictive. However, up until 1991 no single political party has attacked the law directly. They do attack it indirectly, however. For example, the Conservatives suggest that a woman who wants an abortion should be obliged to talk to a counsellor; this in reality would mean a more restrictive law. Another suggestion from Conservatives is that the woman pay the real cost for the abortion. This means that it would not be possible to get an abortion with full help from the national health insurance. There have been no suggestions about how to make the man pay the so-called real costs! Demands for restriction come mainly from the bourgeois parties, and their motives are often of an economic nature.

In the election of September 1991, the Christian Democratic party gained a place in the parliament and in the government for the first time. This is the party in Sweden that is most negative towards abortion. They have a very odd way of arguing. They say "We are against the idea of abortion in principle. However, we also believe that it is inhuman to force a woman to give birth to a child she does not want. In this dilemma we have to accept the woman's right to an abortion." The women's branch of this party has produced a booklet in which they say that legal abortion is unnatural. The Christian Democratic party has declared that life begins at the time of conception. The leader of the party has said that the use of an IUD could be compared to an abortion, and that he has difficulty accepting their use. He has also declared that he is sure that the law will be changed as a result of the debate on premature births and foetal diagnosis. The party wants to make it obligatory for the woman to talk with a counsellor who will persuade the woman to refrain from an abortion. They call it "finding other solutions."

In 1991, the Green party held a congress where they decided to accept the abortion law. However, they want an obligation for counselling, adding that men should be represented at counselling sessions. This is a good example of a confused decision. What does "represented at the sessions" mean? What are the reasons to force a woman to talk to a counsellor when she does not want to? When members of the board of the Green party were questioned about this, they answered that the idea is to support both the man and the woman, and that the law is good, but that there is a need for some changes. This must mean a more restrictive law.

In January 1992 one of the nonsocialist parties in the parliament suggested a change in the abortion act, so that the woman could make the decision only up to the 12th week of pregnancy. They also talked about the importance of keeping the moral and ethical dilemma alive.

It is interesting to note that, during the general election campaign in September 1991, the Christian Democratic party was the only one to put the question of abortion on the agenda. And they were critical of the law. The other parties that agree with their representatives in parliament could vote as they liked if it should come to a new vote. Not to consider abortion as a important political question could be a big mistake. It was a struggle in Sweden to achieve the present abortion law and to get it accepted in people's minds. However, that victory may not last forever, especially not in matters that concern women and sexuality. Since 1975 some important politicians (mainly male) have, from time to time, questioned the law. The following claims have been made: "It is too easy to get an abortion; Many women use abortion as a contraceptive; There are too many abortions; There are too many late abortions."

Most of these statements lack a basis in knowledge. Women in Sweden do not use abortion as a contraceptive. That is an absurd assumption in a country with good contraceptive counselling and cheap and easily available contraceptives. The number of abortions in Sweden is not high, especially when taking into account that the figures show all abortions and that there is no "dark figure." Women have a 30-year period in which they are sexually active and fertile, and there will always be contraceptive failures. Considering this, the figures are not particularly high. Those who criticise the law never tell how high the figures for abortion ought to be. They just say that the figures are too high. A more restrictive law can never be the answer to that problem.

Recent years have seen growing opposition to the abortion act. There is hardly anyone who comes out and says: "Let's change the law and make it more restrictive." This kind of talk emanates from minor religious groups only. In Sweden, with its long tradition in this field, one has to use other methods to make people listen. So new issues have appeared on the scene. At first they may seem important and people who are not against legal abortion accept and use these arguments. But when the different arguments are put together, it is easy to see a pattern much like that of anti-choice groups in, for example, the United States.

These "new" issues are seen in claims such as: "To respect life we have to bury the foetus after an abortion," and "A foetus is a human being with human rights and interests." The last point was brought up by a parliamentary committee looking at the issue of foetal diagnostics. There are groups that claim a woman should not have the right to decide about abortion after foetal diagnostics. The argument for this is that, if she has an abortion, she will choose which child she wants, not whether she will have a child or not. Representatives for disabled people often use this argument; they say that they defend their right to exist. This is also an argument that has been used in other countries.

We also have had discussion of very late abortions, which are rare and performed under strict indications. The argument in this is that there is an important ethical question to be faced when it is possible to have an abortion in the 22nd week, and it could be possible to save a premature baby in the 25th week. However, the time limit is strictly adhered to and there is always at least a two-week margin. But people who fight against abortion often use late abortions as an argument.

Groups called Alternative to Abortion have started, part of an international phenomenon. It is obvious that they want the woman to change her mind and refrain from abortion. They pretend not to be against abortion, but their alternative is often an offer to babysit! Another way the law is being attacked is via the language. For example, instead of the term *pregnant woman*, the word *mother* is used. The foetus is called the *child*, and abortion is called *delivery*. A pregnant woman—especially if she wants to give birth to a child—may call the foetus "my child" from the first day, but it is something else when a society where abortion is accepted says that a foetus is a child with its own rights. This is to send a double message.

In the ideological effort to influence Swedish society we now see growing discussion of natural birth control, a method known as "the method of the Pope." This method is appropriate for perhaps fewer then 5 percent of fertile women—those who have a steady relationship, regular menstruations, and the possibility of taking their temperature at the same hour every day. Sweden is to have access to RU 486, the so-called abortion pill. There is some criticism of this method as making it too easy to have an abortion. It seems as if these groups want to say that, if women must have an abortion, let them at least suffer. When the news about RU 486 was revealed, however, the reaction among the majority was positive.

In the last few years, RFSU have tried to introduce the "emergency pill" or the "morning-after pill." A problem, however, is that even journalists confuse it with RU 486. Those who oppose the morning-after pill argue that the women who takes it does not know if she is causing an abortion or not.

The more extreme groups are small but vocal. It is easy to get the impression that they are bigger than they are. They have a popular singing star among their members, and work mainly through leaflets, meetings, papers, and books, and are rather clever at lobbying. The anti-abortion groups have some influence on decision makers. They have managed to make politicians of all political parties say "this is a difficult question" every time they talk about abortion. Those who want to be acceptable to conservative groups show that they are responsible and wise by giving unclear answers about the abortion law. This could be a sign that anti-choice groups have taken a step forward, with their efforts so far bringing a discussion of the costs for abortions and professional advisory support for the woman, whether she wants it or not.

For the first time in many decades Sweden has seen demonstrations against abortion, with about 3,000 people in attendance. Their arguments include the following: "In Sweden we have restrictions on picking rare flowers, but it is possible to have an abortion." One member of the Right to Life Group recently said that abortion was comparable to the Holocaust during the Second World War.

The anti-choice movement in Sweden concentrates on young people. Yet the younger generation in Sweden does not know what a society with a restrictive abortion law is like, and so they can be reached with emotional messages about murdering babies.

THE FUTURE

There is only one effective way to decrease the number of abortions, and that is with openness on sexual matters, good sex education, easily available and inexpensive contraception, and a society with a positive attitude towards children. Most people in Sweden would agree on that, but not everyone. There will always be some opposition to openness in sexual matters and a woman's right to decide whether to have a child or not. There will always be abortions, even in an open society with good contraception because there are always failures in contraceptive use. Sexuality is a question of emotions, and, at its best, is a question of love. It is not a question of putting out rules and expecting people to follow them. We do not always do the right thing when we are in love.

Changes in attitudes and values result from many years of hard work. Women have had abortions at all times and in all cultures when they have found it impossible to support a child. What differs over time and culture are the medical, economic, social, and psychological risks linked to that abortion. In Sweden we have reached a stage where those risks are minimised.

Throughout history abortion has been a question for women to face. Men have never had to be responsible for their sexual joy in the same way. The cost of an unwanted pregnancy has always been paid by the woman. Women have been the ·ones whom society has put in prison or killed. Women, not men, have been called whores, or worse. Nowadays in Sweden men take a greater part than before, but many still see pregnancy as a woman's question.

According to the law, only the woman can make a decision about abortion. Some men criticise this and demand the chance to try to influence the decision. Men do have this possibility. If their relation with the woman is open-minded and understanding, the woman will discuss the problem, and they will make the decision together. But this may not be the case if the relationship is bad and she has difficulties communicating with him.

It is also important to remember that a man has many ways to influence a decision about abortion. If he just says no and turns his back on the woman, she will in many cases have an abortion because she wants her child to have a father. This is a strong emotional influence.

Men have no rights according to the abortion law. They have to confirm that they are the father if the woman decides to give birth to their child, and they have to pay for the child until it is 18 years old. If they do not do this, the state will pay instead but demand repayment from the father. It is not possible for a man to force a woman to continue a pregnancy; some men feel that this is unfair. In Sweden, the feeling is that it is important to try to involve the man in the decision, but still the final decision must be made by the woman.

The challenge today is to get men more involved in the results of unprotected intercourse, not only to make them more responsible but also to offer a chance to take a more active part in this side of life. That will result in a better relationship between a man and a woman. Now it is common for men to say: "I support you whatever you decide." That may sound nice, but it does not mean much. Thus, even if the anti-abortion movement is well organised, it will have to work hard to change public opinion. If those who defend the right to legal abortion do not join the debate, however, there is a possibility that the anti-abortion movement will grow. Swedish people cannot take sexual politics and the abortion act for granted, allowing the climate to change negatively for women. It is not likely that the abortion act will be changed in the near future, however there will be more intensive debate in the coming years. We have to fight the new religious opposition to abortion and those who moralize over young people and their way of life. We have to stop efforts to reattach shame and guilt to sexuality and unwanted pregnancies. It is often said that young people often do not understand what an abortion is. As proof of this, it is pointed out that they just say that they would ask for an abortion if they needed one. They are not ashamed; they do not seem to feel any guilt. Yet this was one of the important goals of Swedish sex education, and we cannot turn around this progress. It is also important to remember that many teenagers also say that they would never have an abortion.

It is a challenge to give young people a realistic view of abortion and such solid self-esteem that they can make decisions about their own sexuality without guilt and shame and with good protection against unwanted pregnancies and sexually transmitted diseases. An abortion is, after all, a big decision and often difficult to make. Of course, it is better if fewer women have to face this situation.

Anti-abortion groups have never proposed anything to prevent unwanted pregnancies. They never talk about the right to life for all the women in the world who suffer or die from illegal abortions. They are not active in the fight against war. For us who work with sexuality, the challenge has been to defend the right to abortion. We have to work hard to prevent unwanted pregnancies. This we do by offering good contraceptive counselling and sex education, and by defending legal abortion.

APPENDIX: STATISTICS ON ABORTION IN SWEDEN

1860–1920	The proportion of children born outside marriage increased from 9 to 15 percent of all children.
1940s	Fifty-one percent of the women in Stockholm who were refused abortion had illegal abortions.
1944	A parliamentary committee estimated 10,000 to 20,000 illegal abortions per year in Sweden.
1950s and early 1960s	Legal abortions were 2,000 to 3,000 annually. In 1973 the number had increased to 26,000.
1960s	Annually, 10,000 to 20,000 Swedish women went to Poland to have an abortion.
1968	Fifty-seven percent of abortions were carried out after the 12th week. There were 6,000 late abortions.
1982	Five percent of abortions were carried out after the 12th week. Out of 32,500 abortions, there were 1,500 late abortions.
1987	Out of 34,489, 226 abortions were carried out after the 18th week of pregnancy. About 50 percent of those were performed after foetal damage had been diagnosed or because of physical risk for the mother.
1990	More than 95 percent of all abortions are carried out before the end of the 12th week, most of them before the 10th week.
1990	More than 98 percent of abortions are carried out before the end of the 14th week. Between the 18th and 22nd week there are 200 to 300 abortions per year. That is 0.3–0.5 percent of all abortions.

REFERENCES

Abortion. Stockholm: RFSU, 1993 (English version also 1993).

Abortutveckling 1975–1984. Socialstyrelsen redovisar 1987: 1, Stockholm: Socialstyrelsen, 1987.

Callersten-Brunell, M., and M. Lidholm. *Abort. Erfarenheter och teorier.* Stockholm: Liber förlag, 1985.

Davidsson, B., and C. Forsling. *Abort förr och nu—en bok om aborträtten.* Falun: Bokförlag Röda Rummet, 1982.

Den gravida kvinnan och fostret—två individer. Om fosterdiagnostik och aborter. Slutbetänkande av utredningen om det ofödda barnet, Statens offentliga utredningar 1989: 51.

Ethical Aspects of Abortion: Some European Views. London: IPPF Europe Region, 1978.

Familieplanering och abort—erfarenheter av ny lagstiftning. Betänkande av 1980 års abortkommitté, Statens Offentliga Utredningar, 1983: 3.

"Fem år med fri abort," *Särtryck ur Läkartidningen* 77 (1980).

Förslag till abortförebyggande program. Att samordna insatser som rör sexualiteten. Stockholm, Socialstyrelsen, 1990.

Induced Abortion and Family Health: A European View. London: IPPF Europe Region, 1974.

Planned Parenthood in Europe 18, no. 1 (1989) and 20, no. 2 (1991).

Reducing Late Abortions: Access to NHS Services in Early Pregnancy. Proceedings of a Conference organised by the Birth Control Trust, London 1987.

Rätten till abort. 1965 års abortkommitté, Statens Offentliga Utredningar 1971: 58.

The Other Curriculum: European Strategies for School Sex Education. London: IPPF Europe Region, 1989.

Tietze, C. *Induced Abortion: A World Review.* New York: Alan Guttmacher Institute, 1990.

Trost, A-C. *Abort och psykiska besvär.* Västerås: Västerås International Library, 1982.

SWITZERLAND

Anne-Marie Rey

THE HISTORY OF ABORTION LAW

Abortion in the Penal Code

The Swiss abortion law is one of the oldest in Europe. Its enactment in 1942 was preceded by 50 years of discussion. Until then, abortion was ruled by cantonal penal codes, all of which prohibited abortion, accepting only strict medical necessity as a ground for termination of pregnancy. In 1893 the first draft of a federal penal code was produced. According to this draft, abortion was to be punished by imprisonment for up to five years. If the abortionist was a medical person, he or she might be imprisoned for up to 10 years. There was no explicit mention of therapeutic termination of pregnancy, thought by the draft's author, Professor Carl Stooss, to be allowed on the basis of a state of necessity.

After discussion in several expert committees, it was in the draft penal code of 1916 that—following pressure from medical organisations—medical grounds for legal termination of pregnancy were for the first time explicitly mentioned. The wording was less restrictive then than in the current law. In the course of the parliamentary deliberations that started in 1921, the requirement of a written medical consenting opinion was introduced, as a concession to the Catholic conservatives who threatened to oppose the whole penal code if abortion was made legal. Abortion was, together with the death penalty, the most hotly discussed issue in parliament and also during the campaign preceding the referendum in 1938, when the Swiss penal code was adopted by a narrow majority.

In 1912 and repeatedly thereafter, progressive segments of the judiciary and the medical profession, some women's organisations (e.g., the Swiss Working Women's Association), left-wing groups, parties, and parliamentarians had been asking for legal abortion on request within the first two or three months of pregnancy. In 1919, a proposal to introduce abortion on request at the cantonal level was only narrowly defeated in the parliament of Basel City. In the early 1920s, some communist medical doctors attracted thousands of people to hear their speeches in favour of free abortion (Gaillard et al. 1983). Catholic conservatives, the medical establishment, and middle-class women's organisations battled against this demand.

The aim of the new Swiss penal code of 1942 to unify and clarify the law has never been achieved as far as abortion is concerned. The law left a wide range of possible interpretations to doctors (especially after the World Health Organisation defined health as being a state of complete physical, mental, and social well-being), and cantons were free to designate as many doctors to give second opinions as they wished.

The medical practice of termination of pregnancy had already become more open-minded in some urban and Protestant cantons like Zürich and Geneva before the Swiss penal code was enforced. After 1942, this liberalisation process continued, with the result that the number of legal terminations rose sharply and foreign women, especially from France, came to Switzerland in growing numbers to have an abortion. Geneva became a well-known abortion centre. For approximately three decades (1950 to 1980), there were more legal terminations of pregnancy in this canton than live births. In addition, some other cantons like Vaud (with the city of Lausanne), Neuchâtel, Berne, Basel City, and Zürich were soon known for their liberal interpretation of the law.

Attempts to Amend the Penal Code

Only a few years after enactment of the penal code, in the late 1940s and early 1950s, complaints about the "laxity" of the practice of legal abortion led to hot debates in several cantonal parliaments and in the federal parliament. The Catholic conservatives tried to introduce restrictions to the law on the occasion of two partial revisions of the penal code in 1947–50 and again in 1954–71. But on both occasions the articles concerning abortion were excluded from the revisions in order not to endanger enactment of other urgent amendments.

In the late 1960s, progressive medical doctors and the newly formed women's liberation movement began discussing abortion. Legal terminations were estimated at that time at about 22,000 and illegal abortions at about 20,000 to 60,000 per year in Switzerland, as compared to around 100,000 annual births (Stamm 1974).

A scandal involving three doctors in a large number of illegal abortions in the canton of Neuchâtel led to a proposal, in 1971, in the cantonal parliament to address a cantonal initiative to the federal parliament asking for the abolition of Articles 118–121 of the penal code. Three of the authors of this proposal, joined by two persons from the canton of Berne, then formed a committee that launched a federal initiative with the same aim.[1] The initiative was firmly supported by the women's liberation movement and the signatures were collected in a few months. But it had no support in parliament. Instead a proposal to legalise termination of pregnancy at the request of the woman within the first 12 weeks of pregnancy only narrowly missed achieving a majority in the lower house (the National Council). Therefore the group behind the initiative launched a new initiative in 1975 asking precisely for this. The first initiative was withdrawn.

In 1977 the initiative for abortion on request in the first 12 weeks of pregnancy was put to the ballot. It was supported by a broad range of women's organisations, trade unions, and political parties, from left-wing to the right. While the right-wing parties were divided on the question, only the confessionally bound (Catholic and Protestant) parties opted clearly against it. The Catholic Church and organisations near to it took a very strong stance against the initiative, whereas in the Protestant churches there were differing opinions.

The main medical organisations either remained silent or maintained some distance. Among gynaecologists, in 1972, 22 percent favoured abortion on request and 58 percent approved of social grounds for termination of pregnancy. Psychiatrists were a little more favourable, with 38 percent approving of abortion on request. Individual doctors and Christian or left-wing medical organisations were vehemently engaged on either side of the campaign. With 48.3 percent of voters accepting it on the ballot, the initiative only narrowly missed the majority of votes in September 1977. But only in 7 out of the 25 cantons (in 1977 the number of cantons was 25, as against 26 today) did the initiative attract a majority in favour. All the small Catholic cantons voted against. The results of the ballot differed extremely from one canton to the other, with Geneva at the one end (78.7 percent in favour) and Appenzell Inner Rhodes at the other (7.4 percent in favour).

In the meantime parliament had elaborated a compromise that contained a social clause in addition to the medical, juridical, and eugenic grounds for legal termination of pregnancy. But the procedure to be followed by the woman in order to obtain permission for an abortion on social grounds would have been so complicated according to this bill that it clearly would have meant a step backwards for a number of cantons compared to their current practice under the actual law. Consequently, progressive forces joined with reactionaries to start a referendum. In 1978, the bill was swept away by 69 percent of the electorate.

In 1979 the anti-abortion movement in turn launched an initiative asking for the protection of human life from conception to natural death. Again there was a long and heated debate in public, with political parties, organisations, and groups dividing and taking sides in the same way as a few years earlier. The initiative for the right to life was heavily defeated in the ballot in 1985, with 69 percent of the electorate voting against. As in 1977, the results differed greatly from one region to the other. Despite this evident cleavage in public opinion, parliament in 1987 rejected a bill that would have given cantons legislative authority to regulate abortion on their own in accordance with majority opinion in their territory. The bill had been proposed by four of the liberal cantons (Geneva, Vaud, Neuchâtel, and Basel City) and by several parliamentarians.

These debates, which lasted more than 15 years, had very little effect at the legislative level. In 1981 two laws were passed, one obliging cantons to create counselling services for pregnant women, the other stipulating that health insurance had to reimburse without exceptions the costs for legal abortion.

ABORTION: CURRENT LAW AND PRACTICE

The Law of 1942

Abortion in Switzerland is ruled by Articles 118 to 121 of the Swiss penal code, which came into force in 1942. Abortion is forbidden, the only exception being therapeutic termination of pregnancy on medical grounds. Application of the law (procedural and organisational regulations, jurisdiction) lies with each of the 26 cantons.

Article 118 stipulates that a woman who carries out an abortion herself or through another person will be sentenced to imprisonment (from three days to three years). (The person cannot be prosecuted if more than two years have elapsed since the abortion occurred; this is shorter than the normal term that must elapse after a crime, namely five years.) Suspended sentences are possible. The same applies to a person (other than the abortionist) helping the woman. According to several sentences of the federal court, the attempt, even with unsuitable means or upon a woman who was not actually pregnant, is punishable.

Article 119 stipulates that any person performing an abortion on a consenting woman will be sentenced to imprisonment for up to five years. Again a statute of limitations extends for two years after the offence. When an abortion is done on a woman without her consent, the sentence is imprisonment for up to ten years. The minimum sentence is three years in the case of an abortionist who makes a business out of abortion.

Article 120 defines legal termination of pregnancy. A pregnancy may be terminated by a doctor, with the woman's written consent, in order to avoid a danger to her life or a great danger not otherwise avoidable of severe and lasting injury to her health. Before performing the abortion, the doctor must obtain the written consent of a second doctor who is a specialist for the condition of the pregnant woman and who has to be designated by the authorities of the canton where the woman lives or where the abortion will be performed. The cantonal authorities may designate in a general way the specialists authorised to give the second opinion or name a specialist in each particular case. If the woman is not capable of discernment, the written consent of her legal representative is required. In case of emergency, the abortion may be performed without a second consenting opinion. In this case, the doctor has to notify the cantonal authority within 24 hours after the emergency intervention. In the case of any other severe distress of the woman, the judge may commute the sentence.

Article 121 stipulates that a doctor who fails to notify the authorities in case of an emergency termination of pregnancy may be imprisoned for up to three months or fined.

It is noteworthy that Swiss law does not fix a time limit for therapeutic termination of pregnancy nor does it request parental consent for minors. Pregnancy is deemed to start with implantation. Discernment is defined in the Swiss civil code as the capability of acting reasonably, which may be impaired by a child's young age. The law does not stipulate either compulsory counselling or a waiting period before the operation can take place.

Eugenic (foetal) and juridical (rape, incest, etc.) grounds were considered in the legislative process to fall under the medical indications for termination of pregnancy.

The Cleavage Between Law and Practice

Although the law is the same for the whole country and—according to discussion during its passage in parliament and in the early literature—was meant to be very strict, allowing abortion only on severe medical grounds, there was an ever-growing cleavage between law and practice. Because cantons are authorised to designate the doctors allowed to give the second opinion prescribed by Article 120 of the penal code, and because the wording of the law leaves some space for interpretation, soon after enactment of the penal code practice started evolving differently from one canton to the other.

A few years after enactment, six cantons (Basel City, Berne, Geneva, Neuchâtel, Vaud, and Zürich) had already a very liberal practice. They authorised quite a large number of doctors to give the second opinion, among them many psychiatrists, and the woman or her doctor were allowed to choose freely among them. Since 1980, in the canton of Berne any specialist doctor in private practice may give the second opinion. In the canton of Zürich all psychiatrists are allowed to do so. A more and more liberal interpretation of the law was tolerated, so that psychosocial grounds for abortion are now broadly accepted, accounting for over 95 percent of terminations of pregnancy.

In these cantons almost any woman really wanting to terminate her pregnancy will be able to obtain the operation legally. Very seldom will her request be turned down. Over the last 20 years, some more cantons have joined the category of liberal cantons: Aargau, Basel Country, Ticino. Glaris and Jura are also moving in this direction (ASDAC 1990; Dondénaz et al. 1989; Stamm et al. 1990).

In other parts of Switzerland practice is also changing in a more or less liberal direction. Some cantons that counted among the restrictive ones 20 years ago now take an intermediate position: Appenzell Outer Rhodes, Fribourg, Grisons, Lucerne, Saint Gall, Schaffhouse, Thurgovie, Zoug, and of late even the very Catholic canton of Valais. In most of these cantons the second opinion has to be given by a doctor affiliated with a psychiatric hospital or the canton's surgeon general designates in each particular case the private doctor who is to give the second opinion. On the other hand, there still remain a number of small Catholic cantons in central Switzerland where no legal abortions in fact take place: Appenzell Inner Rhodes, Nidwald, Obwald, and Uri.

This inequality leads to what is called "abortion tourism": women from restrictive cantons will travel to more liberal places to have their unwanted pregnancy terminated. According to a judgement of the federal court, cantons are not allowed to restrict abortion to residents.

There is no conscience clause in the Swiss abortion law. Still opinions among medical practitioners and nurses differ greatly. So how the woman will be treated depends very much on whom she will first contact. In a liberal canton, the woman will present her problem to her doctor or a gynaecologist, who will send her to a colleague for the second opinion and then perform the abortion or refer the woman to a colleague or to a hospital for the operation. Some conservative doctors will try to turn her down. Some hospitals refuse altogether to do abortions (e.g., because they are still working with Catholic sisters). But most doctors, if they are not able or not willing to perform the abortion themselves, will refer the woman to a colleague or a hospital where she will be helped (if necessary in another canton).

The pregnant woman may also address herself to one of the counselling or family planning centres existing in most bigger towns, where she will receive first advice, a referral, or even the written consenting opinion. In some towns there also exist women's counselling services, women's health centres, or telephone hotlines that give useful addresses.

There exist great differences not only in the interpretation of the law but also in the way terminations of pregnancy are carried out. In a few cantons, relatively large numbers of terminations are done by doctors (not only gynaecologists but also general practitioners) in their private offices or in private clinics under local anaesthesia and on an outpatient basis. In other cantons, terminations are done mainly or exclusively in public hospitals or private clinics, generally under general anaesthesia, with a hospitalisation of one, two, three, or even more days. In many hospitals, prostaglandins are routinely administered to soften the cervix in the evening of the day before aspiration takes place. All this is not a question of laws or of cantonal regulations (the law, according to a verdict of the federal court, does not allow supplementary cantonal regulations in this field), but depends on hospital rules or the opinion prevailing in the medical establishment.

One special problem is late abortions. Although the Swiss law does not specify any time limits, in practice second-trimester terminations (especially after the 14th or 15th week) are only very reluctantly granted by doctors (e.g., for foetal or severe medical grounds). They are almost always done in a hospital by prostaglandin procedures.

In principle, termination of pregnancy has to be paid for by social insurance. But since health insurance is not compulsory in Switzerland (more than 95 percent of the population do have an insurance, though), some terminations will not be paid by insurance. For poor women, social welfare will have to provide the means in this case. This might be a problem for some women in conservative cantons. There might also be a problem for young girls depending on the family insurance of their parents. Some private doctors will refuse to do terminations at the fees fixed by health insurance, and if a woman has to go to a private doctor in another canton because she cannot obtain the termination at the public hospital in the canton where she lives, her insurance might be insufficient and only reimburse part of the costs.

The Incidence of Abortion

All cantons except Zürich require doctors and hospitals to notify terminations to the cantonal authorities. In some cantons the written consenting opinion has to be sent in (with or without the name of the woman) and is kept in the cantonal archives. Statistics for Switzerland overall do not exist. A group of authors has regularly tried to assemble the cantonal statistics (Dondénaz et al. 1989; Stamm 1974; Stamm et al. 1990), but they had to estimate the total for Switzerland and some underreporting may have to be taken into account.

The number of legal abortions rose sharply after enactment of the penal code. In 1966 and again in 1970, it was estimated at about 22,000 (compared to 110,000 live births in 1966 and 99,000 in 1970). The number began to fall when neighbouring countries introduced abortion on request in the 1970s. Whereas the number of nonresident women having a termination of pregnancy in Switzerland was estimated at over 6,000 in 1973, it was down to 330 in 1986. The number of residents having a termination is also estimated to have dropped since 1980, when it was 17,800, to about 12,900 in 1990 (83,939 live births in 1990).

The abortion rate is estimated to be about 8.6 per 1,000 women ages 15 to 44. The abortion ratio is approximately 154 per 1,000 live births; in other words, for every six births there is one legal abortion, or in every seven pregnancies one is terminated legally.

In 1970, 98 percent of legal abortions were performed in the six liberal cantons of Basel City, Berne, Geneva, Neuchâtel, Vaud, and Zürich (where 53 percent of the Swiss population lived). In 1990 this proportion fell to an estimated 83 percent as a result of more liberal practices in other cantons and therefore has diminished "abortion tourism."

Illegal abortions were estimated at about 20,000 to 60,000 in 1966, at 20,000 to 40,000 in 1970 (Stamm 1974). The incidence dropped to between 5,000 and 12,000 for 1978 (*Revue médicale de Suisse romande* 1979) and 8,000 for 1986 (Stamm et al. 1990). Today one may assume a very low incidence of illegal abortion, most of them, if any, done by doctors without obtaining the second opinion required by law. It seems very unlikely that any illegal abortions are done nowadays by backstreet abortionists; there are no more convictions, no more women seen in hospital with the consequences of botched abortions, and since 1973 there has been no abortion death.

Before the Swiss penal code came into effect, illegal abortion, though widely practiced, was rarely prosecuted. In 1929 there was a total of 72 sentences imposed by courts in Switzerland. After enactment of the code in 1942, the number of convictions rose sharply, attaining an absolute maximum in 1950 (667 convictions). Growing laxity meant the numbers fell to a yearly average of about 380 in the early 1960s. In the late 1960s the number had fallen still further to 150. After the launch of the initiative for decriminalisation of abortion in 1971, the broad public discussions made the number decline to a few convictions per year. Since 1980 there have been only four convictions (one each in 1982 and 1988, two in 1986).

In the 1960s, thousands of Swiss women travelled abroad (Yugoslavia, Italy, England) to have their pregnancies terminated. Today this number has certainly shrunk very much because there is no more need, except for terminations at a later stage of pregnancy, when the operation is difficult to obtain in Switzerland.

The total incidence of abortion may be estimated for 1990 at 14,000 to 20,000 (13,000 legal, the rest illegal or done abroad), as against 42,000 to 82,000 (of which 22,000 were legal) assumed to have taken place in 1966. This dramatic decline of 50 to 80 percent is certainly attributable mainly to the introduction, in the late 1960s, of modern contraceptives; to the creation of family planning centres; and to the progress of sex education in schools. Contraception has largely replaced abortion, and illegal abortion has been replaced by medical termination of pregnancy.

Recent statistics on women having abortions are scarce. The only canton to produce somewhat more sophisticated statistics is Berne. According to their figures (which may be more or less transferable to the whole of Switzerland), among the 1,076 women having a legal abortion in 1990, 40 percent were married, 50 percent were single, and 10 percent were widowed or divorced. Of these women, 54 percent had no child, 18 percent had one child, 20 percent had two children, and 8 percent had three or more children. Sixty-six percent were residents of Swiss nationality, and 34 percent were residents of foreign nationality (as compared to a foreign resident population of about 10 percent). For 84 percent, it was their first abortion, for 13 percent their second, and for 3 percent their third (or more) abortion.

One of the 1,076 women was under age 15, 6.9 percent were ages 15 to 19, 26 percent were 20 to 24 years old, 27.5 percent were 25 to 29, 21 percent were 30 to 34, 12 percent were 35 to 39, and 6.5 percent were 40 and over. Fifty-four percent of the women had not used any form of contraception at the moment of conception, 16 percent had used a condom, 8 percent the rhythm method, 7 percent the pill, 5 percent had interrupted intercourse, 3 percent had an IUD, and the rest had used other methods. Twenty-nine percent of the pregnancies were terminated within eight weeks of the beginning of the last menstrual period, 42 percent in the 9th or 10th week, 21 percent in the 11th or 12th week, and 8 percent after 12 weeks.

In the canton of Berne, only 12 percent of abortions were carried out on an outpatient basis, and 89 percent were done in public hospitals. (These figures are not transferable to other cantons; in Zürich and Geneva in particular the majority of terminations are probably done on an outpatient basis by private doctors.) Several older studies in different cantons (e.g., Kellerhals et al. 1976) showed that Catholic women are relatively more likely to have an abortion than Protestant women.

The Politics of Abortion

Attitudes towards abortion vary as widely as practice in Switzerland. This may best be reflected by the results of the ballots of 1977 and 1985. Opinion polls have shown a trend to more liberal views in the 1970s, but there seems to be stagnation since then, with about two-thirds to four-fifths of respondents approving of the general principle that a woman ought to decide for herself if she needs an abortion or not; and about the same proportion in favour of liberalising the existing law. Yet when it comes to the concrete question of whether abortion on request should be legalised, only about the same proportion as in the ballot of 1977—namely, slightly under 50 percent—agree. Opinion is more liberal in the French-speaking part of Switzerland, in urban areas, and in regions with Protestant majorities. It is more conservative in the German-speaking part, especially in central Switzerland, in the countryside, and in Catholic regions. The cleavage in public opinion coincides almost exactly with the regional differences in abortion practice.

Things are not much different as regards doctors and medical personnel. It is certainly thanks to the changing views of medical doctors that progress has been possible in the practice of abortion during the last 20 years. A recent investigation based on personal interviews with many practitioners directly concerned with abortion (gynaecologists, family planning workers, doctors authorised to deliver the second opinion according to Article 120 of the penal code, cantonal surgeons general) revealed that most think it is up to the women to decide about abortion. But many still believe that some sort of barrier is necessary to protect doctors and help them share their responsibility and to prevent excesses (ASDAC 1990).

Many women are badly informed about the law and practice of abortion. Some think it is prohibited, while some take it for granted that they have a right to access to legal abortion. Although abortion is widely tolerated, nobody likes to talk about it. Professionals prefer to do their work undisturbed as best they can. Many of them have a feeling of acting in a sort of grey zone of semilegality and fear to speak out publicly. Women prefer to keep an abortion secret. Most of them do not talk about it, except to their nearest friends and relatives. When a magazine recently tried to find 100 women prepared to testify that they had had an abortion, with their photograph appearing in the paper, it was impossible to find them.

Sexual morality is considered a private business. Family planning and premarital sex are widely accepted. Most young couples first live together without getting married. Still, when a child is about to be born, most do get married. In 1990, out-of-wedlock births accounted for only 6.1 percent of all births. The acceptance of unwed mothers and their children by society has very much improved, though, over the last 20 years. Nonetheless this segment of the population is particularly stricken by the phenomenon of "new poverty."

Sex education at school is not compulsory in most cantons, but is increasingly becoming generalised, especially in connection with AIDS prevention. Recently high school students in Geneva asked for condom self-service machines to be installed at their school. Family planning centres now exist in almost every canton and in most bigger towns, some of them offering counselling only, some also offering gynaecological checkups and prescribing contraceptives. In most places adolescents can easily obtain contraception either from family planning or school clinics or from doctors in private practice. A family planning association has recently been founded as a branch of the IPPF.

The political forces engaged on either side of the issue of abortion are the same as in the campaign of 1977; left-wing and liberal groups and parties tend to support abortion on request, whereas religiously bound groups and parties would like to make law and practice more restrictive.

The main pro-choice groups acting nationally are the Swiss Union for Decriminalization of Abortion (USPDA), the Swiss Association for the Right to Abortion and Contraception (ASDAC), and some feminist organisations.

Several attempts to get a new initiative for choice started in the 1980s have failed because there remain minor tactical differences among pro-choice groups (e.g., whether social insurance coverage of abortion ought to be included among the claims or not) and because mobilising was too difficult, other problems being politically more acute and difficulties for women in need of abortion having greatly diminished.

Today pro-choice groups concentrate on gathering and distributing information, working for the introduction of the abortion pill RU 486, ameliorating abortion services and procedures, renewing political and media contacts, and building up an international network (e.g., the European Network for Women's Right to Abortion and Contraception—ENWRAC). Some are also involved in the debate about the new reproductive technologies. USPDA and ASDAC also engage in sex education in school and run telephone hotlines giving information about abortion and contraception to women.

Pro-choice arguments have been changing somewhat in the last 10 years since the danger of illegal abortion—once one of the main arguments—has become obsolete. The main arguments today are that there has to be an end to hypocrisy, with abortion taken out of the area of semilegality and vagueness (which also means that practice can suddenly become more restrictive, depending on local doctors, authorities, and political forces); the law has to be adapted to real life and to practice and to the liberal laws of the majority of European countries; and women must be granted the fundamental right to reproductive freedom, which must include abortion as a backup measure when contraception has failed.

The main anti-choice group is Ja zum Leben (Yes to Life), which is mainly Catholic and has several subgroups among doctors and nurses and strong links with fundamentalist groups fighting reproductive technologies. A smaller, mainly Protestant group is called Helfen statt Töten (Help instead of Killing). Several fundamentalist Christian groups are also active in the field of abortion. Most of these groups also fight against sexual freedom, contraception (except natural family planning which they propagate), and sex education at school. They are active in distributing their publications and films (*The Silent Scream*) and working closely together in this respect internationally, especially with their American counterparts. They try to have influence in schools and are also running hotlines for pregnant women seeking help (SOS—futures mères). They are struggling to prevent the chemical firm Roussel Uclaf from introducing the abortion pill RU 486 in Switzerland. Since they have been heavily defeated in the ballot on their initiative in 1985, they keep rather quiet on the political level, and there have been no clinic blockades in Switzerland so far.

The main arguments of the anti-choice movement today are (as they always have been) the right to life from conception, the foetus being a person, and the psychological aftermath of abortion for women. They claim that freer access to abortion will boost the number of operations, undermine morality, destroy the family, and lower respect for life in general.

THE FUTURE

The practice of abortion has clearly moved towards liberalisation over the past 20 years, and there are no signs of regression currently. As regards public opinion, it is hard to say in which way it will move. Sociological studies show a trend to more individualism, which might mean growing adherence to choice; but they also show a tendency to more immaterial values, which might produce the opposite effect. Stagnation seems the most plausible forecast.

Abortion being much less of a problem in day-to-day life nowadays, political interest in the issue is no longer very strong. Most women and professionals directly concerned seem to be able to cope one way or another. New political activities will depend on what is going on in the near future in other countries (e.g., Germany, the United States, England) and on possible changes in political forces. Since it will be difficult for the pro-choice side to obtain the majority of the cantons in a ballot in the foreseeable future, and since the anti-choice movement has only recently been heavily defeated, it is unlikely that any new initiative for a constitutional amendment will be launched soon by either side.

The parliamentary route seems to be more promising. In fact, a proposal was introduced in parliament in April 1993 by a group of 63 parliamentarians belonging to eight different parties. They asked for the penal code to be liberalised to allow abortion on request in the first few months of pregnancy. The proposal will be discussed in 1994. Yet liberalisation of the law will have to jump several hurdles on the way: laws have to pass both houses of parliament, and in the upper house, where every canton has two representatives, the small Catholic cantons have a disproportionate influence. Finally, if a liberal law is passed, anti-choice groups will certainly launch a referendum.[2] However, in this case proponents of the law will have to obtain only the majority of the votes on the ballot (as against the majority of votes *and* of cantons for an initiative proposing a constitutional amendment). The arrival of RU 486 might help prepare the ground for a more rational approach to the issue of abortion. Meanwhile, efforts to alleviate still more the procedures and the practice of abortion will certainly continue on a cantonal level.

NOTES

1. In Switzerland a constitutional amendment is put on the ballot if an initiative is signed by 100,000 (up to 1977 the number was 50,000) citizens having the right to vote. A majority of voters as well as a majority of cantons (the result of the ballot

in each canton counting as this canton's vote) are then needed for the amendment to be adopted. The 1971 initiative was one of the first that women were allowed to sign because up until that year women in Switzerland had not been allowed to vote.

2. An initiative can ask only for a constitutional amendment. There is no way of proposing a law by way of an initiative; a referendum can demand only that a law passed by parliament be put on the ballot.

REFERENCES

ASDAC. *Interruption de grossesse en Suisse: Loi, pratiques et prévention* (German version: Schwangerschaftsabbruch in der Schweiz: Gesetz, Praxis und Prävention). Lausanne: ASDAC, 1990.

Dondénaz, Martine. "Avortement—interruption de grossesse: le cas de la Suisse," *Réalités Sociales* (1987).

Dondénaz, Martine, et al. "Interruption de grossesse en Suisse: chiffres de 1982 à 1986," *Méd. et Hyg.* 47 (1989).

———. "L'interruption de grossesse en Suisse: période 1987–1990," *Méd. et Hyg.* 50 (1992).

Gaillard, Ursula, et al. *Retard de règles*. Lausarre: Ed. d'en bas, 1983.

Kellerhals, J., et al. *Le sens de l'avortement*. Genève: Georg, 1976.

Ketting, Evert, et al. *Schwangerschaftsabbruch: Gesetz und Praxis im internationalen Vergleich*. Tübinger Reihe: DGVT, 1985.

Locher, Jakob. "Landesbericht Schweiz." In Albin Eser (ed.), *Schwangerschaftsabbruch im internationalen Vergleich*. Baden-Baden: Nomos, 1988.

Revue médicale de Suisse romande 12 (1979).

Stamm, Heinrich. "Probleme des legalen Aborts in der Schweiz," *Ars medici*, 1974.

Stamm, Heinrich, et al. "Schwangerschaftsabbruch in der Schweiz 1982 bis 1986," *PRAXIS* 79, no. 9 (1990).

USPDA. *RU 486—Interruption de grossesse précoce: pour le droit de la femme de choisir la méthode* (German version: RU 486—Das Recht der Frauen, beim Abbruch einer Frühschwangerschaft die Methode zu wählen). Zollikofen: USPDA, 1990.

THE USSR

Andrej A. Popov

THE HISTORY OF ABORTION LAW

Pre-1920: Abortion Outlawed

Analysis of the history of family planning in Russia and in the former USSR[1] reveals that the issue of induced abortions cannot be understood apart from the interrelation of state and individual. In addition, freedom of reproductive choice in Russia has always meant freedom of induced abortions.

Traditionally, abortion in Russia was prohibited by law. In this respect Russia was no different from other Western European countries. Capital punishment for inducing abortion was introduced in Russia in 1649 (1523 in England, 1533 in Germany, 1562 in France) (Kyzetcov and Baranova 1982; Sadvokasova 1969). It was in the course of the country's westernization by Peter the Great that all punishment for abortion was reduced and capital punishment was abolished. This change reflected the traditional Russian claim of being not only equal to its neighbours but even more progressive.

Such an aspiration to social progress reflected the nature of Russian social thought rather than the true level of progressiveness. This pretension to progressiveness has been true for the history of abortion legislation in modern Soviet or Russian society as well.

In the Russian Punishment Act of 1895, the juridical status of punishment for induced abortion was established as follows:

Article 1462. Any competent individual consciously acting with the intent to induce abortion in a pregnant woman with her agreement will undergo a loss of all rights and be sentenced to a term of prison of between 5 and 6 years. . . . Any pregnant woman, by her own will or under pressure of any other person, who uses any facility for inducing abortion will undergo loss of all her rights and be sentenced to a term of prison between 4 and 5 years. (Vasilevski' and Vasilevski' 1924, 21)

Despite this law, induced abortion was widespread. In Russia at the end of the 19th century, every fifth pregnancy ended in induced abortion (Sadvokasova 1969, 12). This was an extraordinarily high level for a population with a high birth rate.

Leading the struggle for the legalisation of induced abortion were physicians in the Russian Association of Physicians named in memory of N. I. Pirogov (Pirogov's Association and Congresses). In 1913, at the 12th Pirogov's Congress, the problem of "artificial abortion" was the main topic of the obstetrics and gynaecology section. A resolution was passed recommending elimination of abortion from the list of criminally punishable acts (Vasilevski' and Vasilevski' 1924, 83; Omskoye meditcinskoe obtchestvo 1904). After the congress, an article by V. I. Lenin entitled "The Working Class and Neo-Malthusionism" was published in the Communist party's newspaper *Pravda*. In this article the solutions of the Congress were sharply criticised as being opposed to the Communist party's stand on induced abortion and contraceptive use (so-called neo-Malthusianism) (Sadvokasova 1969, 13).

The position of the party was summed up as follows:

Free access to contraceptives and abortion constitutes the ABCs of the democratic rights of citizens, but . . . as the working class is growing up and becoming stronger in its fight, it demands a high birth rate in order to improve the battle their fathers have waged and complete the building of the new society. . . . This is why, and only why, we are the formal enemies of neo-Malthusianism. (Sadvokasova 1969, 13)

Such was the line of the Communist party: pro-natalism and the cynical manipulation of the population. The fundamental principle of the party's social policy was to relate to the individual and to the population solely as instruments for attaining their own goals. Importantly, however, these true aims were always disguised by populist slogans, and so remained attractive to marginal strata of the population.

The beginning of the 20th century was characterised by the continued political activity of the entire Russian intelligentsia for legalisation of induced abortion. For example, in 1914 at the 10th Congress of the Russian section of the International Criminology Union, a call was made "to remove induced abortions from the list of criminally punished actions" (Vasilevski' and Vasilevski' 1924, 86). One of the most outstanding Russian philosophers of the time, V. V. Rozanov, in response to the resolution of the 10th Congress of Criminologists, wrote:

It is impossible for the state to listen to speculation that the foetus is not yet a living essence and that therefore its killing shouldn't be punished. How stupid! A foetus is state property, the national instrument. . . . And for the damaging of national property—whether living or dead—there are strong punishments. (Vasilevski' and Vasilevski' 1924, 87)

In 1917, the Soviet era of abortion began. The fight for legalisation of induced abortions was now continued by the Communist party. Their goal was not new: to use abortion for the destruction of the old social bases of life, the traditional family and religion.

1920: Legalisation of Abortion

On November 16, 1920, the first law of Narcomzdrav (Narodnyi' Commissariat Zdravoohraneniya, or People's Commissariat of Public Health Services) and Narcomjust (Narodnyi' Commissariat Yustitzii, or People's Commissariat of Justice) was published, abolishing altogether any punishment for inducing abortions either for the woman or for the physicians involved.[2] According to this law:

1. Abortions would be provided free of charge in Soviet hospitals.
2. No one except licensed physicians could provide induced abortions.
3. Those guilty of inducing illegal abortions—paramedics or traditional physicians— must be punished by losing their rights to practice medicine and will be criminally prosecuted.
4. A physician who induces an abortion by way of private practice or for a charge will be prosecuted by trial.

The introduction to this law talked of "the dangers of abortion for society," upheld "the principles of protecting motherhood and childhood," and predicted "the gradual elimination of this phenomenon." But in reality the law ushered in the second stage of the history of abortion. This lasted from 1920 to 1924 and was characterised by (1) a considerable increase in the number of abortions owing to a decrease in the number of illegal abortions; (2) an increase in the deficit of abortion beds in the hospitals; and (3) moves by obstetricians and gynaecologists that immediately began to sabotage the 1920 law (Vasilevski' and Vasilevski' 1924).

Particularly strong was the negative attitude of obstetricians and gynaecologists towards the social-indications clause for abortion. As a result of this resistance, on November 3, 1924, the second decree of Narcomzsdrav and Narcomjust appeared, limiting induced abortions that were free of charge and organising special commissions to determine eligibility for free abortions (Aboptye v 1925 gogy 1927, 21).

At the same time, in 1924 in Moscow and Leningrad, some private commercial clinics were established, providing induced abortions for a fee. Moreover, in 1924, in the majority of Gybsdravotdel (Gybernski' otdel zsravoochranenia, or Provincial Department of Public Health), a fee for induced abortions was introduced. Such commercialisation resulted in two very important consequences: (1) an abortion industry was created in Russia; and (2) there was an adaptation and re-orientatation of health services with the inducement of abortion becoming the principal and cheapest method of family planning. Simultaneously, the population adapted to regularly induced abortions as the most simple and available method of birth control.

1936: Abortion Prohibited

On May 25, 1936, the draft of a law prohibiting abortion was submitted for public discussion (Sadvokasova 1969, 29). This propaganda campaign passed successfully. This draft was supported by the Soviet population and scientists, and two months later induced abortions were entirely prohibited. But the occurrence of organised public discussion was unprecedented and would not be repeated in the future. It is evidence that the authorities were seriously afraid of the reaction of the population to this law.

On July 27, 1936, the decree of CIK and SNK of the USSR (Centralnyi' Ispolnitelnyi Komitet i Soviet Narodnych Komissarov, or Central Executive Committee and Soviet People's Commissaries) was published.[3] What the authorities had in mind when publishing this law was simply to prohibit abortion completely. The principal conditions of this law were as follows:

1. To prohibit abortions under almost every circumstance; abortions were permitted only for life-threatening and eugenic reasons.

2. Physicians were penalised for inducing abortions in hospital by one- to two-year prison terms; for abortions induced by physicians in outpatient conditions or by nonmedical persons, the term was three years in jail.

3. Anyone (for example, a husband) pressuring a woman into having an abortion faced a sentence of up to two years imprisonment.

4. The pregnant woman herself was to be prosecuted or fined up to 3,000 roubles in the case of repeated abortions.

The following 20 years were characterised by an unsuccessful fight against illegal abortions. To decrease the abortion rate was not the only goal of Narcomzdrav. At the same time it tried to prevent infringements of the law. This latter goal, from the point of view of totalitarian logic, was more important than asserting the concerns and health of women.

Illegal abortions constituted a serious problem for Soviet public health services, and the instructions to fight abortions appeared regularly up to 1957.[4] However, it was exactly this widespread inducement of illegal abortions that was cited as the principal cause for legalising abortion again in 1955. However, in 1939, the year after publication of Narkomzdrav's next directive,[5] an unusual event occurred. The authorities understood the failure of all attempts to end illegal abortions, so the only possible solution was to make the problem appear less. This was done in 1939.[6] Narkomzdrav ordered that all collection of statistical information about induced abortions be stopped. The collection of statistics on abortion was renewed only after legalisation of induced abortion in 1955, two decades later.

1955: Abortion Re-legalised

On November 23, 1955, a declaration of the Soviet government was published that marked the beginning of a new stage in the history of induced abortions in the USSR: "The Presidium of the Supreme Soviet of the USSR, aiming to give women the opportunity to solve the question of their motherhood by themselves, and also with the purpose of preventing any harm to the health of women by abortions outside of hospitals . . . decrees to abolish the bill prohibiting abortions."[7]

Subsequent events between 1955 and 1969 reflected the generally more democratic context of social life in the country. In March 1956, statistical forms were again introduced and the collection of information about induced abortions began (Sadvokasova 1969, 117). However, publication of this information occurred for the first time only in 1988 (Naseleniye SSSP 1988; Zdorovie naseleniya 1989). Up until 1988 this information was secret, available only to clerks of Minzdravs (Ministerstvo Zdravoochranenia, or Ministry of Public Health Services) of the USSR and union republics.

From 1956 to 1970 there were attempts to replace abortions with effective contraceptives. Significantly, this decision was only the restoration of a strategy of developing family planning that had existed prior to the prohibition of abortion in 1936 (Sadvokasova 1969). In 1960, at the first All-Union Congress of Obstetricians and Gynaecologists, resolutions were passed concerning the necessity of decreasing the abortion rate and increasing the distribution of contraception (Sadvokasova 1969, 126). And on October 9, 1970, an instructive letter of extraordinary importance was published by the Minzdrav of the USSR. It recommended the mass use of oral contraception, but only under medical observation and with a physician's prescription.[8]

1974 and After: Manipulating the Statistics

In 1974, the Minzdrav published a further instructive letter that basically prohibited the mass use of oral hormonal contraception.[9] What did the Minzdrav suggest instead? In 1975 it suggested that women be encouraged to give birth to more children rather than inducing abortions (Poltcthanova 1975). Such a reorientation in public policy—the shift from allowing free

reproductive choice to pro-natalist propaganda and reproductive compul-
sion—was not accidental. This was only one particular consequence of the
general move away from democratic positions that had begun in the 1960s.
The result was a new increase in illegal abortions because effective contraception and public abortion services were not available. In these circumstances criminal abortions provided the only accessible choice for Soviet
women.

The Minzdrav tried to fight these illegal abortions in the old, familiar way
by regulating the procedure for legal abortion. However, having the same
experience of failing to prohibit abortion totally, the Minzdrav selected another way. The de jure granting of legal abortions was broadened. In 1976
an order by Minsdrav of the USSR was published in which the final date
for induced abortion was extended from 9 weeks to 12 weeks.[10] (Let us note
that this and many subsequent changes broadening the grounds on which
abortion was legal were only formal de jure steps. They were not followed
by the simultaneous increase of actual de facto accessibility of induced abortions for the population.)

The effect of the prohibition of oral contraception, together with the de
jure extension of legal induced abortion, was an unprecedented rise in the
rate of abortion inducement between 1980 and 1984: the out-of-hospital
inducement of early, safe, abortions (so-called mini-abortions). Although
enormous numbers of mini-abortions were being performed, it is crucial to
note that they were neither legalised by the Public Health Ministry nor were
they registered.

When such registration finally began in 1988, mini-abortions accounted
for more than 10 percent of all induced abortions in the country (Zdorovie
naseleniya 1989; Demograficesky ezhegodnik 1990). The mini-abortions reflected a search for a better and safe alternative to abortions, but within the
limits of the abortion paradigm of the Soviet health service. Abortion paradigm indicates not only the presence of an abortion industry but also the
technological adaptation of the whole public health system to abortion production. The essential element was the mental adaptation by physicians and
most of the population to induced abortion as a regular method of family
planning.

Moreover, illegal abortions continued to present a serious problem. Minzdrav tried to solve this by optimizing the procedure of registering induced
abortions and making formal an increase in their accessibility. It is important
to note that these measures failed. And yet most of these attempts to eliminate illegal abortions were quite serious. In 1982 an Order of Minzdrav was
published in which women were given the right to choose the hospital and
physician by themselves, with the agreement of a special commission of local
doctors. Final gestation age for abortions on medical grounds was extended
up to 28 weeks.[11]

Simultaneously, the trend prohibiting contraception was continued. Minzdrav, in 1983, published an instructive letter recommending the use of oral contraceptives only for the purposes of medical treatment.[12] Moreover, between 1984 and 1986, the widespread provision of mini-abortions continued, albeit without official sanction (Kalchenko and Sutta 1984; Bloshanskii and Zhukowskii 1985; Ponochevnaya 1985; Sadayskas and Chigrehe 1985; Kavkasidze, n.d.). In 1986, the commercial provision of mini-abortions in profit-earning clinics began, as did their commercial provision by state hospitals.

It was not until June 5, 1987, that official permission for mini-abortions was granted. According to this official instruction, the induced mini-abortions included abortions provided during the earliest stage (not more than 20 days) by the method of vacuum aspiration with the obligatory laboratory or instrumental testing of pregnancy. In 1989, the formulation was changed to "menstrual regulation by vacuum aspiration during the early gestation period" (Zdorovie naseleniya 1989). This change was only an attempt by Minzdrav to decrease artificially the level of induced abortions by way of statistical manipulations.

Obviously, the official discourse is about only one type of induced abortions because in both the mini and conventional abortions there is the need for either instrumental or laboratory confirmation of pregnancy with the ultrasound echolocation or determination of the level of chorional honadotropini. The main difference between Soviet mini-abortions and contraceptive routine vacuum aspiration in Western countries lies in the necessity to confirm pregnancy (Homasuridze 1985).

Two subsequent steps in the abortion policy of Minzdrav were extraordinary, even on a world scale. First, continuing the traditional trend of fighting against illegal abortion through maximum formal accessibility to abortion, under a Minzdrav order of December 31, 1987, Soviet physicians received official permission to provide artificial abortions up to the gestation age of 28 weeks on juridical, genetic, vital, broad medical, sociomedical, and just simply social grounds. The second step was a decree of December 1988 that prohibited induced abortions provided in commercial nonstate hospitals. This amounted to the restoration of the state monopoly on induced abortion provision.

Thus was formed the unparalleled features of the Soviet national model of family planning, based solely on the provision of induced abortions. The essential features of this national model are as follows:

- An extremely high level of widespread provisioning of induced abortions
- An extremely low level of use of modern contraceptive methods (IUD, pills, voluntary sterilisation)
- Essential prevalence of induced abortion usage in the composition of family planning methods

- Widespread induced abortion not only for limiting the number of births but for birth spacing as well

- Widespread provisioning of illegal abortions

- Low quality of abortion services, including long waiting periods, poor anaesthesia, and other problems

- Inaccessibility of modern contraceptives, information, and services

- High level of cultural and mental resistance to the introduction of alternative contraception-based models and their diffusion

- High level of acceptability of family planning models based on post hoc or post factum reproductive behaviour and reproductive decision making

- High level of commercialisation of family planning services

The main historical dates and changes in legislative acts about induced abortions in the USSR are briefly demonstrated in Table 1.

The Politics of Abortion

Why were legalised induced abortions selected in Russia at the beginning of this century as an instrument for destruction of the traditional bases of the state? Legalisation of abortion seemed the most rapid way to create changes in traditional family relations and in women's social position. The family became an important object of attention for the new Soviet authorities. Traditional family life and religion were the most basic bearers of the old culture. They were the most serious targets of destruction in the attempt to achieve the principal aims of the new Soviet authorities: "the construction of a New Society" and "the creation of a New Soviet Man."

Thus, abortion policy was one among many instruments in the purposeful destruction of the prerevolutionary Russian family and Russian culture. Artificial marginalisation, ruralisation, and urbanisation of the country were other equally important means, each dramatic in its consequences. At the same time, adoption in 1920 of the law legalising abortion was the continuation of a prerevolutionary trend towards humanistic reform. Thus legalisation was presented as the achievement of social movements advocating this policy. In reality, social activity was manifested only by the official social structure and institutions. Social opinion, social movements, and social discussions were absent up to the end of the 1980s, in line with the general trait of totalitarian society.

This is the reason why, in an analysis of the abortion phenomenon, we can see only the interrelations of different interests in different national structures and institutes: central and peripheral Minzdraves, practical physicians, departmental researchers, the scientists of the USSR Academy of Sciences, other state departments, and so on. The only exception to this rule

Table 1
Grounds on Which Abortions Are Legal, USSR, 1920–1987

Year		Narrow	Broad	Eug-enic	Rape/Incest	Social-Medical	On Request	Gestation Age	Condition	Cost
1920	(L)	-	-	-	-	-	x	-	Clinic	Free
1924	(I)	-	-	-	-	x	-	-	Clinic	Free
1924	(L)	-	-	-	-	-	x	-	Prv. cl.	Fees
1924	(I)	-	-	-	-	x	-	-	Clinic	Fees
1926	(I,a)	-	-	-	-	x	-	12 wks	Clinic	Fees
1936	(L)	x	x	x	x	-	-	-	Clinic	Free
1955	(L)	x	x	x	x	-	-	12-28 wks	Clinic	Free
1955	(L)	-	-	-	-	x	x	12 wks	Clinic	Fees
1962	(I,a)	-	-	-	-	x	x	12 wks	Clinic	F/C*
1976	(I,a)	-	-	-	-	-	x	12 wks	Clinic	F/C**
1982	(I,a)	-	-	-	-	-	x	12 wks	Clinic*	F/C**
1982	(I,a)	x	x	x	x	-	-	12-28 wks	Clinic*	F/C**
1987	(I,a)	-	-	-	-	-	x	20 days	Amb	F/C**
1986	(L)	-	-	-	-	-	-	20 days	Com.cl	Fees
1987	(I,a)	x	x	x	x	x	x	12-28 wks	Clinic*	F/C**

Key:

L - State U.S.S.R. laws
I - Instructions of Ministry of Public Health of the U.S.S.R.
a - amendment to previous Law or Instruction
Clinic - only in area Clinics or Hospitals
Clinic* - change of area abortion clinic or hospital is available
Prv.Cl. - abortions available in private clinics
Com.Cl. - abortions available in commercial clinics
Amb - abortions available in outpatient hospitals
F/C* - abortions free of charge and money compensation is available for employed women only
F/Com** abortions free of charge for all women, money compensation available in case of complications for all women

Sources: Sadvokasova 1969; Vasilevski' and Vasilevski' 1924; *Ob iskysstvennom preryevanii beremennosti 1958; O sapreshenii abortov, yvelicenii material'noi' pomotchi rogenitsam, ystanovlenii gosydarstvennoi' pomotchi mnogocemeinyem, raschirenii seti rodil'nyeh domov, detskih yaslei' i detskih domov, ysilenii ygolovnogo nakasaniya sa neplatyogh alimentov i o necotoryh ismeneniyah v sakonodatel'stve o rasvodah 1958; O otmene obyasetel'nogo sapolneniya kart ytcheta aborta 1939;* USSR, Ministerstvo zdravookhraneniya SSSR, 1962, 1976, 1982 and 1987; *Metoditceskie ykasaniya po vyepolneniyu postanovleniya Soveta Ministrov SSSR ot 29.12.88,* 1988.

was the role of the intelligentsia. The voices of most women in this chorus were inaudible. This has been the most characteristic trait of the discourse.

Already in 1919, the Narkomzdrav of RSFSR and physicians blocked adoption of the law legalising abortions (Vasilevski' and Vasilevski' 1924, 96). Even after the law took effect, abortion was usually unavailable owing to the efforts of physicians who introduced payment for services for the majority of women. Thus, through the efforts of physicians, abortions became de facto unavailable even before adoption of the law of 1936, in which the complete de jure prohibition of abortion was established (Vasilevski' and Vasilevski' 1924, 108). Soviet physicians actively supported both the draft of the law of 1936 and the law itself.

A typical example of the reaction of Soviet physicians to the law of 1936 was the article by Narodny' Commissar Zdravoohrahehiya (State Commissioner of Health) N. A. Semachko, "What a Wonderful Law!" published in 1937 on the first anniversary of the law. The law was also ostensibly supported by the population, as expressed in women's letters and responses. These were widely published while propagandistic discussions of the proposed law were being conducted. Such titles included: "The Tragedy of My Life," "Abortion Brings Illness," "Let Children Live," "Every Woman Must Have a Child," "To Be a Happy Mother," "Motherhood—It Is a Special Feeling, It Is Wonderful." Of course, all these responses were the result of propaganda campaigns; we can only guess the true reaction of the population to the law.

On the other hand, for the most part these responses may have reflected the feelings of the people, who have always been conforming and socially apathetic. Even in modern times the reactions of Soviet women to state family planning matters has been absent.

The adoption of the law of 1920 not only meant the legalisation of induced abortions but, more important, it signalled the beginning of a national monopoly on the provision of induced abortions. In fact, it was a departmental monopoly of physicians on the provision of abortion and decision making in this area. The authorities and physicians were able to pursue their special pro-natalist, eugenic, and economic aims. This was the point of view of the main theoretician and author of the abortion law of 1920, Dr. A. B. Gens, who wrote in 1927:

Before us stands the wide and quite timely opportunity to use the achievement of eugenics for the real sanitation of the population . . . releasing our future society from man's genetically transmitted diseases. We have already obtained, in relation to this, a wonderful method [abortions]. . . . It is just the time for us to adopt the drafted law initiating compulsory surgical sterilisation [as selected by A. B. Gens] for all men and women with mental disease. (Aboptye v 1925 gogy 1927, 28)

The state's purpose consisted of creating a common centralised medical department and submitting its activity to state tasks. In fact, monopolisation of abortion services was a result of and an important stage in the monopolisation of health services in Soviet Russia, actively carried out at the beginning of the 1920s. Manifested in this process was the regulatory aspiration of the new totalitarian state to control not only the health services but also the health of the population. The innovations in the centralized public health structures would mean control of the family and its reproductive functions—birth and the socialisation of children.

Publication of the 1955 law re-legalising abortion led the way for a new stage. The law came about because of the continued failure of the state to enforce compulsory reproduction among women, leading it to return reproductive freedom to women. In this, the paradox of abortion in the USSR is revealed: on the one hand, the state's ambition to control the reproductive behavior of the population as a whole, and on the other hand, the impossibility of enacting such control.[13]

The return of reproductive freedom came at a routine moment in democratic reforms coming at the end of more than 50 years. And with this action yet another aspect of abortion in the former USSR is revealed: just as changes in reproductive and sexual freedom have been perfect indicators of changes in the general social freedom of society, so these changes in abortion policy reflect broader changes in the social and political life of the country.

At the beginning of the 1970s, there was a dramatic shift in family planning, a consequence of the political coup in the mid-1960s and the country's return to Stalinist policies at the beginning of the 1970s. Reproductive freedom, as well as all other personal freedoms, were the first victims of this coup. By prohibiting oral contraception and gradually extending the grounds for legal provision of induced abortions, the Soviet Public Health Services formulated the final stage of a national model of family planning, based solely on induced abortions. As a result, at the beginning of the 1980s, the Soviet Public Health Service established its own logic of development and potential for the expansive provision of new kinds of abortion services. This was manifested in the history of mini-abortions.

From the beginning of the 1980s, family planning in the USSR was characterised by the following parallel elements: diffuse provision of mini-abortions; continuation of the fight against illegal abortion; local attempts to make modern contraceptives available; continuation of official efforts to block widespread availability of modern contraceptives; commercialisation of an abortion industry; gradual loss of power by the Minzdrav of the former USSR; and transfer of initiative to the local territorial Public Health Service departments.

Up to the end of the 1980s, the Minzdrav and its local branches continued to be subject to the politics of family planning. New substructures of Minzdrav appeared with their interests in the induced abortion and family planning: the Soviet National Association called Family and Health (Thomas

1990), Minzdravs of the union republics, medical and commercial hospitals, and independent associations of commercial clinics. Naturally, these structures aspired to become new subjects of family planning policy and abortion provision. Nonetheless, their activities have remained verbal in character; none of these institutions has had the opportunity to conduct politics truly independently from Minzdrav or from central authorities.

The policies of other social institutions to abortion were determined by their general political positions. But the problem of family planning and artificial abortion was the principal object of political manipulation at all times. The abortion problem by itself in all cases was not the independent object of their attention, but only a comfortable occasion for political manipulation. The position of Minzdrav and its substructures was the only exception to this rule. For example, at the end of the 1980s, Muslim authorities in the former Central Asian republics were spared much attention on family planning and abortion because of widespread pro-natalist propaganda within Islamic fundamentalism. The sharply negative reaction of the Catholic Church in the Baltic republics may be explained by their general tendency towards political independence and the Western orientation of the Roman Catholic Church. This ensured the actualisation of the most traditionalist Catholic positions.

The relation of the Russian (so-called Red) Orthodox Church to family planning and induced abortions up to this time had not been officially declared, since this church has traditionally escaped dealing with modern problems. It is a fact that in the process of subsequent reform, the Russian Orthodox Church will give this problem more attention. But this is unlikely in the near future, provided abortion is not used for any nationalist, traditional, pro-natalist, or other political objectives.

The motives of these different institutions are important. They were at the foundation of their attitudes toward abortion policy in the former USSR. These institutions were involved in the issue only inasfar as it suited their wider political ends. Therefore, taking into account the changing political situation in the former USSR and in the union republics, to consider the institutions as serious subjects in the politics of family planning and abortion is premature.

Women themselves must also be counted, not only as the objects of politics but as full and active subjects in this politics. However, visible social activity by women is still absent in the fields of family planning and abortion. As a result, at the present time only Minzdrav and its different Public Health substructures have interest in the administration of abortions. As a consequence, only they can be counted as real political players in this issue.

On January 13, 1989, the Soviet National Association of Family Planning was officially instituted. Later in 1989, the former USSR became a formal member of IPPF (Thomas 1990). The country moved from being the first in the world to legalise induced abortions to being the only member of the

IPPF that based its national model of family planning on the broadest provision of induced abortion.

ABORTION: CURRENT LAW AND PRACTICE

The Legacy of History

The right to family planning, or "free and responsible parenthood," is the internationally acknowledged and inherent right of each person. Moreover, realisation of the right of each person to family planning serves as the legal and organisational basis for the guarantee of many other fundamental human rights—women's rights in general, women's right to choose, children's rights, the right of a person to health, and so on. Family planning is given this important status in a number of UNO documents ratified by the former USSR.

However, in our country the right to family planning was unrealised and inaccessible. This can be explained by the lack of information, of specialised and qualified medical assistance in family planning, and of modern contraceptives. In practice, only the right to induced abortions on social indications was realised, and this is reflected in its actual use by the population.

In the USSR, fertility shifted from high to low by the middle of the 1970s; this entailed a sharp rise in the level of induced abortions. The character of the current correlation between the birthrate and level of abortion is similar to that in Western European countries and Japan in the first and second thirds of the century. But the substitution of induced abortions with effective methods and means of contraception, which occurred in subsequent years in these other countries, did not take place in the USSR. Induced abortions are still the main method of family planning in the former USSR.

At present, the former USSR is one of the few countries among the economically developed nations of the world in which abortions prevail over the use of contraceptives in family planning. In the USSR, the transition from abortions to effective contraception, frequently called "the contraception revolution," has not come yet; in some regions it has not even begun. The problem of availability of effective methods and means of contraception is still unsolved, as well as the availability of information and special medical care in relation to family planning. The family planning services have not yet been created.

The difference between the former USSR and all Western countries lies not only in the temporal lag but also in the total absence of social reflection on and, consequently, underestimation of the scale of the problem. It is presumed that the situation will change as a result of changes in sexual behaviour, especially among young people; as a consequence of AIDS; as an effect of the changing demographic situation in Middle Asia; and because of increasing social and demographical stratification in the process of western-ization of the society.

The Incidence of Abortion

Another important event was the abolition in 1989 of Glavlit (Glavnoe Literaturnoe Ypravlenie, or Central Literary [Censorship] Board). In September, the statistical collection entitled *The Population of the USSR, 1987* was published (Naseleniye SSSP 1988). This was the first time in 60 years that official data on induced abortions had been published. This publication of official statistics on induced abortions represented a new opportunity to reflect on the principal focus of Soviet methods of family planning.

The annual 6 to 7 million abortions taking place in the Soviet Union by the end of the 1980s accounted for 20 to 25 percent of the world's annual total, which is estimated at 26 to 31 million abortions (Thomas 1990). Taking into account all types of illegal abortions (criminal, out-of-hospital, self-induced, or unregistered), the general number of abortions in the USSR can be increased by at least 50 percent. As a result, the true level of abortions is estimated at 11 million, or 181 abortions for 1,000 women ages 15 to 49 (Henshaw 1990).

Starting in 1970, both the absolute number of abortions and indices of abortion were lowered (see Table 2). Despite that, by 1985 the level of abortion in the USSR exceeded that in most Eastern European countries by 2 to 4 times and the level in Western European countries by 6 to 10 times. The main problem is that it is impossible to evaluate absolutely and precisely either the true number of induced abortions or the other epidemiological characteristics involved: their prevalence at the present time, the dynamics in the past, and the prognosis for the near future.

In 1988, the number of illegal abortions performed in the Soviet Union (criminal, self-induced, unregistered) officially accounted for 13 percent of all abortions (see Tables 3 and 7). This differed among the republics, ranging from 11 percent in the RSFSR to 40 percent in Tajikistan. Evidently, the numbers are underestimated. Using official terminology, the discourse is about "abortions that were started and/or performed outside the hospital," but which led to complications that required in-patient treatment.

Thus, more than 700,000 illegal abortions were officially registered in the USSR in 1988, and the same number in 1989. However, only 172 persons were prosecuted in the 1989 for providing illegal abortions, and only 92 persons were prosecuted for women's deaths following illegal abortions. In the same year, 447 women died following illegal abortions (Vestnik statistiki 1991). This is only one example of the difference between the de jure and de facto situation of induced abortions in the USSR.

Local evaluations based on selective surveys at the beginning of the 1980s reveal the real number of illegal abortions to be 50 to 70 percent higher (Po-

Table 2
Number of Abortions, Abortion Rate, and Abortion Ratio, USSR, 1954–1989

Year	Number of Abortions (thousands)	Abortion Rate	Abortion Ratio
1954	-	134.5	-
1955	-	176.1	-
1956	-	244.5	-
1957	-	151.9	-
1958	-	154.4	-
1959	-	140.4	-
1960	-	147.9	-
1961	-	141.9	-
1962	-	140.4	-
1963	-	139.2	-
1964	-	139.2	-
1970	7276	114.2	170
1975	7135	105.7	153
1976	7293	107.4	155
1977	7238	106.1	154
1978	7160	104.7	150
1979	7009	102.4	146
1980	7003	102.3	143
1981	6834	99.6	137
1982	6912	100.3	135
1983	6765	97.7	124
1984	6780	97.2	125
1985	7034	100.3	127
1986	7116	101.2	126
1987	6818	97.0	121
1988	7228*	103.2	112
	6504**	92.6	118
	6068***	86.6	112
1989	6974*	99.8	136

Notes:
* - includes mini-abortions and abortions in departmental public health services.
** - includes mini-abortions.
*** - excludes mini-abortions and abortions in departmental public health services.

Sources: Sadvokasova 1969; Naseleniye SSSP v 1987, 1988; Zdorovie naseleniya SSSR i deyatelnost uchrezdenii zsravookhraneniya v 1988, 1989; Demograficesky ezhegodnik SSSR, 1990; Remennik 1988; Abortions v 1926, 1929; Zdravookhranenie v SSSR v 1989, 1990.

pov 1990; Popov 1982). But in respect to the whole Soviet Union, the above-mentioned numbers are still underestimated and as a result the true number of criminal abortions remains terra incognita even for specialists. Thus, the total number of induced abortions in the former USSR is still unknown. The informed estimate is that at the end of the 1980s, there were between 10 and 11 million, of which 6.97 million were officially recognized (Popov 1990).

The dynamics of induced abortion show only the the visible part of a proverbial iceberg. Its invisible part is significant, the interaction between

Table 3
Illegal Abortions in the USSR and Soviet Republics, 1988

Republics	Illegal Abortions (total)	Percent of Illegal Abortions			Deaths from all Abortions
		All Abortions	Abortions of First-Time Pregnant Women	Abortions of Women Younger than 17	
USSR	737107	12.8	20.4	15.2	67.7
RSFSR	418147	12.8	20.4	15.2	67.7
Ukraine	88742	11.5	19.6	14.8	55.3
Byelorussia	21159	15.6	23.8	21.6	66.7
Uzbekistan	63901	27.3	60.3	44.4	64.7
Kazakhstan	47637	16.2	28.8	24.1	90.9
Georgia	8769	11.9	46.3	17.7	100.0
Azerbaijan	9498	23.8	75.1	100.0	100.0
Lithuania	5050	14.5	27.3	16.6	100.0
Moldavia	12192	12.8	21.8	17.9	16.7
Latvia	7039	13.9	23.9	23.4	100.0
Kirgizia	17888	26.3	40.0	14.8	36.7
Tajikistan	17357	39.9	61.4	23.8	29.4
Armenia	5929	22.2	75.2	70.6	100.0
Turkmenia	9254	26.1	45.1	27.4	33.3
Estonia	4495	15.1	18.9	16.8	-

Note: Excludes abortions performed in departmental health service.

Sources: Zdorovie naseleniya SSSR i deyatelnost uchrezdenii zsravookhraneniya v 1988; Zdravookhranenie v SSSR v 1989.

the following elements: (1) the availability of legal abortions; (2) the availability of nonlegal abortions; and (3) the availability of modern contraceptives—oral and intrauterine devices. During the last 10 years, only the first factor underwent real change: the availability of legal induced abortions, connected with a wide use of so-called mini-abortions.

Mini-abortions today present a phenomenon of statistical significance, averaging in 1988–89 almost 8 percent of the total number of induced abortions in the former USSR, ranging from 0.1 percent in Moldavia to 25 percent in Tajikistan (see Table 4). Despite such a range, mini-abortions serve as an integral component in family planning in all republics. Moreover, the growth in the number of mini-abortions and at the same time their incomplete registration can explain the reduction in all induced abortions in the USSR in the 1980s (see Table 2). It is also considered that the registration of mini-abortions even after 1988 was extremely incomplete. To evaluate the numbers of unregistered mini-abortions is rather difficult. In some republics the number and level of induced abortions increased significantly owing to mini-abortions, particularly in the RSFSR, Byelorussia, Ukraine, Lithuania, and Tajikistan (see Table 5). Judging from the available data, the majority of mini-abortions are performed in outpatient conditions—that is, they have become a routine, everyday procedure.

Taking into account these remarks, we can assume that the true level of abortions in the Soviet Union from 1970 to 1988 fluctuated very little, if at all. Between 1975 and 1983, the rate of abortion in various republics varied by a factor of 4 (see Table 6).

The main news of induced abortions in the former Soviet Union in 1989 concerned the growth of their indices in the USSR as a whole and in some republics: RSFSR, Ukraine, Byelorussia, Kazakhstan, Azerbaijan, Lithuania, Kirgizia, Turkmenistan, Tajikistan, and Armenia. The greatest increase in the level of abortions up (to 50 percent) was in the Byelorussian SSR, the Ukrainian SSR, RSFSR, and Lithuania. The increases probably resulted from a conjuncture of factors. In the RSFSR, Ukraine, and Byelorussia, for example, the increase was intensified by the reproductive consequences of radiophobia and teratophobia following the Chernobyl catastrophe. Moreover, at the same time the increase in the abortion rate was influenced by the large-scale introduction of mini-abortions, especially typical for RSFSR, Ukraine, and Byelorussia (Kalchenko et al. 1984; Bloshanskii and Zhukowskii 1985; Ponochevnaya 1985; Kavkasidze n.d.) as well as for Turkmenia, but this was presented only for the first time in official statistics in 1989 (see Table 7).

The population devoid of effective contraceptives was obliged to use induced abortions as the main instrument for reproductive independence. This is substantiated by slower growth in abortions in the Ukrainian SSR compared to the Byelorussian SSR. In the Ukraine, starting in 1986, intrauterine devices were introduced as a response to the Chernobyl catastrophe. A high

Table 4
Mini-Abortions, USSR, 1980–1989

	Number of abortions (thousands)				Number of Abortions per 1,000 Women ages 15-49			
	1980	1985	1988	1989	1980	1985	1988	1989
Induced abortions (excluding mini-abortions)	7003	7034	6968	5214	102.3	100.3	82.6	74.7
Induced abortions (including mini-abortions)	7003	7034	6504	6672	102.3	100.3	92.6	95.6
Mini-abortions	-	-	464	1457	-	-	6.7*	20.9

* - estimate

Sources: Zdorovie naseleniya SSSR i deyatelnost uchrezdenii zsravookhraneniya v 1988; Demograficesky ezhegodnik SSSR, 1990; Zdravookhranenie v SSSR v 1989.

Table 5
Mini-Abortions in the Former USSR and Soviet Republics, 1988–1989

Republic	Number of abortions	Mini-abortions		Percentage of Mini-abortions in
		per 100 Abortions	per 1,000 Women ages 15-49	Outpatient Conditions
USSR	5767,221	7.6	20.9	73.8
RSFSR	3832,240	6.1	22.9	71.3
Ukraine	773,792	7.1	25.9	74.2
Byelorussia	135,493	2.6	53.3	84.1
Uzbekistan	233,986	7.3	2.1	100.0
Kazakhstan	294,596	8.0	20.0	75.5
Georgia	73,773	3.5	3.2	77.7
Azerbaijan	39,885	9.6	2.3	12.7
Lithuania	34,845	–	20.8	100.0
Moldavia	94,998	0.08	12.9	76.5
Latvia	50,587	1.6	2.6	55.3
Kirgizia	67,667	5.9	22.1	57.5
Tajikistan	43,463	2.3	13.9	86.8
Armenia	26,670	9.3	1.3	0
Turkmenia	35,514	5.4	5.2	91.2
Estonia	29,712	3.3	6.7	91.8

*Sources: Zdorovie naseleniya SSSR i deyatelnost uchrezdenii zsravookhraneniya v 1988;
Demograficesky ezhegodnik SSSR, 1990; Zdravookhranenie v SSSR v 1989.*

Table 6
Number of Abortions per 1,000 Women Ages 15–49, USSR and Soviet Republics, 1975–1989

Republic	1975	1980	1985	1988*	1989*
USSR	105.7	102.3	100.3	82.3	95.5
RSFSR	126.3	122.8	123.6	105.2	117.7
Ukraine	88.3	94.1	92.2	61.9	86.1
Byelorussia	78.7	81.1	80.0	54.1	101.7
Uzbekistan	51.9	43.8	46.9	50.8	48.0
Kazakhstan	108.7	99.2	90.7	72.2	86.2
Georgia	74.0	67.7	52.4	54.5	51.3
Azerbaijan	43.1	39.0	30.8	22.4	23.3
Lithuania	53.0	50.9	46.3	38.0	53.9
Moldavia	89.7	90.7	96.0	88.4	82.8
Latvia	91.4	92.5	88.7	76.8	75.2
Kirgizia	84.1	76.6	73.8	67.7	85.9
Tajikistan	53.4	45.3	39.5	38.6	46.5
Armenia	60.5	38.8	38.4	30.2	31.3
Turkmenia	60.8	51.1	40.9	43.1	45.4
Estonia	107.1	96.7	91.4	77.3	73.8

* - Including departmental health services

Sources: Naseleniye SSSP v 1987, 1988; Zdorovie naseleniya SSSR i deyatelnost uchrezdenii zsravookhraneniya v 1988; Demograficesky ezhegodnik SSSR, 1990; Zdravookhranenie v SSSR v 1989.

Table 7

Some Features of the Use of Induced Abortions, USSR and Soviet Republics, 1988

Republics	Total number of abortions	Per 100 of all abortions				
		Illegal Abortions	Abortions of First Time Pregnant Women	Abortions of Women Younger than 17	Lethal Cases	Mini-Abortions
USSR	5,767,221	12.8	4.78	0.56	0.01	7.6
RSFSR	3,832,240	10.9	4.87	0.6	0.01	6.1
Ukraine	773,792	11.5	4.73	0.56	0.01	17.1
Byelorussia	135,493	15.6	6.87	0.49	0.01	2.6
Uzbekistan	233,986	27.3	4.18	0.05	0.007	7.3
Kazakhstan	294,596	16.2	3.30	0.38	0.01	8.0
Georgia	73,773	11.9	1.67	0.05	0.001	3.5
Azerbaijan	39,885	23.8	2.96	0.007	0.018	9.6
Lithuania	34,845	14.5	12.23	0.50	0.003	–
Moldavia	94,998	12.8	4.76	0.46	0.013	0.08
Latvia	50,587	13.9	7.05	0.002	0.002	1.6
Kirgizia	67,667	26.4	2.78	0.37	0.044	5.9
Tajikistan	43,463	39.9	3.93	0.14	0.039	2.3
Armenia	26,670	22.2	4.02	0.06	0.011	9.3
Turkmenia	35,514	26.1	3.95	0.33	0.009	25.4
Estonia	29,712	15.1	8.13	0.94	–	3.3

* - excluding abortions performed in departmental health service

Sources: Zdorovie naseleniya SSSR i deyatelnost uchrezdenii zsravookhraneniya v 1988; Zdravookhranenie v SSSR v 1989.

Table 8
Indices of the Provision of Contraceptives, USSR, 1988

Indices of Provision	1975			1980			1985			1989		
	CN	IUD	PL	CN	IUD	PL	CN	IUD	PL	CN	IUD	PL
Needs of the population	100	100	100	100	100	100	100	100	100	100	100	100
Availability in drug stores	16	11	-	34	10	9	15	30	9	39	39	2
Funds	14	11	-	18	10	4	8	19	9	11	30	2

Abbreviations: CN - condoms, IUD - intrauterine device, PL - oral hormonal contraceptives (pills)

Source: Popov, n.d.

level of abortions can be seen in the Central Asian republics, and recently it was comparable to or even above the level of abortions in the Baltic republics. In addition, the high level of nonhospital abortions presents a typical modern feature of family planning in the Central Asian republics: the average level of registered nonhospital (illegal) abortions in the USSR is 13 percent, but in Tajikistan it is 30 percent.

Without a doubt, differences in the abortion rates of the Baltic republics and the former Soviet Middle Asian republics were the result of cultural differences, or attitudes toward abortion and reproductive choice in Muslim versus Christian societies.

Contraception and Health

The prevalence of induced abortions in the USSR is explained by the low availability of contraceptive information, medical assistance in the use of contraception, and contraceptive devices themselves. Figures from the Ministry of Public Health show that provision of contraceptives in 1989 was only 11 to 30 percent (see Table 8). Using this data, it is necessary to consider that production of the main contraceptive was minimal. As a result, in 1990 changes in contraceptive usage occurred (see Table 9).

That 80 to 90 percent of women responding to a survey claimed that it was not difficult to buy contraceptives ("Problemye molodegi" 1990) is not surprising. It indicates that they are uninformed because they do not use any contraceptives. The recent state of oral contraception can be summarised as follows:

1. By the mid-1980s, oral contraceptives were used by 1 to 3 percent of Moscow women (Popov 1986). The same rate seems to hold in other European regions of

Table 9
Contraceptive Use in the Former USSR and Soviet Republics, 1990

Union Republic	Percentage of all women			
	using now	not using	using sometimes	Don't know
USSR	18.7	57.7	9.3	8.9
RSFSR	21.8	56.8	9.7	6.0
Ukraine	14.5	61.9	8.9	9.6
Byelorussia	13.0	60.4	9.8	11.8
Uzbekistan	18.8	49.7	9.3	17.2
Kazakhstan	22.1	55.0	7.9	9.0
Georgia	8.4	59.1	8.7	20.4
Azerbaijan	6.5	41.9	10.7	35.3
Lithuania	12.1	68.7	7.4	6.5
Moldavia	15.2	63.2	6.6	11.4
Latvia	18.6	57.8	12.9	5.1
Kirgizia	24.6	51.3	5.9	13.4
Tajikistan	14.5	59.3	6.3	17.7
Armenia	12.0	59.5	9.6	16.7
Turkmenia	12.1	54.7	7.7	22.9
Estonia	26.4	53.5	9.1	3.1

Sources: Vestnik Statistiki 1991; Problemye molodegi i molodoi cem'i, 1990.

the former USSR. This reveals a fundamental change that took place recently: the availability of oral contraceptives and a crucial change in public opinion as well as in the position of doctors.

2. Almost 80 percent of respondents knew about oral contraceptives, which is a significant fact, especially for a country with such an extremely low percentage of people using them (Antonov and Medkov 1987; Zotin and Mytil' 1985).

3. No more than 20 percent of respondents considered oral contraception to be the most effective means of family planning. Compared to other contraceptive methods, oral contraceptives are used least, the most frequently used methods being condoms and coitus interruptus (Zotin and Mytil' 1985).

4. Oral contraceptives were considered the most convenient by no more than 40 percent of respondents. On the other hand, use of contraception in itself was considered as the best method of family planning only by a minority of respondents; about 10 percent in Russia and 25 percent in Moscow preferred induced abortion as the main means of family planning (Popov 1986). Oral contraceptives are considered as the most safe form of family planning by only 5 to 6 percent of respondents. This is a direct consequence of the negative attitude of Soviet doctors, who conducted an anti–oral-contraceptive war during the last 20 years (Homasuridze 1985).

The present situation has deep roots in the late 1960s and early 1970s, when oral contraceptives appeared on the Soviet market. The conflict between the traditional Soviet model based on induced abortions and the alternative modernist model based on the use of modern contraceptives ended in the utter defeat of the contraception model (Homasuridze 1985).

The decisive factor in this conflict was the instructive letter of the Ministry of Health, which prohibited de facto the use of oral contraceptives in the USSR. The document contained a list of 10 diseases identified as direct contra-indications to oral contraceptives, and in addition a lot of indirect contra-indications.[14] Considering the present high rate of sickness, some 80 to 90 percent of women had either indirect or direct contra-indications to oral contraception.

As a result, even now the majority of doctors hold negative attitudes towards oral contraceptives, confirmed by leading specialists (Poltcthavnova 1975). The problem is complicated by the monopoly held by the former USSR Ministry of Health in the importation and dissemination of medicines, including oral contraceptives. As for public opinion, apprehension in relation to oral contraceptives is a direct consequence of the attitude of Soviet doctors. Consequently, the dissemination of oral contraceptives in the Soviet market is just beginning. The population and the majority of doctors have accepted their use and are potentially ready to change behaviour. That makes us believe that the main limiting factor for greater use of oral contraceptives is availability. The future situation will be determined by the activity of Western pharmaceutical firms.

Among the direct results of the inaccessibility of contraception is a high level of illegal abortions and abortions for women pregnant for the first time (see Table 7). As was stated before, this is a widespread phenomenon.

The most dramatic consequence of the high level of induced abortion is maternal mortality, which is high in comparison with other European countries and economically developed countries of the world in general (see Table 10). It should be noted that, despite the general absence of the family planning services, there is unequal maternal mortality, with a fourfold difference between the least affected and most affected republics (see Table 11).

Moreover, there was a great divergence between maternal mortality in any republic of the USSR and selected foreign countries (see Table 12). Such divergence can be attributed to peculiarities and imperfections in the Soviet social and public health services.

THE FUTURE

What can we say now about the future of abortion in contemporary Russia and the CIS? We may state that the dynamics of induced abortions are and will be determined by the spread of mini-abortions. Mini-abortions may turn into the main method of family planning in the former USSR. But for a better prognosis, it is necessary to consider the following circumstances: adaptation of the public health services to mini-abortions; adaptation of the population to induced abortions; genuine availability of contraceptives, information, and services aimed at the use of contraception; and absence of an adequate service of family planning.

Taking into account all of these factors, we can suppose that in the immediate future induced abortions will be substituted, not by modern contraception, but by safer and more convenient mini-abortions or by another advanced technology providing safe, early induced abortions. Probably vacuum aspiration during the earliest gestation period (mini-abortions) will become the main method of family planning in Russia. The future may also see availability of the morning-after pill and of RU 486. These can be considered as possible substitutions where the social system is already largely adapted to induced abortion technology and after-the-fact considerations of family planning.

The prognosis is extremely unfavourable because the transition from induced abortions to contraceptive use will hardly be possible. As a result, if there is any contraceptive revolution in the CIS or Russia, it will happen far in the future. But any possible change in family planning policy, contraceptive use, or abortion policy will be connected to political changes and to successful westernization. In the present political circumstances, any prognosis is unreliable, but it is most probable that little will change in the next five years.

Table 10
Causes of Maternal Mortality, USSR and Soviet Republics

Union Republic	All Causes (100%)	As Percentage of all:		
		Extrauterine Pregnancy	Spontaneous Abortions	Illegal Abortions
USSR	2,312	5.0	2.4	23.2
RSFSR	1,175	6.3	2.6	30.9
Ukraine	284	6.7	2.8	27.1
Byelorussia	40	15.0	5.0	25.0
Uzbekistan	270	0.4	1.1	4.8
Kazakhstan	198	4.0	3.5	17.7
Georgia	21	0	0	0
Azerbaijan	40	10.0	0	7.5
Lithuania	11	0	0	27.3
Moldavia	31	3.2	3.2	32.3
Latvia	12	0	0	25.0
Kirgizia	72	6.9	1.4	9.7
Tajikistan	88	3.4	1.1	3.4
Armenia	22	4.6	4.6	9.1
Turkmenia	42	2.4	0	14.2
Estonia	6	0	0	0

Sources: Zdorovie naseleniya SSSR i deyatelnost uchrezdenii zsravookhraneniya v 1988; Zdravookhranenie v SSSR v 1989.

Table 11
Maternal Mortality in the USSR and Soviet Republics, 1980 and 1988

Republic	1980	1988
USSR	56.4	43.0
RSFSR	68.0	50.0
Ukraine	44.8	38.2
Byelorussia	29.1	24.5
Uzbekistan	46.3	38.9
Kazakhstan	55.6	48.6
Georgia	25.7	22.8
Azerbaijan	38.7	21.7
Lithuania	27.0	19.4
Moldavia	64.1	35.0
Latvia	25.3	29.1
Kirgizia	49.4	53.8
Tajikistan	94.2	48.6
Armenia	27.0	29.4
Turkmenia	40.8	33.4
Estonia	27.0	23.9

*Sources: Zdorovie naseleniya SSSR
i deyatelnost uchrezdenii zsravookhraneniya
v 1988; Zdravookhranenie v SSSR v 1989.*

Table 12
Maternal Mortality Associated with Induced Abortions, USSR, Soviet
Republics, and Selected Countries, 1985–1988

Republic	Deaths per 100,000 Abortions	Countries	Deaths per 100,000 Abortions
Soviet Union	10	Bulgaria	1.3
RSFSR	10	Czechoslovakia	0.4
Lithuania	3	Denmark	0.7
Estonia	0	England and Wales	1.3
Tadjikistan	39	Hungary	0.8
Kirgizia	44	Sweden	0.4
		United States	0.6

*Sources: Zdorovie naseleniya SSSR i deyatelnost uchrezdanii zsravookhraneniya v
1988; Henshaw and Morrow 1990; Zdravookhranenie v SSSR v 1989.*

NOTES

1. This chapter covers the situation that existed in the former USSR and Soviet
Union republics until 1991. The principal characteristics of family planning in contemporary Russia and the Commonwealth of Independent States (CIS) remain unchanged.

2. *Ob iskysstvennom preryevanii beremnnosti* (About artificial interruption of preg-

nancy), Postanovlenie Narodnogo Komissariata sdravoochraneniya i Narodnogo komissariata justicii ot 16 noyabrya 1920 goda (The Order of People's Commissariat of Public Health Services and People's Commissariat of Justice); Postanovleniya KPSS i Sovetskogo Pravitelstva ob okhrane zdorov'ya naroda (The Orders of KPSU and Soviet Government about Public Health Defence), (Moscow: Medgiz, 1958).

3. *O sapreshenii abortov, yvelicenii material'noi' pomotchi rogenitsam, ystanovlenii gosydarstvennoi' pomotchi mnogocemeinyem, raschirenii seti rodil'nyeh domov, detskih yaslei' i detskih domov, ysilenii ygolovnogo nakasaniya sa neplatyogh alimentov i o necotoryh ismeneniyah v sakonodatel'stve o rasvodah* (Concerning the prohibition of abortion, the increase of financial help to mothers, the establishment of state help for large families, the broadening of the network of maternity hospitals, day-care centres, the amplification of juridical penalty for deviation from alimentary fees and about certain changes in legislation on divorce), Postanovleniya KPSS i Sovetskogo Pravitelstva ob okhrane zdorov'ya naroda (The Orders of KPSU and Soviet Government about Public Health Defence), (Moscow: Medgiz, 1958).

4. "O resyl'tatah obsledovaniya sostoyaniya dela bor'bye s abortami, ytceta i otchetnosti po abortam v YSSR, BSSR i ryade oblastei RSFSR" (About the outcome of the inspection of results of the fight against abortion, abortion registration and reporting in YSSR, BSSR and some provinces of RSFSR), *Oficial'nyei' sbornik NKZdrava SSSR i RSFR* (Official issue of PCP Health of the USSR and RSFSR) 20 (1937): pp.4–6. Also *Instructcia o provedenii bor'bye s prestupnyemi abortami* (Instruction about the fight developing against criminal abortions), NKZdrav SSR, Moscow, 1939; *Sanitarno-prosvetitel'naya pabota po bor'be s abortom* (Public prevention of abortion), Instruktivno-metoditceskoe pic'mo (Instructive and methodological letter), (Moscow: ISP MS SSSR, 1957).

5. *Instructcia o provedenii bor'bye s prestupnyemi abortami* (Instruction about the fight developing against criminal abortions), 1939, op. cit.

6. "Ob otmene obyasatel'nogo sapolneniya kart ytcheta aborta," forma no. 6 (About the elimination of abortion registration forms obligatory complication, statistical order no. 6), *Official'nyei' sbornik NKZdrava SSSR* (Official issue of PCP Health of the USSR) 9 (1939): 14.

7. *O otmene saprescheniya abortov* (About the elimination of abortion prohibition), Ykaz Prezidiyma Verhovnogo Soveta SSSR ot 23 noyabrya 1955 g., (The Bill of the Presidium of the High Council of the USSR), Postanovleniya KPSS i Sovetskogo Pravitelstva ob okhrane zdorov'ya naroda (The Orders of KPSU and the Soviet Government about Public Health Defence), (Moscow: Medgiz, 1958).

8. *Reshenije simpoziuma po gormonal'noj kontracepcii* (Decisions of symposium on hormonal contraception), MZ SSSR Gl. Upr. lech.-prof. pomoshchi detyam i materyam MZ SSSR. Vses. NII akusherstva i ginecologii (USSR Ministry of Health. All-Union Scientific Research Institute of Obstetrics and Gynaecology). Moscow, September 9, 1970.

9. *O pobochnom dejstvii i oslozhnenijah pri primenenii oral'nych kontraceptivov. Informacionoje pis'mo* (On side effects of oral contraceptive use. Information paper), MZ SSSR. Upravlenije po vnedreniju novyh lekarstvennyh sredstv i medtehniki. Vsesojuznyj centr po izucheniju pobochnogo dejstvija lekarstvennyh sredstv. (USSR Ministry of Health. Department for introduction of new medicines and medical equipment. All-Union center of research on side-effects of medicines), Moscow, 1974.

10. USSR. Ministerstvo zdravookhraneniya SSSR (The Order of the Minister of Public Health) M. 1976. No 08-23/11. *O poryadke resrecheniya operatcii iskusstvennogo prerivaniya beremennosti* (About the permission for the operation of induced interruption of pregnancy), July 8, 1976, Moscow, 1976.

11. USSR, Ministerstvo zdravookhraneniya SSSR (The Order of the Minister of Public Health) M. 1982. No 234. *Ob utverzdenii instryktsii o poryadke provedeniya iskusstvennogo prerivaniya beremennosti* (About the confirmation of the instruction on the operation of induced interruption of pregnancy), March 16, 1982, Moscow, 1982.

12. *Methody preduprezhdenija beremennosti* (Methods of birth control), Metodicheskije recomendacii (Recommendations) /MZ SSSR. Glavnoje upravlenije lechebno-profilakticheskoi pomoshchi materyam i detyam MZ SSSR (Main department of medical and prophylactic treatment for mothers and children of USSR Ministry of Health), Moscow, 1983.

13. *O otmene saprescheniya abortov* (About the elimination of abortion prohibition), 1958, op. cit.

14. *O pobochnom dejstvii i oslozhnenijah pri primenenii oral'nych kontraceptivov* (On side effects of oral contraceptive use), 1974, op. cit.

REFERENCES

Abortions v 1926 g (Abortions in 1926). Moscow: Statisdat, 1929.

Aboptye v 1925 gogy (Abortions in 1925). Moscow: Statizdat, 1927.

Antonov, A. I., and V. M. Medkov. *Vtoroi' rebenok* (Second child). Moscow: Mysl', 1987.

Bloshanskii, Yr. M., and Ya. G. Zhukowskii. "Vacuum-aspiratsiya soderzhimogo matki pri zaderzhke menstryatsii" (Vacuum aspiration with menstrual delay). *Akysherrstvo i ginekologiya* (Obstetrics and Gynaecology) 7 (1985): 55–58.

Demograficesky ezhegodnik SSSR, 1990 (Demographic yearbook, USSR, 1990). Moscow: Financi i statistica (Finances and statistics), 1990.

Henshaw, S. K. "Induced Abortion: A World Review, 1990," *International Family Planning Perspectives* 12, no. 2 (June 1990): 59–65.

Henshaw, S. K., and Morrow, E. *Induced Abortion: A World Review—1990 Supplement.* New York: Alan Guttmacher Institute, 1990.

Homasuridze, A. G. "Osnovnyje rezul'taty i puti razvitija gormonal'noj kontracepcii" (Main aspects of hormonal contraception), *Medico-social'nyje aspekty rozhdajemosti: Sbornik nauchnych trudov* (Some medical and social aspects of birth rate: Collection of papers). Tbilisi: Metznilereba, 1985: 50–61.

Kalchenko, E. I., and F. V. Sutta. "Nekotorie aspekti rperivaniya beremennosti metodom vacuum-aspiratii" (Some aspects of pregnancy interruption by the method of vacuum aspiration), *Akusherstvo i ginekologiya* (Obstetrics and gynaecology) 12 (1984): 43–44.

Kavkasidze, G. Menstrual Regulation Procedures in the USSR Report 22, UNFPA-WHO/EURO-IPPF-ZHORDANIA Institute Meeting, From Abortion to Contraception, Tbilisi, October 10–13.

Kyznetcov, V. K., and E. V. Baranova, "Abort kak problema meditcinskoi' demografii" (Abortion as a medical demography problem), *Obzor* (Review) VNIIMI MS SSSR 1 (1982).

Metoditceskie ykasaniya po vyepolneniyu postanovleniya Soveta Ministrov SSSR ot 29.12.88 (Instruction for realisation of Soviet of Ministry of the USSR Bill from December 29, 1988), Moscow, Mir.

Naseleniye SSSP v 1987: Statisticheskyi' sbornik (Population of the USSR in 1987: Statistical yearbook). Moscow: Financi i statistica (Finances and statistics), 1988.

Omskoye meditcinskoe obtchestvo (Omsk Medical Association), Komissiya po bop'be s isskystvennyemi vyekidyechami (Commission against Induced Abortions). *Doklad komissii po bor'be s isskystvennyemi vyekidyechami Omskomy meditcinskomy obtchestvy* (Report of the Commission against Induced Abortions of Omsk Medical Association), Moscow, 1904.

Poltcthanova, S. L. *Propoganda mer predupregdenija aborta v sovremennyeh ysloviyah: Metodicheskije recomendacii* (The propaganda of abortion-preventing measures in modern conditions: Methodological recommendations). MZ SSSR, Glavnoje upravlenije lechebno-profilakticheskoi pomoshchi materyam i detyam MZ SSSR, Glavnoe sanitarno-epidemiologitceskoe ypravlenie (Main department of medical and prophylactic treatment for mothers and children of the USSR Ministry of Health, Main department of epidemiology and health), Moscow, 1975.

Ponochevnaya, S. P. "Prerivanie beremennosti v rannie sroki vacuum-aspiratiei" (Pregnancy interruption in the early stages by vacuum aspiration), *Sdravookchranenie* (Public Health Services) Kishinev 5 (1985): 26–28.

Popov, A. A. "O chastote i prichinakh vnebolnichnickh abortov: Obzor literatyri" (About the frequency and reasons of nonhospital abortions: Review of literature), *Zdravookhranenie Rossiiskoi Federatsii* (Public Health of the Russian Federation) 6 (1982): 27–30.

———. "Regulirovanije rozhdenij v sovremennyh semjah" (Birth control in modern families), *Semi'ya-sdorovi'e-obtchestvo* (Family-Health-Society). Moscow: Mysl', 1986.

———. "Sky-High Abortion Rates Reflect Dire Lack of Choice," *Entre Nous* (European Family Planning Magazine) 16 (September 1990): 5–7.

———. "Iskysstvennye abortye i planirovanie semi'i v SSSR" (Induced abortions and family planning in the USSR), *Sem'ya i semeinaya politika* (Family and Family Policy), ISEPN AN SSSP, n.d.

"Problemye molodegi i molodoi cem'i" (Problems of youth and young families), *Statisticeski' sbornik* (Statistical collection). Moscow: Goskomstat SSSR, 1990: 216–23.

Remennik, L. I. "Mesto aborta v structure metodov kontrolya rogdaemosti v SSSR i sa rybegom" (The role of abortion in the structure of birth control measures in the USSR and abroad), *Problemye demograficeskogo rasvitiya* (Problems of Demography Development). Moscow: Academy of Sciences of the USSR, 1988: 86–99.

Sadayskas, V. M., and V. Yu Chigrehe. "Sravnenie metodov prerivaniya beremennosti" (An estimation of pregnancy interruption procedures), *Akusherstvo i ginecologiya* (Obstetrics and gynaecology) 3 (1985): 37–39.

Sadvokasova, E. A. *Social'no-gigienitceskie acpektye regylirovaniya razmerov sem'i* (Social and hygienic aspects of birth control). Moscow: Meditcina, 1969.

Thomas, L. "Family Planning First Birthday," *Entre Nous* (European Family Planning Magazine) 16 (September 1990): 6.

USSR, Ministerstvo zdravookhraneniya SSSR (The Order of the Minister of Public Health) M. 1962. No 377, *O merah po ycileniyu bop'bye s abortami* (About measures to fight against abortion), Moscow, 1962.

———. M. 1981. No 430, *Ob utverzdenii instryktivno-metoditceskih ykasani' po organisatcii pabotye gensko' konsyl'tacii* (About the confirmation of the instruction on the women's clinic working organization), April 22, 1981, Moscow, 1982.

———. M. 1987. No 757, *Ob utverzhdenii instruktsii o poryadke provedeniya operatsii iskysstvennogo prerivaniya berenennosti rannikh srokov metodom varyym-aspiratsii* (On the instruction and order of induced interruption of pregnancy in the early stages, using the method of vacuum aspiration), May 6, 1987, Moscow, 1987.

———. M. 1987. No 1342, *O poryadke resrecheniya operatcii iskusstvennogo prerivaniya beremennosti po nemedetcinskim pokasaniyam* (About the permission for the operation of induced interruption of pregnancy on nonmedical grounds), December 31, 1987, Moscow, 1987.

Vestnik statistiki (Statistical Courier) 3 (1991).

Vasilevski', L. V., and L. M. Vasilevski'. *Abort kak social'noe yavlenie* (Abortion as a social phenomenon). Moscow-Leningrad: Frenkel, 1924.

Zdravookhranenie v SSSR v 1989 (Public Health in the USSR in 1989). Statisticheskie materiali (Statistical materials), Moscow, 1990.

Zdorovie naseleniya SSSR i deyatelnost uchrezdenii zsravookhraneniya v 1988 (Health of the population in the USSR and public health services activities in 1988). Moscow: Ministry of Public Health, 1989.

Zotin, V., and A. Mytil'. "Oswedomlennost vstupajushchih v brak o metodah i sredstvah kontracepcii" (Awareness of newly married couples about means and devices of contraception), *Molodozheny* (Newly married couples). Moscow: Mysl', 1985.

FOR FURTHER READING

Cook, R. J. "Abortion Laws and Policies: Challenges and Opportunities," *International Journal of Gynecology and Obstetrics*, Supplement 3, (1989): 61–87.

———. "International Dimensions of the Department of Justice Arguments in the Webster Case," *Law, Medicine and Health Care* 17, no. 4 (1989): 384–94.

———. "International Protection of Women's Reproductive Rights," *New York University Journal of International Law and Politics* 24, no. 2 (1992): 645–727.

Cook, R. J., and B. M. Dickens. *Issues in Reproductive Health Law in the Commonwealth*. London: Commenwealth Secretariat, 1986.

———. "International Developments in Abortion Laws: 1977–1988," *American Journal of Public Health* 78 (1988).

Cook, R. J., and P. Senanayake, (ed.). *The Human Problem of Abortion: Medical and Legal Dimensions*. London: IPPF, 1979.

Eser, A., and H-G. Koch, (eds.). *Schwangerschaftaabbruch im Internationalen Vergleich*. Baden-Baden: Nomos Verlagsgesellschaft, 1988.

Francome, C. *Abortion Freedom: A Worldwide Movement*. London: Allen and Unwin, 1984.

Frankowski, S. J., and G. F. Cole, (eds.). *Abortion and Protection of the Human Fetus: Legal Problems in a Cross-Cultural Perspective*. Lancaster: Martinus Nijhoff, 1987.

Glendon, M. A. *Abortion and Divorce in Western Law: American Failures, European Responses*. Cambridge, Mass.: Harvard University Press, 1987.

Henshaw, S. K. "Induced Abortion: A World Review, 1990," *International Family Planning Perspectives* 12, no. 2 (1990): 59–65.

Henshaw, S. K., and E. Morrow. *Induced Abortion: A World Review—1990 Supplement*. New York: Alan Guttmacher Institute, 1990.

Hodgson, J. E. (ed.). *Abortion and Sterilization: Medical and Social Aspects*. London: Academic Press, 1981.

IPPF Europe Region. *Late Abortion in Europe: Report of a Colloquium.* London: IPPF, 1989.

Jacobson, J. *The Global Politics of Abortion.* Worldwatch Paper 97, Washington, D.C.: Worldwatch Institute, 1990.

Jones, E. F., J. D. Forrest, N. Goldman, et al., *Teenage Pregnancy in Industrialized Countries.* New Haven: Yale Univ. Press, 1986.

Jones, E. F., J. D. Forrest, and S. K. Henshaw. "Unintended Pregnancy, Contraceptive Practice and Family Planning in Developed Countries," *Family Planning Perspectives* 20, no. 2 (1988): 53–67.

Ketting, E. "Induced Abortion in Europe: An Overview," *Planned Parenthood in Europe* 18 (1989): 2–4.

Ketting, E., and P. Van Praag. *Schwangerschaftaabbruch: Gesetz und Praxis im Internationalen Vergleich.* Verlag Tübingen: DGVT, 1985.

Knoppers, B. M., J. Brault, and E. Sloss. "Abortion in Francophone Countries," *American Journal of Comparative Law* 38, no. 4 (1990): 889–922.

Lovenduski, J., and J. Outshoorn. *The New Politics of Abortion.* London: Sage, 1986.

McLaurin, K., C. Hord, and M. Wolf. *Health Systems' Role in Abortion Care: The Need for a Pro-active Approach.* Carrboro, N.C.: International Projects Assistance Services, 1991.

Petchesky, R. *Abortion and Women's Choice: The State, Sexuality and Reproductive Freedom.* London: Verso, 1986.

Rossi, A., and B. Sitaraman. "Abortion in Context: Historical Trends and Future Changes," *Family Planning Perspectives* 20, no. 6 (1988): 273–281.

Rubin, E. R. *Abortion, Politics and the Courts: Roe v. Wade and Its Aftermath.* Westport, Ct.: Greenwood Press, 1987.

Sachdev, P. (ed.). *International Handbook on Abortion.* Westport, Ct.: Greenwood Press, 1988.

Spinelli, A. (ed.). *Late Abortion in Europe: Report of a Colloquium.* London: IPPF Europe Region, 1989.

Stassenborg, S. *The Pro-Choice Movement: Organization and Activism in the Abortion Conflict.* New York: Oxford University Press, 1991.

Taule, N., and S. Cohen, (eds.). *Reproductive Laws for the 1990s: A Briefing Handbook.* New Jersey: Humana Press, 1988.

Tietze, C., and S. K. Henshaw. *Induced Abortion: A World Review.* 6th ed. New York: Alan Guttmacher Institute, 1986.

INDEX

ABOUT THE CONTRIBUTORS

ÁDÁM BALOGH, M.D., Ph.D., is an associate professor in the Department of Obstetrics and Gynaecology at the University Medical School of Debrecen, Hungary. He is head of the Diagnostic and Reproductive Endocrinology Research Laboratory, a consultant to the Family Planning Centre, and a lecturer. His special interest is obstetrics and gynaecology and laboratory (clinical chemistry) investigations. He has produced 76 publications on contraception, infertility, family planning, reproductive pharmocology, menopause and osteoporosis, and induced and spontaneous abortion. He is a member of the board of the Hungarian Society for Osteoporosis, and was a WHO adviser in 1978, 1986, 1989, and 1990.

VICKY CLAEYS has been Executive Director of the Belgian Family Planning Association (FCGSO), Flemish branch, since 1981. FCGSO is a member of the International Planned Parenthood Federation, Europe Region. Vicky has published articles on sexuality and on relationships in women's magazines and the *CGSO Yearbook*. She is also author of *The Belgian Abortion Story*, FCGSO, Brussels, 1985.

ANNA EGGERT is a teacher by profession and now works with unemployed adults. She started researching the issue of abortion in 1983, when the constitutional referendum in the Republic of Ireland prompted her to write her undergraduate dissertation on abortion in Ireland (Essen University, 1984). She moved to Belfast the same year and became a member of the Northern Ireland Abortion Campaign, and then a founder member of the Northern Ireland Abortion Law Reform Association. She has published on the issue of abortion with Bill Rolston. She is a mother of two, a feminist, and a fighter for women's rights.

COLETTE GALLARD spent her first 15 years in Algeria. When her family returned to France in 1949, she earned her baccalaureate, took a degree in law, and had four children. She joined the French Family Planning Movement in 1972, where she trained and has been working as a counsellor and group leader since. She was elected to the national board of the French Family Planning Movement in 1978, and two years later became a member of the Executive Committee. In 1984, with another member, she set up the Movement's International Commission. She has been extensively involved in staff training in France (prevention of child sex abuse) and recently in training schemes on contraceptive education in Romania (1990), Zaire (1991), and Poland (1992). Early in 1992 she was elected to the International Planned Parenthood Federation's European Regional Council Executive Committee.

ENCARNA BODELÓN GONZÁLEZ studied law at the University of Barcelona and worked in the field of criminology at the Erasmus University, Rotterdam, and in the Women's Studies Department at Utrecht. Currently she teaches the sociology of penal control at the Institute of Criminology in Barcelona. Her main interest is in the area of feminist theory, and she is preparing her dissertation on the "Feminism of the Difference and the Concept of Rights."

BRITA GULLI is a political scientist living in Oslo. She is currently working on a research project on new genetic and reproductive techniques and their impact on women, in particular their implications for women's self-determination. This research is funded by the Norwegian Research Council. She has recently published a book on equality policies in Norway, in particular the problem of sexually neutral laws and public policies. She is active in the women's movement.

EVERT KETTING studied sociology at the universities of Leiden and Utrecht in the Netherlands. In 1978 he finished a thesis on the liberalisation of abortion in the Netherlands ("From Crime to Assistance"). He was coordinator of research in STIMEZO, the Dutch national abortion organization. Currently he is Deputy Director of the Netherlands Institute of Social Sexological Research (NISSO), a consultant to the International Planned Parenthood Federation, and to the International Health Foundation. He has published more than 100 articles and books on family planning, induced abortion, sexuality, and mental health.

SABINE KLEIN-SCHONNEFELD studied law, sociology, and psychology at the universities of Bochum and Münster and has worked since in the fields of criminal law, political criminal procedure, criminology, and the evaluation of legal education. She has been an activist in the women's movement for the last 20 years, and for the last 10 years has been engaged in women's studies. Her main research interests are in women's integration in the labour market and the different structures of social control of women, including violence against women and children. She is currently setting up a training and counselling department against sexual harassment in the workplace within the civil service in Bremen. She lectures at the University of Bremen.

LÁSZLO G. LAMPÉ, M.D., Ph.D., F.R.C.O.G., is a professor and the chair of the Department of Obstetrics and Gynaecology at the University Medical School of Debrecen, Hungary. His clinical and research specialties have been in the areas of foetal endocrinology, reproductive physiology, perinatology, gynaecologic oncology, abortion issues, and reproductive research ethics. He has published 248 publications on these issues, including three textbooks. He is a fellow of the Royal College of Obstetrics and Gynaecology, as well as president or board member of the following Hungarian societies: Oncology, Obstetrics/Gynaecology, Endocrinology and Metabolism, Family Planning, as well as the International Society for Gynaecology and Obstetrics (Ethics Committee).

OSKAR LEHNER has studied law and works as an assistant professor at the University of Linz, Austria, lecturing on Austrian legal history. His main specialties are in the areas of family law, women's law, and the history of constitutional law. During the 1980s he worked as a freelance reporter in Latin America. His main publications are *Familie-Recht-Politik: Die Entwicklung des österreichischen Familienrechts im 19. und 20. Jahrhundert* (Wien 1987) and *Österreichische Verfasungs- und Verwaltungsgeschichte* (Linz 1992).

KATARINA LINDAHL is Executive Director of RFSU, the Swedish Association for Sex Education. RFSU is involved in education, information, and shaping public opinion on issues concerning sexual politics. Katarina Lindahl does a lot of educational work and is very active in the debate in Sweden. She has been engaged in the movement for women's rights for a long time and has paid a great deal of attention to the question of abortion rights. Before she started work with RFSU she was a journalist, a social worker, and an information officer. She is a graduate of the University of Stockholm and also a qualified social worker. She lives in Stockholm and has a seven-year-old daughter.

JOLANTA PLAKWICZ is an English teacher and literary translator in Warsaw. She was a founding member of the Polish Feminist Association, which dates back to the beginning of the 1980s. She is actively involved in the struggle for women's rights in Poland, including the right of women to decide on abortion. She is co-founder of the Federation for Women and Family Planning. As well as having written numerous commentaries and reports on the situation of Polish women for the United Nations and the Council of Europe, among others, she is the author of a chapter on Poland in *Superwomen and the Double Burden*, a book on women in Eastern and Central Europe and the former Soviet Union (London 1992). She is a member of a number of international women's organisations and networks.

ANDREJ A. POPOV, M.D., Ph.D., is a research associate at the Centre of Demography and Human Ecology of the Institute of Employment Studies of the Russian Academy of Sciences and the director of the Transnational Family Research Institute in Moscow. His doctorate was on the demographic characteristics of birth control in the Russian Soviet Republic. He continued his studies in family planning at the Institute of Sociological Studies and the Institute of Socio-Economic Studies, both in the USSR Academy of Sciences. He has published over 40 articles on abortion, reproductive health, and contraceptive behaviour in the former Soviet Union. In 1991–92 he was a Population Council Fellow at the Office of Population Research at Princeton University, United States.

NELL RASMUSSEN is a graduate in law and criminology. From 1977 to 1989 she was a professor at the Copenhagen School for Social Workers and a researcher and part-time teacher at the University of Copenhagen. She is co-author of a book on rape and of numerous articles on criminological and legal questions with specific reference to women. She is also the author of books on family and children's law. From 1989 until 1991 she was a principle in the Danish Council of Ethics of the Danish Parliament. She is presently employed as a management consultant to the Danish Family Planning Association.

ANNE-MARIE REY is President of Union Suisse pour décriminaliser l'avortement (USPDA), the Swiss Union for the Decriminalization of Abortion. She has been involved in the Swiss pro-choice movement since 1970. Happily married since 1962, she has three grown children. She has been a member of the parliament of the canton of Berne for the Social Democratic party since 1988 and is engaged in politics on women's and environmental issues.

MARKETTA RITAMIES is a research associate at the Population Research Institute, the Finnish Population and Family Welfare Federation. She has a master's degree from the University of Helsinki (1964). After graduation, she started to work at the Population Research Institute as a researcher, concentrating on issues of fertility and abortion. Her recent publications have dealt with persons living alone in Finland, Finnish development co-operation in relation to population questions, family policy in Western Europe, and consensual unions in Finland.

BILL ROLSTON was raised in Belfast. After a six-year sojourn in the United States, he returned to Belfast where he graduated in sociology in 1974. He received his doctorate in sociology in 1977, and since that time has taught at the University of Ulster (previously the Ulster Polytechnic), where he is now a senior lecturer. He has written extensively on politics and society in Northern Ireland. In 1984 he was one of the founder members of the Northern Ireland Abortion Law Reform Association.

MADELEINE SIMMS, M.A., M.Sc., is the author of many books and papers on the social and political aspects of abortion in Britain. She has been Senior Research Officer at the Institute for Social Studies in Medical Care since 1977 and, with Christopher Smith, wrote *Teenage Mothers and Their Partners* (London 1986).

RADIM UZEL, M.D., CSc., is associated in his capacity of research worker in gynaecology and sexology with the Institute of Mother and Child Care in Prague. His professional interest is mainly with the problems of family planning and sex education. He is well known not only as a specialist but also as a speaker, broadcaster, and author of a number of articles in both the popular and specialised press. He is author of several books on family planning and sex education. Currently he is the Scientific Secretary of the Czech Sexological Society and Executive Director of the Family Planning Association of the Czech Republic.

DIMITER VASSILEV graduated from university in 1956 and practiced as a general practitioner, surgeon, public health officer, and, for the last 28 years, gynaecologist. He founded the Bulgarian Family Planning Association in 1973 and is a member of the Central Council of the International Planned Parenthood Federation. Apart from being the author of the first manual on contraception in Bulgaria, *Contemporary Contraception* (1979), he has written more than 200 publications.

DUARTE VILAR is a sociologist who has been working since 1979 in the Portuguese Family Planning Association, specifically in the areas of community and school sex education. Since 1988 he has been the Executive Director of the Portuguese Family Planning Association. He has participated in a number of studies of adolescence and sexuality in Portugal.

ELEONORA ZIELIŃSKA is a professor at the University School of Law in Warsaw, Poland, and Director of the Institute of Penal Law. She is a specialist in comparative criminal law and medical law, and has published numerous comparative studies, primarily on alternatives to imprisonment, on the legal responsibility of physicians, and on abortion-related subjects. She acts as an expert in the Polish parliament and works as a law consultant for the Warsaw Chamber of Physicians.

ISBN 0-313-28723-6

9 780313 287237

90000>

HARDCOVER BAR CODE